Environmentally Induced Illnesses

Environmentally Induced Illnesses

Ethics, Risk Assessment and Human Rights

THOMAS KERNS

McFarland & Company, Inc., Publishers
Jefferson, North Carolina, and London

Library of Congress Cataloguing-in-Publication Data

Kerns, Thomas A., 1942–
    Environmentally induced illnesses : ethics, risk assessment, and
human rights / Thomas Kerns.
      p.   cm.
    Includes bibliographical references and index.
    ISBN 0-7864-0827-8 (softcover : 50# alkaline paper) ∞
    1. Environmentally induced diseases. 2. Environmentally
induced diseases—Moral and ethical aspects. 3. Environmental
health—Moral and ethical aspects. 4. Human rights—Health
aspects. I. Title.
RA566.K465   2001
615.9'02—dc21   00-66235

British Library cataloguing data are available

Manufactured in the United States of America

Cover image ©2001 Artville

McFarland & Company, Inc., Publishers
  Box 611, Jefferson, North Carolina 28640
  www.mcfarlandpub.com

Acknowledgments

In many ways, I am like the turtle on the fencepost. I did not get here without a great deal of help.

I had constant support and help from my dear parents, Dr. Thomas A. Kerns and Tops Kerns, from siblings, Jane, Patsy, Bob, Mary K., Will, John and Pete, and from my children, Tom, Lisa and Roxanne. In addition, I must express deep gratitude to my teaching colleague, Karen Stuhldreher, and the students in the Coordinated Studies Program *World's Health World's Women*, winter 1998; and to my good friend and deeply respected colleague, Jim Harnish, for his comments on an early draft of this book, and the students in the Coordinated Studies Program Jim and I taught, *Ethics, Rights and Religion: Questions of Conscience for the New Millennium*, spring 1998.

Contents

Contents

Preface

At 10 o'clock on Sunday morning July 2, 1995, sitting comfortably in my study preparing to do some work on a biostatistics assignment, a sharp metallic, acidic taste suddenly emerged on my tongue and on the roof of my mouth. It was a sensation I had never felt before. Within less than six months I would be diagnosed with a toxicant induced chemical sensitivity disorder and my 52 year old life would be dramatically changed in ways I would never have guessed. I would find it virtually impossible to be in any of the carpeted rooms at the college where I am a professor (and almost all the college rooms were carpeted), my marriage would end, I would have to find a chemically safer place to live, I would be unable to get into my vehicle without becoming sick, I could not go out to restaurants, theaters, and many stores because they made me ill, I would not be able to go to church because of the chemicals in artificial fragrances that people wore, and I would sometimes find it almost impossible to be around even my own grown children because of a hypersensitivity to some of the chemicals in their homes and on their clothing.

Before this diagnosis I had been an almost perfectly healthy man in his prime years, who exercised and ran at least two miles every day (sometimes five miles or more), who had virtually no medical complaints, who loved his work teaching philosophy and who was considered quite good at it, who loved his family deeply, who enjoyed several hobbies, who was completing the writing of two books, and whose life was generally rather good.

In fact, at the age of 51, I had decided that I wanted to go back to graduate school and earn another postgraduate degree, this time a master's in public health (MPH). My degrees in philosophy had been earned 25 years earlier, and I was now eagerly anticipating the challenge of taking on an entirely new enterprise to complement my teaching and writing. In addition to teaching regular philosophy courses, I had been teaching courses in medical ethics and HIV/AIDS for approximately ten years and was enjoying it. It seemed like a good idea to earn a degree in public health, and it also seemed like it would be great fun. I applied to the University of Washington School of Public Health and was accepted.

Classes for the MPH started in mid–June 1995, just two weeks before the metallic taste began. I was enjoying the classes thoroughly, although they were challenging, and I liked my classmates a lot. I was relishing the experience of being a student again, and having fun working with peers to understand new concepts and to complete challenging homework assignments.

That Sunday morning, July 2, my wife was gone for a few days of traveling with friends, and I was cherishing the peace. I had just settled in, with a mug of hot coffee in one hand, my feet up on the desk, and a heavy textbook in my lap, to do some homework for the biostatistics and epidemiology courses we were all working through that summer.

The unusual metallic taste was sharp enough to be not only distinctive, but also immensely distracting. It was difficult to concentrate on the biostatistics assignment without wondering about what was going on in my body that would cause such an odd taste. "I wonder if it's the coffee," I thought. "Something foul about this particular cup." So I went out to the kitchen and made another mug, adding just the right amount of creamer and my usual two tablets of NutraSweet.[1]

After several hours of personal observation and experimentation, I discovered that the taste did not seem to be related to the coffee at all. Nor could I make it go away even when I went outside and sat on the front porch. It seemed to come and go on its own whim, regardless of where I was or what I was doing.

The next day in epidemiology class, I asked a few MD friends if they knew what might cause a metallic taste like that. Had I changed my diet lately, they asked. I had not. Was I on any medications? No.

Well, it's probably nothing, they said. Wait for a few days, and it will probably go away on its own.

Unfortunately the taste did not go away. I could not make it go away. I was also, I now noticed, often feeling dizzy in the mornings after taking a shower. Sinuses and nasal passages were closing up during the shower, and just being in our bedroom for any length of time made my nasal passages close up so severely that I literally could not breathe through my nose at all.

During the next weeks, as the taste continued to come and go, I noticed a variety of other symptoms, particularly while in the classroom building where the MPH classes were being held; symptoms such as slight nausea, mental confusion, difficulty concentrating, an odd raspiness in my voice that sometimes led to coughing and choking, and occasionally sudden great fatigue. I eventually made an appointment with my regular family physician. She also seemed puzzled, though not terribly concerned. She ordered some routine blood work and, when the results came back a week later, all the tests seemed to be within normal limits. I eventually saw another physician in my HMO who specialized in occupational medicine and she too declared that nothing was discernibly wrong.

Over the next weeks I explored a variety of different hypotheses to explain what was happening to my body, one of which was that I had perhaps developed some kind of allergy. Allergy tests all proved negative, however. I eventually visited a physician who specializes in environmental medicine. After taking a thorough medical history, doing an examination of recent blood work, asking about what symptoms I generally experienced in relation to various exposures, and recommending more lab tests, he eventually diagnosed me with multiple chemical sensitivity (MCS), probably developed as a result of chemical injury.

As a diagnosis, MCS is considered somewhat controversial among conventional medical practitioners. However, since these physicians as a rule have received no medical training in low dose toxicant induced pathologies, either while in medical school or in postgraduate education, it is not surprising that they would find the diagnosis to be outside the limits of their expertise.

This, as societies will soon realize, is a significant weakness in medical training that sorely needs to be remedied. As the number of people suffering from toxicant induced pathologies continues to grow with each passing year, and as their impact on society begins to take an increasingly serious toll, it will become more and more important that our physicians be trained to recognize and treat such conditions.

This book examines some of the ethical issues associated with the increasing emergence of low dose toxicant induced illnesses.

I have written two other books on ethical issues in public health,[2] but this one is different. In each of those I took great pains to argue both sides of the relevant issues, to explain the thinking on both sides, and to show the legitimate tensions between the two opposing positions.

This book is different from those in that it takes a clear position and argues for it. The position taken is this: today's public policy regarding the manufacture, marketing and use of toxics is inadequate. It fails to adequately protect the health of the world's citizens. Significant changes need to be made, and in Chapter Three I recommend several.

I am entirely aware that there is another side to this question: namely, that position represented by the chemical manufacturing corporations and by the recent crop of optimists who claim that today's environmental policies are entirely adequate to protect the environment and public health. I believe their position to be mistaken, and much of this book explains why.

The book is arranged (after the Introduction) in four chapters which have a logical progression. It argues that, given certain facts about toxicant induced illnesses (Chapter One, Data), and given certain ethical principles (Chapter Two, Principles), some definite changes will need to be made (Chapter Three, Modest Proposals), despite some serious obstacles and challenges (Chapter Four, Brick Walls). The recommended changes are momentous, and the challenges heroic. But, as we will soon see, they must be faced if we hope to avoid some very serious threats to our physical health, to our mental capacities, and to the future well-being of our children, our grandchildren, and the generations to come.

Notes

1. A brand name for the artificial sweetener aspartame.

2. T.A. Kerns, *Ethical Issues in HIV Vaccine Trials* (New York: St. Martin's Press [Macmillan, Ltd., in the UK], 1997) 244 + xvi; and T.A. Kerns, *Jenner on Trial: An Ethical Examination of Vaccine Research in the Age of Smallpox and the Age of AIDS* (Lanham, MD: University Press of America, 1997) 104.

Introduction

A 1988 article by Robert Gould in *Cosmopolitan*, a magazine targeted primarily at women, reassured readers that:

> [There] is practically no risk of becoming HIV-infected through ordinary vaginal or oral sex even with an HIV-infected male. The vaginal secretions produced during sexual arousal keep the virus from penetrating the vaginal walls. [The author's] explanation: "Nature has arranged this so that sex will feel good and be good for you."[1]

This claim is absurd, of course, and it was known even in 1988 to be absurd. Nineteen eighty-eight is hardly so early in the HIV/AIDS epidemic that holding or publishing such an irresponsible opinion could be considered excusable.

Cosmopolitan, of course, is not a medical journal. Still, we might expect that its editors have a journalistic and perhaps even ethical obligation to their readers to refrain from publishing an opinion that could have such potentially devastating health consequences.

Now, more than a decade later, it is widely recognized that claims such as those made in the *Cosmopolitan* article were highly irresponsible, and that the failure to prevent such articles from being published was ethically problematic and showed appalling journalistic standards.

Today, when we are witnessing the emergence of another epidemic,

5

this time an epidemic of toxicant induced illnesses, similar misrepresentations of these disorders have appeared in the popular press,[2] misrepresentations which are often abetted by corporate interests that do not wish to see their chemicals given a bad name. Only with the knowledge and understanding which come with time will we eventually be able to look back on this era and recognize the level of journalistic standards (and corporate influence) that have allowed such stories to be published. Even with all that is currently known about the health effects of long term exposure to low doses of toxicants, much more still needs to be discovered. In addition, communities need to be made more aware of the health risks to which they are daily being exposed without their knowledge and without their consent. John Wargo, in the penultimate chapter of his book, *Our Children's Toxic Legacy: How Science and Law Fail to Protect Us from Pesticides*, says (and provides persuasive evidence to the effect) that there is "little hope that we are even aware of the magnitude and distribution of significant threats to environmental health."[3]

This Book's Scope

This book focuses essentially on a small portion of the field of environmental health, and on an even smaller portion of the field of environmental ethics. In order to more precisely delineate the concerns examined here, we shall now look briefly at each of those two fields.

ENVIRONMENTAL HEALTH

Environmental and occupational health is a broad field encompassing a wide variety of subdisciplines, but this book is primarily concerned only with the following areas of environmental health.

It discusses the *human* health effects more than the health effects on wildlife, although it clearly recognizes that effects on wildlife may be strongly suggestive of potential effects in human beings.

It discusses the human health effects of exposure to toxicants that are relatively *ubiquitous* in the environment. These include a wide variety of chemicals: for example, many solvents, aldehydes (e.g., formaldehyde), pesticides, room "deodorizers," artificial fragrances, as well as all the byproducts of industrial waste and the burning of fossil fuels (including those used in internal combustion engines).

Let us look briefly at three chemicals, chosen almost at random, to which we are commonly exposed in daily life.

Formaldehyde is a toxicant found in a bewildering number of consumer products,[4] including bed mattresses, boxsprings, padded furniture, as well as in a wide variety of everyday articles such as some new clothing,[5] much carpeting,[6] and most of the plywood and fiberboard with which most homes, cabinets, and some furniture are built. If formaldehyde were to somehow stay locked in those products it might not result in adverse human health effects, but it does not stay locked in. It volatilizes, sometimes for years, into indoor environments where it is then inhaled by the inhabitants.

Artificial fragrances are simply mixtures of volatile organic chemicals and solvents, often over 100 of them in any one fragrance product, and most of those chemicals are petroleum derivatives. Some of the most common chemicals found in these artificial fragrances include toluene, xylene, acetone, benzene derivatives, and various aldehydes.[7] These chemicals are simply compounded in such a way as to trick the brain into thinking that it is smelling something pleasant. Artificial fragrances are found in an enormously wide variety of products besides the perfumes, colognes, aftershaves and lotions that are applied directly to the skin (and thereby given relatively direct access to the bloodstream). Fragrances are also found in many home cleaning products, and in most laundry detergents, dryer sheets, toilet paper, fabric softeners, and so on. For months after clothing, bed sheets, and other materials are washed in these products, their fumes can pass onto the skin (and thence into the bloodstream) and into the indoor environment where they are then inhaled.[8]

Pesticides (i.e., insecticides, fungicides, herbicides, microbicides) are also found almost everywhere in the environment, both indoors and outdoors.[9] Many homes, most schools, virtually all grocery stores, restaurants, malls, department stores, and most public office buildings are regularly fumigated with insecticides. Most public parks and other public areas are regularly sprayed with herbicides, and sometimes with insecticides. Almost all federal, state, and county roadways are regularly sprayed with herbicides. Large areas of agricultural crops and private timberlands are sprayed regularly with herbicides and insecticides.[10] Some of the worst pesticide spraying takes place on golf courses,[11] in cemeteries, and on private neighborhood lawns.

These three classes of toxicants (and many others) can thus be found almost everywhere in the environment; in fact, it is almost impossible to avoid exposure to them daily by breathing, by ingestion, and by absorption through the skin and mucus membranes. The focus of this book will be on the human health effects of exposure to chemicals such as these.

This book discusses the human health effects of *long-term* exposure to these ubiquitous toxicants. Virtually everyone has endured and is continuing to endure long-term exposure, even when they wish to avoid it, to many of these toxicants.

It discusses the human health effects of long-term exposure to what we still call *low* doses of these ubiquitous toxicants; that is, to levels of these toxicants which have heretofore been considered acceptable, or "generally regarded as safe" (GRAS).

Toxicologists often like to quote Paracelsus' famous dictum to the effect that "the dose makes the poison," by which they mean to suggest that nothing is actually toxic in itself, but that things instead become toxic depending on the dose which is absorbed by the organism. Everything, even water, they say, is toxic in some dose. And, by extension, they also suggest that almost every substance is *not* poisonous at some very low dose.

In reality, however, Paracelsus' dictum is incomplete. He should rather have said that it is the dose *plus the host* which makes the poison.[12] That is, the quantity and quality of the toxic substance, and the characteristics—both inherited and acquired—of the exposed host are the two factors which truly determine whether a substance will prove toxic to a particular organism. Moreover, there is the phenomenon of bioaccumulation which must be factored in as well. When small, seemingly nontoxic doses of a substance accumulate in an organism over time, the cumulative dose can become seriously large and clearly toxic. Furthermore, these built-up quantities are often not easily or accurately measurable with current technologies. (In addition, the *mixtures* of these chemicals which bioaccumulate within an organism in low doses may have toxic effects many times those of any one chemical.[13])

Finally, this book discusses the *chronic* effects of these exposures rather than the immediate, acute health effects. We will be less concerned, therefore, with the immediate symptoms people might exhibit after exposure to a large chemical spill, for example: symptoms such as abdominal pain, vomiting, dizziness, constriction or dilation of the pupils, sweating, muscle twitching, seizures or even respiratory arrest and death. We will instead be more concerned with the long-term adverse health effects that people might experience as a result of such an exposure.

For example, a story in the Seattle news media on January 20, 1998, reported that a large dose of extra chlorine had been accidentally added to the water supply of one of Seattle's large neighborhoods the previous day. The story concluded by reporting that fortunately no one had suffered any serious, long-term, or irremediable harm. How the writer could have determined within one day that no one would suffer any long-term or irreversible adverse effects was not explained. Indeed it could not have been explained because it could not have been determined. If there were adverse health effects which may not have become evident for days, weeks or months after exposure, it was clearly premature for the news media to announce that no one had been harmed. Yet the media do this regularly, assuring us that no one has been chronically or seriously harmed by an accidental local exposure to toxicants.

Thus, while the medical specialists in toxicology may be interested in the immediate acute adverse health effects of exposure to toxics, in this book we will be more concerned with the *chronic* effects, some of which may not become clinically evident until quite some time after the exposure has occurred.

In summary, this book will primarily focus on the chronic human health effects that may result from long-term exposure to low doses of toxicants that are ubiquitous in the environment, and which have, in the past, been generally regarded as safe.

Arriving at a name for some of the disorders that seem to be caused by long-term exposure to low doses of ambient chemicals has been somewhat problematic.[14] The following names, among others, have been suggested for some of these conditions: Allergic Hypersensitivity induced by chemicals (a term the World Health Organization has recently chosen to use),[15] Multiple Chemical Sensitivity (MCS),[16] Chemical Sensitivity (CS),[17] Environmental Illness (EI), Sick Building Syndrome, and Toxicant Induced Loss of Tolerance (TILT).[18] These disorders have in the past been sometimes referred to as a kind of "allergic" reaction, or even as "total allergy syndrome." Although many modern allergists prefer to use the term "allergy" in its much narrower designation—to indicate only those conditions characterized by certain kinds of antibody reactions (viz., IgE mediated) induced by specific antigens—when the term allergy was first coined (by Von Pirquet in 1906) it was used to mean "'altered reactivity' of whatever origin."[19] Nevertheless, by consensus the term allergy is not now commonly used to designate the symptoms of certain toxicant induced illnesses.

Although I will use the somewhat broad term Toxicant Induced Pathology, or Toxicant Induced Illness in referring to this class of conditions, the terms MCS and CS are more descriptive of the symptoms of some of these conditions. Environmental Illness, though it does say something about the etiology of toxicant induced illnesses, seems perhaps a little too broad. And "chemical sensitivity" does not adequately express the sometimes dramatically disabling nature of many of these conditions. As physician and researcher Claudia Miller says, "Although chemical sensitivity certainly sounds like an inconvenient problem to have, the words fail to convey the potentially disabling nature of the condition and its postulated origins in a toxic exposure."[20] I particularly like her use of the term TILT (Toxicant Induced Loss of Tolerance) because it indicates both something about the etiology and something about the disabling symptoms experienced by sufferers. She draws an analogy here with the tilt, or "game over," message of a pinball machine:

> [With] a pinball machine, a player has just so much latitude—he can jiggle the machine, nudge it, bump it, rock it, but when he exceeds the limit for that machine, the "TILT" message appears, the lights go out, and the ball cascades to the bottom. The machine's tolerance has been exceeded and no amount of effort will make the bumpers or flippers operate as they did before. The game is over.[21]

This name, then, at least has the additional virtue (which the term "sensitivity" does not have) of hinting at some of the disabling and incapacitating nature of toxicant induced illnesses. This term would probably be appreciated by the toughened old truck driver who, after he had been badly disabled by a chemical sensitivity disorder, said "Chemical sensitivity? Hell, let's cut this sensitivity BS. If your kid runs out in the street and gets hit by a truck and his body is broken and crippled, you don't say, poor child, he's sensitive to trucks. Let's quit with this sensitivity crap. These chemicals are *poison*."

This fellow simply wanted the name of the disorder which had disabled him to at least hint at its intensely destructive nature.

In any case, chemical sensitivity disorders probably constitute quite an extensive class, and not just one uniform disorder. If Miller and others are correct, chemical sensitivity disorders (or TILT) may represent a whole new disease mechanism, much as the germ theory did in the 18th century. Microbe-induced diseases—what we now refer to as infectious diseases—were certainly not all of the same kind, nor did they all exhibit the same symptomology. They did, however, all fall into the same class of conditions in the sense that they were all caused by microbes. Toxicant induced pathologies likewise do not all exhibit the same symptoms (though there do seem to be some intriguing similarities among many of them). But, even if the illnesses do not present themselves in a physician's office in the same way, it may well be that they all have the same cause, namely pathogenic toxicants.[22]

In any case, this is the class of conditions we will be examining in this book: those chronic conditions that appear to have been brought on by exposure to low doses of ubiquitous environmental toxicants at levels which have in the past been generally regarded as safe.

ENVIRONMENTAL ETHICS

Like environmental health, environmental ethics is a broad field comprising numerous subdisciplines. And we will also be examining only a small segment of it. This book discusses only those portions of the field of environmental ethics which consider the ethical issues surrounding the human health effects that result from exposure to what have been considered nonsignificant levels of ambient environmental toxicants. These ethical issues, as we will see in Chapters Two and Three, are quite complex, and can be approached from at least two different perspectives outlined by ethicists: the teleological and the deontological. We will examine both the teleological-consequentialist method of environmental health risk assessment, and the deontological approach represented in human rights documents. Before we do that, however, we will, in Chapter One, look at the array of adverse human health effects associated with exposure to environmental toxicants.

The Problem

Why is the threat of low dose exposure to environmental toxicants so dangerous and so problematic? There are actually several reasons.

One of the simplest and most important reasons these exposures are problematic is that low doses of toxicants are completely

invisible, often completely unsmellable (i.e., they often occur in concentrations well below the olfactory threshold), and thus are virtually undetectable by all normal human abilities to perceive. There is
thus no simple way to determine when and whether one is being
exposed to these chemicals. One function of our long-evolved sensory apparatus is to warn us of the presence of dangers and threats,
so that we can take action to protect ourselves. In the case of exposure to low doses of environmental toxicants, however, our senses
are often not able to detect any clues that would alert us to danger,
so we remain completely unaware that we are being exposed to dangerous substances.

Of course *high* doses of airborne chemical fumes sometimes are
visible (appearing perhaps as a cloud) and may even be readily
detected by smell and other sensations. High doses of chemical contaminants in water might be detected by a bitter or chemical taste
or smell. In addition, some occupational settings where high doses
of airborne chemicals might be found—for example, in areas where
those chemicals are stored and used—are often required by law to
be clearly labeled. Thus, even though high concentrations may not
actually be visible to the naked eye or sensible in other ways, they
are in a sense made visible by clear notification and labeling practices. People in these situations are verbally warned about the presence of toxic substances, so they have the opportunity to know what
they are being exposed to. But low doses of chemicals, because they
are legally considered to be at negligible levels, have no such
notification or labeling requirements. Since they are usually well
below our normal sensory threshold detection limits, and are therefore invisible and insensible to us, they pose a hazard that may be
more insidious than other risks which might be more readily detected
by human senses.

Because many of these environmental toxicants are invisible and
sometimes difficult to detect (especially without the use of expensive
technical environmental assays) we sometimes must rely on written
records of chemical dispersal or pollution in a given locale in order
to know what people in that locale might be exposed to. Written
records can sometimes help by documenting the dispersal of toxicants into a given region. Unfortunately, the records documenting
these chemical dispersals sometimes disappear or are lost, so that
the toxicants remaining in an environment can last much longer than
their records. This can happen particularly in the case of highly persistent toxicants, such as the organochlorine pesticides, PCBs, and

dioxins, as well as many of the chemicals and heavy metals associated with mining and smelting.[23]

Another significant problem is that many of these toxicants are ubiquitous. They can actually be found virtually everywhere around us in our air, in our buildings, in our water,[24] in our soil, on our food, embedded in the fabrics from which our clothing is made, embedded in many of the materials that we encounter in everyday life, and can be found as well on the surfaces of furniture, bedding, walls, floors, lawns, streets and roadways.

Besides the chemicals we manufacture and deliberately put into our consumer products each year, there are also industrial chemical byproducts that are unintentionally put into the environment each year.

An example of the former is formaldehyde, which is deliberately added to so many of our consumer products; millions of pounds of pesticides[25] are applied in virtually all public places, indoors and outdoors, in the United States every year; a high volume[26] of artificial fragrance chemicals is added to our water and air space in the form of laundry detergents, perfumes, colognes, aftershaves, hairsprays, lotions and handsoaps, in addition to the artificial scents often added to pesticides. All these chemicals have been *deliberately* put into our daily environment each year. Industrial waste chemical byproducts are also released by American (and other) manufacturers, mostly unintentionally, and are dispersed into our air, our water, and over our land, and sometimes underground. According to an Environmental Protection Agency (EPA) report, in 1995 the most recent year for which data are currently available:

> [The] volume of toxic waste containing all TRI [toxic release inventory] chemicals ... was over 35 billion pounds. Since 1991, when EPA first began collecting TRI waste data, there has been a 7 percent increase in [chemical] waste generation.[27]

Thirty-five billion pounds of toxic industrial byproducts certainly seems like a significant quantity of toxicants to be adding to the environment each year, the environment which human beings and other life forms need in order to live, to live well, and to reproduce. This quantity of toxic industrial waste is added *each year*. Moreover, this number does not come close, unfortunately, to indicating the total quantity of industrial chemical byproducts dumped into our environment. It represents only those individual environmental pollutants that are formally listed on the federal Toxics Release

Inventory (TRI), i.e., only the reportable toxicants, and even then only that portion of those designated toxicants which American industry chooses to report.

Though we might hope that these data covered all the toxics released by industry each year, we sadly know they do not. There are approximately 80,000 chemicals in common industrial use today (almost none of which existed before World War II). Only 600 or so—those pollutants currently recognized to be the most highly toxic chemical byproducts of major industrial processes—are designated on the TRI.[28] Thus, we might expect that some quantity of environmental toxicants greater than 35 billion pounds is actually released each year. Furthermore, these data cover only toxic releases by American manufacturers; they do not include data on toxics released by non–American manufacturers in other parts of the world. Nor do these data cover small businesses, since they have been legally exempted from any TRI reporting. In addition, there was only a 66 percent compliance rate for reporting in 1995; i.e., only 66 percent of those industries that were required to report their TRI releases actually did report them.[29] Furthermore, since TRI data rely entirely on self-reporting by industry, and the "EPA has never assigned any staff to check the quality of the self-reported data,"[30] we might well wonder whether even these 66 percent of manufacturers have been forthcoming about the full extent of their toxic byproduct releases. We should probably not be surprised to learn that many industries have underreported their actual releases.

These industrial toxic byproducts and the chemicals (like formaldehyde, pesticides and artificial fragrance chemicals) which are deliberately added to our environment in consumer products, foods and so on, add up to a huge quantity of environmental toxicants circulating every day in our air, water and soil. They have become an inherent part of the vegetable and animal food chain. In their work *Toxic Deception*, Fagin and Lavelle state:

> Nearly six trillion pounds [of chemicals are] produced annually for plastics, glues, fuels, dyes, and other chemical products. In 1995, the 100 largest U.S.-based chemical manufacturers sold more than $234 billion worth of chemical products—a 17 percent increase over the previous year—and made $35 billion in profits. Their products have become such a pervasive part of American life, in fact, that an estimated 98 percent of all families now use pesticides at least once a year. Every year more than a billion pounds of pesticides are used in the United States [alone].[31]

We can see, therefore, that these toxicants are inescapably ubiquitous in the environment. They are perhaps somewhat more concentrated in certain locations than in others, but they are nonetheless present almost everywhere in our lives.

The ubiquity of these toxicants creates yet another problem: exposure to them is virtually unavoidable. Almost every piece of clothing we purchase, every piece of furniture, all carpeting, most of our food, much of our water, many of our building and remodeling materials, all of our office machines and our home computers, in fact, practically all of our manufactured consumer products are contaminated to some degree with a variety of chemical compounds, some of them intentionally applied or added, and some of them present only as accidental contaminants and byproducts. Much of the air we breathe—in our office buildings, in our homes and apartment buildings, in urban areas, in areas where there is industry and the large scale use of fossil fuels, in agricultural areas (where pesticides are used), in forest lands (again, due to pesticide use), in our city, county, and state parks (pesticide use), on our golf courses (heavy pesticide use),[32] in our neighborhoods (toxic lawncare products and pesticides) in our stores and malls (pesticides), and along virtually all of our roadways (again, pesticide use as well as lead and other byproducts of auto and diesel exhaust)—much of our air is contaminated with detectable levels of a wide variety of synthetic chemical pollutants.

If a person tries to avoid exposure to these synthetic toxicants, as sufferers of multiple chemical sensitivity must, they will find it virtually impossible to do so. The most that a person will be able to accomplish is to somewhat *reduce* their level of toxicant exposure. Most of the 75,000 to 80,000 synthetic chemical compounds in common industrial use today were not even in existence before the middle of the 20th century, and approximately 1,000 new chemicals are being added to that number each year.[33] Many of these chemicals are so widespread that no one can successfully avoid breathing, touching, absorbing, eating or drinking at least some of them. Exposure to a wide variety of these newly developed xenobiotic toxicants is virtually inevitable.

Yet another problem is that adequate information about the full extent to which we are exposed to these toxicants, and about what the potential health effects of all these exposures are likely to be, has not been adequately developed, and what little is known is not readily available.

Because testing for the health effects of most of these new chemical compounds has never been done, almost nothing is known about their health effects, even their acute effects, and especially not about their long-term chronic effects on human tissues, organs and systems. In fact, some of the little information which is known—the full list of ingredients in insecticide and herbicide compounds, for example, or the chemical ingredients in artificial fragrance products—has actually been deliberately hidden from public view by the manufacturers of these products. These manufacturers believe that they have a financial interest in people *not* knowing the full list of chemicals (and their health effects) which make up their products. Even if people knew to ask for Material Safety Data Sheets (MSDS) for each of the chemicals to which they thought they might be exposed, and even if those MSDSs were made readily available to them, they would soon discover that the information on those sheets is seldom complete, and is sometimes actually wrong.[34] What they may not discover, moreover, because this fact is not disclosed on an MSDS, is that the information on it is provided entirely by the manufacturer of that chemical. That is, the information is not provided by any independent third party who might be expected to have a somewhat more objective and complete view of the character, toxicity, and exposure effects of the compound, but by a corporation which has a large financial interest in the widespread distribution and use of the chemical product.

More importantly, no information at all is made available (because so little exists as yet) about the health effects of exposure to the *mixtures* of chemicals to which we are all exposed. We all know very well that some pharmaceutical products can have dangerous additive or multiplicative effects when mixed. In the same way, ambient environmental chemicals can have adverse additive, multiplicative or synergistic effects when mixed together in our air, water and food, and then again mixed together in or bodies. If it is true that the average person, on an average day, comes into contact with between 200 and 300 different synthetic chemicals[35] (and that number is growing each year with the continued manufacture and proliferation of synthetic chemicals), then the number of possible interactions between mixtures of chemicals, for any given person, is very large. Because exposure to toxic mixtures has been so little studied, and because so little attention has been given to the potential interactions among the various toxicants in this daily chemical milieu, hardly anything is known about the possible health effects of those potential interactions.

We are thus operating in a very serious knowledge vacuum.[36] We do not yet have anything even resembling an adequate understanding of the long-term (or even near-term) health effects of exposure to the chemical combinations that we encounter daily.

Because these chemicals are ubiquitous, because there is so little available information about the health effects of these chemicals, and because we are given even less information than is known about them, we are therefore, in effect, no longer free to decide whether we wish to expose ourselves, our families, and our children to these toxicants. The freedom to choose whether we wish to be exposed to these toxicants or not based on knowledge of the potential risks and potential benefits of such exposures has in effect escaped us. We have lost that freedom. We have given it up. Or it has, perhaps, been taken from us. In any event, we do not have the freedom to choose. Informed consent, the moral foundation of all medical-, health- and research-related ethical activity, is no longer ours to give.

Yet another significant problem concerns the near impossibility of detecting the early stages of some of these long-term health effects from exposure to toxicants. We know, for example, that the growth, development, and eventual emergence of some cancers can be a very long-term process, sometimes occurring over a period of years or decades. The same is true of certain cardiovascular diseases, some endocrine disruption effects, and other conditions as well. We know also that sometimes the early stages of these disorders are virtually undetectable, and that sometimes we are made aware of them only after significant damage has already been done, perhaps only after the condition has become untreatable and irreversible.

There is something of an analogy here with the early days of the HIV/AIDS pandemic, and the problems that developed as a result of a virally contaminated blood supply. It was probably as early as 1978 that HIV had entered the blood supply, well before the first AIDS case was recognized in 1981, when blood donors, who had no idea they carried any dangerous infectious diseases, donated HIV infected blood. *The American Journal of Public Health* said:

> In the seven years that elapsed before antibody screening effectively created the possibility of blood safety, tens of thousands became infected. Seventy-five percent to 85% of hemophiliacs dependent upon clotting factor derived from thousands of blood units became infected. Approximately 30,000 transfusion recipients were infected as well. The seeds of this iatrogenic tragedy were sown even before the first cases of acquired immunodeficiency syndrome (AIDS) ... were reported.[37]

Just as this tragedy was already well under way many years before anyone recognized there was even a problem, let alone one of global proportions, so today's dispersal of these enormous quantities of toxicants into the air and water, into the food supply, and into the consumer products we use in our daily lives, may also be making for a tragedy of global proportions. The main difference between the case of HIV in the blood supply and toxicant dispersal into our environment is this: with HIV there was no warning and no way that public health officials could have prevented it. Human Immunodeficiency Virus, as the causative agent of AIDS, wasn't even detected, after all, until 1984—three years after the first cases of AIDS were discovered—so officials could hardly have tested for the presence of HIV in the blood supply. But with the toxicants we are daily releasing into the environment, we already have had numerous warnings. Scientists and activists have been warning for decades, even well before Rachel Carson's classic *Silent Spring* was first published in 1962, about the toxic effects on human health and on the environment of our almost indiscriminate release of chemicals. Unfortunately, as with poor Cassandra in Greek mythology, the warnings have gone almost completely unheeded. And the potential adverse human health effects of exposure to these toxicants go well beyond cancer, as we will see in Chapter One.

Some of the adverse neurologic, immunologic, reproductive and endocrinologic effects of long-term exposure to low doses of toxicants may unfortunately develop in a long-term manner: slow and invisible in their early stages; serious, untreatable, and irreversible in their ultimate consequences. Many cancers, as we well know, may not become clinically evident until 20 to 40 years after exposure to a triggering carcinogen. And since we already know that many of these toxicants bioaccumulate in human tissues over time,[38] it should not come as any great surprise to learn that the total body load of these toxicants in every human population on earth is continuing to increase. And as the total body load of these toxicants increases, so too does the likelihood of pathology eventually emerging. We already know, for example, that endocrine system disruption, and the consequent effects on reproductive development, can take many years to become fully evident after young children (or fetuses) have been exposed to chemicals.[39]

Yet another problem with exposure to these toxicants is that the long-term neurologic, immunologic, or endocrinologic effects of some of them (not to mention their carcinogenic effects) can often be irreversible. Serious and irreversible adverse effects deserve particularly special care, and the agents which can cause them require the most stringent regulation. But U.S. regulatory policy, and international policy even more so, has so far been inadequate in this regard.

Furthermore, some of these chemical compounds—particularly the insecticides, herbicides, fungicides, rodenticides, and microbicides (many of which can be found in use in most households)—are specifically and intentionally designed to be biotoxic. "Designer poisons," one author terms them.[40] Thus, many of the chemical toxicants that we encounter on a daily basis are specifically intended to be damaging to biological systems. It should come, then, as no great surprise to learn that they may also do damage to human biological systems.

And finally, it should be noted that the problem of toxicant induced illnesses is global in its extent. In addition to the growing worldwide incidence of cancers and other toxicant induced illnesses, two recent reports have clearly and independently documented the worldwide extent of chemical sensitivity disorders. According to one report, chemical intolerance illnesses were reported in every country studied, including Algeria, Argentina, Australia, Austria, Bahamas, Belgium, Brazil, Canada, Chile, Colombia, Costa Rica, Croatia, Denmark, England, Finland, France, Germany, Greece, Guam, Kenya, Luxembourg, Malaysia, Mauritius, Mexico, New Zealand, the Netherlands, Northern Ireland, Norway, the Philippines, Puerto Rico, Russia, Senegal, South Africa, Sweden, the United States, and Venezuela.[41]

Toxicant induced illnesses have been found and documented in both industrialized and developing nations.

Given some of the challenging characteristics of commonly encountered chemical pollutants and the illnesses associated with them, we might expect that government regulatory agencies around the world would be highly vigilant in protecting their people from these pollutants. We might even naively hope to see some corporate manufacturers exhibiting an appropriate level of concern about people's health. Unfortunately, though, we see too little done. Parents, for example (a group often concerned about their children's potential exposures), are simply too overwhelmed with the myriad of other responsibilities that come with being a good parent in the modern world to take much political action. Government regulatory agencies are overworked and underfunded, and they simply have not been given the kind of legal and popular mandate to strictly test, regulate, and police the manufacture and release of toxicants. And manufacturers, of course, have not wished to police themselves, especially when such self-regulation could have a significant negative impact on their financial returns. They have instead fought vigorously and successfully to avoid having their activities and processes monitored and regulated by government agencies.

Meaningful changes, therefore, if any are to come, will probably need to begin—as has been the case with tobacco policy—with an increase in popular awareness of toxicant induced illnesses, and with eventual recognition by the medical community that long-term exposure to even low levels of toxicants can indeed cause serious human disease. Government monitoring, regulation, and control of low levels of toxicant exposure will need to become an essential component of protecting our families, children, and future generations from these potentially dangerous contaminants.

That the levels of synthetic toxicants ubiquitous in today's world may have adverse human health effects is still considered by some—particularly by those with corporate and financial interests in the matter—to be controversial. Corporate tobacco interests also, of course, consider claims about the adverse health effects of tobacco to be controversial. They regularly dispute scientific claims that tobacco is an addictive drug, that it is a carcinogen, and that smoking tobacco is a serious contributor to respiratory and cardiovascular disease as well as to male erectile dysfunction. Confirmation of the potential adverse health effects of ambient environmental toxicants may not yet be as overwhelming as the evidence supporting tobacco's addictiveness or carcinogenicity, but there is a large and growing body of well-designed scientific studies (a few will be described in Chapter One) which strongly support the claims against these contaminants.

There are some significant differences, of course, between the risks of adverse health effects due to tobacco use and the risks of adverse health effects due to exposure to ambient environmental toxicants. One of the key differences is the degree to which a person has control over, and thus is able to avoid, exposure to these toxicants. Setting aside for a moment the issue of tobacco's addictiveness, a person may effectively choose to avoid the negative consequences of smoking tobacco by simply not smoking it and by avoiding situations in which others are smoking it. And yet, that same person will find it virtually impossible to avoid exposure to ambient environmental toxicants, even including pesticides. These chemicals are so ubiquitous in the outdoor and indoor air, in our water, food, and soil, and so common in our clothing, our furniture, and in our public and private buildings, and (as we have said) are so invisible and undetectable, that it is virtually impossible for a person to avoid exposure to them. Thus, the adverse health consequences that may result from breathing local air (or drinking local water, or eating local food) contaminated with pesticide residues, for example, may also be virtually inescapable. Our governments and public health agencies have allowed these chemical toxicants to be so widely dispersed in the environment in the second half of the 20th century that exposure to them is a virtual certainty, whether a person wishes to avoid them or not.

Given these realities, it will be argued later in this book, it should be the responsibility of policymakers and lawmakers to ensure that citizens are able, if they so wish, to protect themselves from overexposure to these toxicants. Steps in this direction can be taken by legislation and regulation, or even by simply requiring full disclosure about the potential risks to which people are presently being exposed.

In Chapter One of this book, we will look at some of the evidence that supports the recognition of the pathogenicity of long-term exposure to low levels of commonly used synthetic chemical products and byproducts. In Chapter Two some of the key ethical principles will be outlined which, it will be argued, should guide our thinking about how best to deal with the plethora of environmental toxicants to which we are exposed. Chapter Three details some broad (and quite modest) policy recommendations that I believe clearly follow from recognizing the data in Chapter One and the principles in Chapter Two. Chapter Four, then, explores some of the obstacles and challenges that will have to be met and dealt with in the process of implementing the proposals recommended in Chapter Three.

We begin now with the data on human health effects.

Notes

1. G. Stine, *Acquired Immune Deficiency Syndrome: Biological, Medical, Social and Legal Issues*, 1st ed. (Englewood Cliffs, NJ: Prentice Hall, 1993) 462+xxxii. p. 347.

2. See, for example, M. Fumento, "Allergic to Life," *Reason*, June 1996, 20–26, and John Stossel, "Allergic to the World," ABC's 20/20, 1997.

3. J. Wargo, *Our Children's Toxic Legacy: How Science and Law Fail to Protect Us from Pesticides*, (New Haven, CT: Yale University Press, 1996) 380+xvi.

4. D.J. Rapp, *Is This Your Child's World? How You Can Fix the Schools and Homes That Are Making Your Children Sick* (New York: Bantam, 1996) 635+xix. pp. 525–27.

5. *Ibid.*, p. 14.

6. Besides formaldehyde, chemicals commonly found in carpets include acetone, benzene, hexane, styrene, decane, toluene, diisocyanate, xylene, and numerous others. See *ibid.*, p. 260.

7. See Appendix VI for the 20 most common chemicals found in artificial fragrances.

8. It may also be true that even some products labeled as "natural" fragrance products can include, as part of their make-up, synthetic chemical ingredients. Consider: "[A]rtificial fragrances, i.e., compounds not yet regarded as natural substances, may be present in products claimed to be based on natural ingredients." See S.C. Rastogi, J.D. Johansen and T. Mennde, "Natural ingredients based cosmetics: content of selected fragrance sensitizers," *Contact Dermatitis*, 34, Number 6 (June 1996) 423–26.

9. One German study found chlordane and other pesticides in the vacuum bags of many homes.

10. See C. Van Strum, *A Bitter Fog: Herbicides and Human Rights* (San Francisco: Sierra Club Books, 1983) 288+x.

11. "A 30-year-old navy lieutenant develops a rash, then basketball-sized blisters, then internal organ damage, and dies in 1982 after a game of golf on a course that had just been sprayed with the fungicide Daconil 2787, which is still on the market." D. Fagin and M. Lavelle, *Toxic Deception: How the Chemical Industry Manipulates Science, Bends the Law, and Endangers Your Health* (Secaucus, NJ: Carol Publishing, 1997) 294+xxvi. p. 6.

12. C.S. Miller, "Chemical Sensitivity: symptom, syndrome or mechanism for disease?" *Toxicology*, 111 (1996) 69–86. p. 80.

13. For more on mixtures of chemicals, see Chapter Two.

14. "When I use a word," Humpty Dumpty said, in rather a scornful tone, "it means just what I choose it to mean—neither more nor less." "The question is," said Alice, "whether you can make words mean so many different things." "The question is," said Humpty Dumpty, "which is to be master—that's all." L Carroll, *Through the Looking Glass* (New York: Bantam, 1871, 1981) 98–218. p. 169

15. J.G. Vos, M. Younes and E. Smith, eds., *Allergic Hypersensitivities Induced by Chemicals: Recommendations for Prevention* (London: CRC Press on behalf of the World Health Organization Regional Office for Europe, 1996) 348.

16. N. Ashford and C. Miller, *Chemical Exposures: Low Levels, High Stakes*, 1st ed. (New York: Van Nostrand Reinhold, 1991) 214.

17. W. Rea, MD, *Chemical Sensitivity*, 4 (Boca Raton, FL: Lewis Publishers, and CRC Press, 1992–97) 2924.

18. C. Miller, "White Paper: Chemical Sensitivity: History and Phenomenology," *Toxicology and Industrial Health*, 10, Number 4/5 (1994) 253–76.

19. C.S. Miller, "Chemical Sensitivity: symptom, syndrome or mechanism for disease?" *Toxicology*, 111 (1996) 69–86. p. 81. Emphasis in original.

20. C.S. Miller, "Toxicant-induced Loss of Tolerance—An Emerging Theory of Disease?" *Environmental Health Perspectives*, 105, Supplement 2 (March 1997) 445–53. p. 445.

21. C.S. Miller, "Chemical Sensitivity: symptom, syndrome or mechanism for disease?" *Toxicology*, 111 (1996) 69–86. p. 81.

22. C. Miller, "White Paper: Chemical Sensitivity: History and Phenomenology," *Toxicology and Industrial Health*, 10, Number 4/5 (1994) 253–76. p. 8.

23. See, for example, the news story about a defunct smelter in Everett, Washington, that has "levels of arsenic, lead and cadmium higher than in residential areas around the old Tacoma smelter that Asarco shut down in 1985." AP. "State seeking records for defunct smelter," *The Eugene Register-Guard*, March 26, 1997. Documents that recorded these pollutants were largely lost.

24. "The number of public-health advisories warning people not to eat the fish they catch in lakes, rivers and bays has increased 72 percent nationwide in recent years, the Natural Resources Defense Council said yesterday. States issued 2,194 fish warnings in 1996—up from 1,278 in 1993, the report said, citing data from the Environmental Protection Agency. The numbers include statewide advisories as well as advisories for individual bodies of water.... 'We don't want to be unduly alarmist,' Chasis said. 'We're not saying people should not fish or eat what they catch. We're saying that people need to be aware of the public-health advisories and not just assume that their favorite fishing hole is OK.'" E. Kelly, "Fillet of methylmercury: Fish health warnings rise," *Seattle Times*, April 9 1998. A8.

25. The actual amount of pesticide use is probably in the billions of pounds, not millions, every year, but no data are collected anywhere tallying the total volume of pesticides used in the nation. It is literally the case that no one knows how much pesticide is used.

26. Data on total volume of artificial chemical fragrances used are also not recorded by any agency anywhere. Literally, no one knows the total volume of artificial fragrance chemicals added to our environment every year, but it too is probably at least in the millions of pounds.

27. D. Kearns, *EPA's 1995 Toxics Release Data Include First-Ever Reporting on 286 New Chemicals*. EPA, May 20, 1997. The actual total release for 1995 of all chemicals on the TRI was 35,027,058,218 pounds, according to data on the EPA's TRI homepage (http://www.epa.gov/opptintr/tri/pdr95/drover01.htm).

28. D. Kearns, *EPA's 1995 Toxics Release Data Include First-Ever Reporting on 286 New Chemicals*. EPA, May 20, 1997. See also S. Steingraber, *Living Downstream: An Ecologist Looks at Cancer and the Environment* (Reading, MA: Addison-Wesley, 1997) 357+xvi. p. 101.

29. S. Steingraber, *Living Downstream: An Ecologist Looks at Cancer*

and the Environment (Reading, MA: Addison-Wesley, 1997) 357+xvi. p. 101.

30. P. Montague, "Childhood Cancer and Pollution," *Rachel's Environment and Health Weekly*, #559 (August 14, 1997).

31. D. Fagin and M. Lavelle, *Toxic Deception: How the Chemical Industry Manipulates Science, Bends the Law, and Endangers Your Health* (Secaucus, NJ: Carol Publishing, 1997) 294+xxvi. p. xvii. The pesticide figure is an estimate, of course.

32. Some few golf courses have begun to maintain their grounds with no or minimal use of pesticides and chemical fertilizers. See J. Stuller, "Golf gets back to nature, inviting everyone to play," *Smithsonian*, April 1997, 56–66.

33. These estimates are found in many sources, including L. Lawson, *Staying Well in a Toxic World* (Chicago: Noble Press, 1993) 488.

34. MSDSs "often contain deficiencies that preclude the prudent physician from relying exclusively on them." S. Lerman and H. Kipen, "Material Safety Data Sheets: Caveat Emptor," *Archives of Internal Medicine*, 150, #5 (May 1990) 981–4. p. 981.

35. L. Lawson, *Staying Well in a Toxic World* (Chicago: Noble Press, 1993) 488.

36. For documentation of the extent of this knowledge vacuum, see D. Fagin and M. Lavelle, *Toxic Deception: How the Chemical Industry Manipulates Science, Bends the Law, and Endangers Your Health* (Secaucus, NJ: Carol Publishing, 1997) 294+xxvi.

37. "Book review of *HIV and the Blood Supply*," *American Journal of Public Health*, 87, Number 3 (March 1997) 474.

38. See Chapter One.

39. Much of this work is summarized in T. Colburn, D. Dumanoski and J.P. Myers, *Our Stolen Future: Are We Threatening Our Fertility, Intelligence and Survival?—A Scientific Detective Story* (New York: Penguin Books USA, 1996) 306+xii.

40. M. Moses, *Designer Poisons: How to Protect Your Health and Home from Toxic Pesticides* (San Francisco: Pesticide Education Center, 1995) 415.

41. C. Duehring, "The global problem of MCS part one: overview of investigative reports' findings," *Medical and Legal Briefs*, 2, Number 5 (March/April 1997) 1–5. p. 1.

ONE

———— Data ————

"Exposure to many chemicals results in allergic hyper-sensitivity which causes conditions such as contact dermatitis and asthma."
—World Health Organization[1]

Here in Chapter One we will review research findings that give some indication of the variety of adverse human health effects which can result from long-term exposure to what have in the past been considered low doses of ubiquitous environmental toxicants. After detailing some of these findings, and after (in Chapter Two) articulating some fundamental ethical principles, we will then (in Chapter Three) make policy recommendations that are intended to minimize human exposure to such toxicants.

We begin with an overview.

1. Health Effects Overview

Human populations worldwide have been shown to suffer a wide variety of adverse health effects as a result of exposure to levels of toxicants that have heretofore been considered low.

No one in the medical and toxicology communities, of course, has any doubt that exposure to *large* doses of synthetic industrial solvents, chlorinated chemical compounds, organophosphate pesticides, and other industrial reagents, solvents, and byproducts can cause people to suffer significant adverse health effects, sometimes including death. Incidents such as the explosion at Bhopal and other large chemical spills have only served to underscore the dangerous adverse effects of exposure to high doses of industrial chemicals.

However, in addition to adverse health effects from exposure to large doses of toxicants, a significant percentage of people also suffer adverse health effects, with varying degrees of severity, as a result of long-term exposure to low levels of environmental toxicants.

We should probably not be surprised to learn that low doses of toxicants can have quite dramatic effects on a human body. The common drug aspirin (acetylsalicylic acid), for example, exerts its effect on the body at doses measured in parts per million (ppm). Lester and Gibbs write, in *A Citizen's Guide to Risk Studies*:

> One part per million means that there is one milligram of that substance for every kilogram of body weight. For ... an adult weighing 59 kilograms (130 pounds), a dose of 1 ppm equals 59 milligrams. The average aspirin contains 325 milligrams of active ingredient, so that two tablets would be approximately the equivalent of 11 ppm in a 130 pound adult. This dosage can stop pain and reduce fever.[2]

At even smaller doses—one-quarter of the amount commonly used for pain relief—aspirin can also have effects on the body that reduce the risk of cardiovascular disease. We should probably, therefore, not consider it surprising that small doses of chemicals, even in the range of parts per million or less, can cause relatively large effects in an organism as complex and finely tuned as the human body.

Some of the adverse health effects from long-term exposure to low doses of toxicants include (as we will see below) carcinogenicity; reproductive disorders; immune system dysregulation; respiratory disorders such as inflammation in the nasal mucosa and airway passages, and Reactive Airways Disease Syndrome; neurological disorders such as dizziness, decreased ability to concentrate and learn, and various other forms of cerebral dysfunction; sleep disorders; gastrointestinal tract disorders such as nausea, gastritis and diarrhea; reproductive disorders[3]; endocrine system dysregulation[4]; chronic fatigue syndrome; Gulf War Illness[5]; dermatologic disorders such as chloracne[6] and dermagraphia; fibromyalgia; and Multiple Chemical Sensitivity (MCS).[7]

While chloracne may be a less common consequence of chemical exposures, chemical sensitivity disorders are a much more common occurrence. Chemical sensitivity symptoms can range from moderate rhinitis, sinusitis, tinnitus (ringing in the ears), increased and irregular heart rate, metallic taste sensations, various paraesthesias (unusual neural sensations), and ocular disorders, to more serious memory loss, inability to concentrate, severely impaired mentation, nausea, severe migraines, and even potentially fatal asthma and reactive airway disease.

Much of the research in the past three or four decades on adverse health effects of low level chemical exposures has focused primarily, if not exclusively, on carcinogenicity. Even a recent study of adverse health effects in sawmill workers exposed to chlorophenate wood preservatives focused only on carcinogenicity,[8] though it is clear that such wood workers may also suffer from immune system dysfunction, neurological problems, endocrine disruption, respiratory disorders, toxicant induced behavioral disorders, and any number of other health effects.[9] Fortunately, such occupational and environmental health research is beginning to expand its field of interest to include other kinds of health effects besides cancer.

Immune system dysregulation, for example, has also been shown to result from exposure to toxicants,[10] as have some kinds of behavioral disorders,[11] and measurable mental deficits in children whose mothers have been exposed to even small doses of PCBs.[12] A wide range of body systems can be affected.

One potential adverse consequence of both acute high-dose exposures and chronic low-dose exposures to toxics is the risk of becoming "sensitized" to (or intolerant of) future exposures to low levels of ambient toxicants. This condition, usually referred to as chemical sensitivity,[13] MCS, or chemical intolerance, renders a person symptomatically reactive to very low levels of a wide spectrum of toxicants.[14] Sensitized persons can become reactive to a wide variety of chemical residues, including common air and water pollutants, and even small residues of pesticides found, for example, in food, water, air, new clothing, bedding and furniture. They can go on to develop a hypersensitivity to formaldehyde residues (in building materials, bedding, furniture, and many fabrics), as well as to industrial solvents, chemical byproducts of industrial processes, and other chemicals that may exist in residual quantities in the environment. The personal and social consequences of having become sensitized in this way can range from relatively mild to so severe as to be completely disabling.

In a 1995 study commissioned by the European Union to examine the prevalence of MCS in member nations, MCS-like illnesses were reported to be widespread throughout Europe. The report that resulted from this study, released in November 1995, was prepared by a group of individuals and agencies from around the world. Researchers involved in the study included Nicholas Ashford, professor at the Massachusetts Institute of Technology, researchers from Ergonomia Ltd. in Athens, the Institute of Environmental Toxicology in Germany, the Institute of Environmental and Occupational Medicine in Denmark, the University of Athens (Greece) Department of Analytical Chemistry, and the Occupational Health Program of the University of Massachusetts Medical Center in Worcester, Massachusetts.[15]

In this report, MCS was defined as:

> [A] sensitivity, such as that induced by toluene diisocyanate (TDI) which begins as specific hypersensitivity to a single agent (or class of substances) but which may evolve into non-specific hyper-responsiveness described as ... the heightened, extraordinary, or unusual response of individuals to known or unknown exposures whose symptoms do not completely resolve upon removal from the exposures and/or whose "sensitivities" seem to spread to other agents. These individuals may experience: a heightened response to agents at the same exposure levels as other individuals; a response at lower levels than those that affect other individuals; [or] a response at an earlier time than that experienced by other individuals.[16]

Nor do those who suffer from these conditions fit neatly into any discernible risk group. Those with MCS in this study included:

> [A] French botanist, a Croatian chemical engineer, an 18-year-old boy in Greece ... a safety engineer at a petroleum refinery in Brazil, and rural South Africans in an isolated undeveloped area where professional medical attention is scarce and a pastor operating a make-shift clinic sees several new cases of chemical sensitivity every week.[17]

The report cited a variety of chemical substances as initiators of these conditions:

> [P]esticides (including pyrethroids and lindane), solvents, paints and lacquers, and formaldehyde. Other initiating substances and events included carpets, carpet glue, anesthesia, antibiotics and other pharmaceuticals, hairdressing chemicals, pentachlorophenol and wood preservatives, mercury amalgams, heavy metals, diesel exhaust,

industrial degreasers, methyl methacrylate, new buildings, newly renovated buildings, inks, stress, PCBs, chemical labs, drycleaning fluids (trichloroethylene), household chemicals (especially those containing chlorine), industrial chemicals, and pesticide and fertilizer residues in food and water.[18]

In other words, quite a wide variety of chemicals can induce quite a wide range of symptoms, in the same way that quite a wide variety of microbial organisms can cause quite a wide range of infectious diseases. One virus may cause an internal cancer, for example, while another may cause a runny nose or skin eruptions. Furthermore, just as these chemical compounds can be found in literally every nation on earth (and even in both polar ice caps), so can these chemically induced diseases.

We turn now to a more detailed examination of some of the specific adverse health effects that can result from long-term exposure to low doses of ambient toxicants.

2. Cancers

Cancers are probably the pathologies most commonly recognized as associated with exposure to environmental toxicants. "WHO [the World Health Organization] has concluded that at least 80% of all cancer is attributable to environmental influences."[19] Though this book will not primarily focus on cancer as one of the health consequences of exposure to ambient environmental contaminants (which many cancers clearly are), it does need to be mentioned as one of the prime examples of toxicant induced illnesses. After all, cancer does kill one in five Americans.[20] "More than a thousand of us die every day [in the U.S.] from cancer. Millions of us are suffering with it now, and millions of our children are already fated to be the future's cancer victims."[21] Furthermore, the incidence of cancer continues to grow. In just the past 50 years, "cancer has galloped from ninth to second place in claiming the lives of American people."[22] If WHO's figures are correct, the large majority of those cancers are attributable to environmental toxicants.

Cancer, therefore, "is not just another degenerative and unavoidable disease of the aging process. It has distinct and identifiable causes, and these are mainly exposures to chemical or physical agents in the environment."[23] Even the National Cancer Institute, an organization which (for political reasons[24]) has historically been rather slow to acknowledge the environmental dimensions of cancer etiology, has stated that:

> We are just beginning to understand the full range of health effects resulting from the exposure to occupational and environmental agents and factors.... Lack of appreciation of the potential hazards of environmental and food source contaminants, and laws, policies and regulations protecting and promoting tobacco use, worsen the cancer problem and drive up health care costs.[25]

The recognition of environmental contaminants as contributing to the cause of various cancers goes back at least to World War II.[26] Moreover, the increase since World War II in the incidence of many cancers clearly parallels the rapid increase in chemical production, use, and dispersal into the environment since the mid–1940s. It is significant that between 1950 and 1991 the incidence of cancer (all types combined) increased 49.3 percent.[27] Or, as Steingraber stated in *Living Downstream*:

> At mid-century a cancer diagnosis was the expected fate of about 25 percent of Americans—a ratio [Rachel] Carson found so shocking that it inspired the title of one of her chapters[28]—while today, about 40 percent of us (38.3 percent of women and 48.2 percent of men) will contract the disease sometime within our lifespans. Cancer is now the second leading cause of death overall, and the leading cause of death among Americans aged thirty-five to sixty-four.
> More of the overall upsurge has occurred in the past two decades than in the previous two, and increases in cancer incidence are seen in all age groups—from infants to the elderly.[29]

Some of the increased incidence of cancer in older adults, of course, can be attributed to tobacco smoking, but the incidence of "cancer not tied to smoking has increased down the generations" as well.[30] The incidence of childhood cancers alone, according to the National Cancer Institute, is increasing at the rate of approximately 1 percent per year,[31] and probably very few of these cancers are directly related to tobacco smoking. Some oncologists estimate that "a newborn child faces a risk of about 1 in 600 of contracting cancer by age 10."[32] This degree of increased incidence, say researchers, is "big enough that better diagnosis and reporting of the diseases are unlikely to be the principal explanation...; childhood cancer is such a serious ailment that it is usually detected."[33] It is much more likely, say these experts, that "toxins in the air, food, dust, soil and drinking water" are the significant factors.[34] Several studies, in fact, have found a clear and significant association between home use of insecticides and herbicides and an increased risk of childhood cancers.[35]

Childhood cancers, of course, are not the only cancers that are increasing in the population. According to public health researcher Devra Davis,

> U.S. white women born in the 1940s have had 30 percent more non-smoking-related cancers than did women of their grandmothers' generation (women born between 1888 and 1897). Among men, the differences were even starker. White men born in the 1940s have had more than twice as much non-tobacco-related cancer than [sic] their grandfathers did at the same age. What this is telling us is that there is something going on here in addition to smoking, and we need to figure out what that is.[36]

What that is, of course, is a growing global chemicalization, which translates into enormous increases in human exposure to synthetic environmental carcinogens (and the U.S. National Cancer Institute takes the position that there is no level of exposure to a carcinogen that is small enough to be safe).[37] Looking at pesticides alone, for example,

> Many of the most common lawn pesticides used in America, including the weed-killer 2,4-D, the fungicide chlorothalonil, and the insecticide chlorpyrifos (Dursban), have been shown to cause cancer or birth defects in lab animals.[38]

Other herbicides have been shown to be associated with an increased risk of breast cancer.[39] Insecticides may also be responsible for an increased risk of certain cancers, even (perhaps especially) in children. To cite just one recent study, the use of flea and tick treatments in the home has been shown to correlate with an increase in brain tumors in children exposed to those products.[40]

And yet it is still possible to manufacture and sell all these products legally.

Pesticides are not the only class of carcinogenic chemicals that have been widely, regularly and legally, dispersed into our environment since World War II. To get some idea of the quantity of such carcinogens, we can turn to the *Biennial Report on Carcinogens*, a document produced biannually by the National Toxicology Program of the U.S. Department of Health and Human Services.

The report exists because the National Toxicology Program is charged
by law with publishing "a list of all substances (i) which either are known
to be carcinogens or may reasonably be anticipated to be carcinogens,
and (ii) to which a significant number of persons residing in the United
States are exposed." The edition that stands next to the Toxics Release
Inventory ... is 473 pages long and features nearly 200 entries.[41]

What the existence of such a list of carcinogens means, of course,
is that "trading in cancer-causing chemicals is still a perfectly legal
activity."[42] Furthermore, this list represents only those chemicals that
have both a) been identified as actual or probable carcinogens' and
b) have been identified as carcinogens to which a large number of
U.S. citizens are regularly exposed. Researchers have estimated that
of the 75,000 to 80,000 chemicals in common commercial use today,
something between five and ten percent of them are probably carcinogenic. This means that approximately 3,750 to 8,000 carcinogenic chemicals exist and are in common commercial use today[43]
(even though the *Biennial Report on Carcinogens* lists only 200). The
increased incidence of cancers, therefore, should come as no great
surprise, given the quantity of carcinogens to which we are regularly
exposed in our environment.

Tragic as this is, carcinogenicity will not be the only, or even
the primary, focus of this book. The well documented connection
between the increased incidence of many human (and other animal)
cancers and the huge increase in the production, transportation, use
and dispersal of synthetic chemicals has been well explored in other
works,[44] so it will not be a central focus in this book. Instead, while
it clearly is important to recognize that the incidence of certain cancers is positively associated with increased exposure to environmental
carcinogens, this book will focus primarily on adverse health effects
other than cancer which are attributable to long-term and widespread exposure to environmental contaminants. Adverse health
effects such as damage to the respiratory system and (in the next section but one) to the immune system.

3. Respiratory Disorders

Like cancers, many forms of asthma and Reactive Airways Dysfunction Syndrome (RADS) have long been recognized as being clearly
associated with exposure to environmental pollutants. "Physicians
have long warned their asthmatic patients to avoid irritants such as
cigarette smoke, perfume, and strong cleaning agents, suggesting

that such exposures might further irritate vulnerable airways, making their asthma worse."[45] After all, "asthma is inflammation, and inflammation can be caused by irritants, chemical or otherwise.... Indeed, some feel that recent upward trends in asthma morbidity and mortality parallel increases in atmospheric pollution."[46]

To note just one example, the mother below describes how her seven year old son was exposed to methyl isocyanate (MIC) in the normal course of simply attending elementary school. (MIC is the chemical that was responsible for so many deaths and injuries in Bhopal in 1984; it is highly reactive and highly volatile.) Her child's school was located not far from a corporation that used and had stores of MIC, and on one day a drum of it was accidentally spilled in the factory. Fumes eventually wafted to the elementary school and were blown into its ventilation system. The mother writes:

> Not unlike those studied in Bhopal, my son Aaron experienced a severe asthma attack five months after his exposure to MIC. Since then, on numerous occasions, he has been rushed to the hospital or a doctor's office for emergency treatments. I have watched my son's health deteriorate to the point of requiring an air filter in his bedroom, a breathing machine at his bedside, a pocket bronchodilator for use in school and during severe bouts, and prescriptions of prednisone.[47]

Her son's health had been dramatically and irreversibly affected by a chemical that she did not even know he was at risk of being exposed to. He had become one of the "increased incidence of asthma" statistics detailed in current medical journals, and the prognosis is that he will probably continue to struggle with it for the rest of his life. Unfortunately, an increase in asthma *mortality* is also being regularly documented in the public health literature, so this young man's hopes of living a full and complete life have also been put at substantial risk.

This family sadly discovered what many are still discovering, that what we do not know can indeed hurt us.

Just as environmental toxicants can cause severe and chronic damage to the respiratory system, so they can also cause long-term damage to the immune system.

4. The Immune System

Medical researchers are increasingly recognizing that the human immune system can also be measurably damaged by long-term, low dose exposure to ambient toxicants.

According to Rachel's Environment and Health Weekly, as early as 1984, the U.S. National Toxicology Program (NTP), within the U.S. Department of Health and Human Services, observed that:

> [C]hemical damage to the immune system could result in "hypersensitivity or allergy" to specific chemicals or to chemicals in general. NTP said damage to the immune system can have far-reaching consequences for an individual, leaving him or her vulnerable to attack by bacteria and viruses, at heightened risk of cancer, and even predisposed to develop AIDS.[48]

Persuasive evidence showing that commonly used pesticides, for instance, do cause significant immune system compromise has continued to accumulate. In 1996 the World Resources Institute (WRI) published a report which examined the growing body of literature documenting pesticide-induced immune system damage in laboratory animals, wildlife, and human beings.[49] The three major classes of pesticides examined in the studies reviewed by WRI included the organochlorines such as DDT, chlordane, and lindane, the organophosphates such as melathion and chlorpyrifos, and the carbamates, such as aldicarb. Organochlorines, because of their high toxicity and their long persistence in the environment and in human tissues, deserve special mention.

There are approximately eleven thousand different synthetic organochlorines in existence,[50] and virtually all of them are highly persistent, highly reactive with human tissues, and very frequently associated with human cancers. These chemicals derive their name from the simple fact that their molecules include both chlorine and carbon atoms, resulting in a chemical bond that is strong and difficult to break. Polychlorinated biphenyls—PCBs—are some of the oldest of the organochlorine chemicals, though we may be more familiar with organochlorines such as DDT, lindane, chlordane, dieldrin and others that have been used as insecticides. When organochlorine chemicals volatilize, because they are so persistent in air, water, and on airborne particulates, they can easily drift on wind currents for thousands of miles,[51] afterwards being deposited in water and on soil and vegetation. From there they enter the food chain, and diet is believed to be a major source of human (and other animal) exposure.[52]

In one controlled experiment, undertaken by Dutch virologist Albert D. M. E. Osterhaus of Erasmus University in Rotterdam, two groups of harbor seals—subjects and controls—were fed fish from two different sources. One group of seals, the controls, were fed fish from the less polluted waters of the North Atlantic, and the other group, the subjects, were fed fish from the heavily polluted Baltic sea, fish which "contained 10 times as much organochlorine pollution (for example DDT and PCBs) as the Atlantic fish."[53] The researchers emphasized that "both kinds of fish were taken from catches destined for (and considered legally fit for) human consumption."[54] Important findings emerged from this study concerning the impact on the mammalian immune system of eating polluted fish.

Osterhaus's methodology was described in *Rachel's Environment and Health Weekly.*

> [For two years, he] sampled blood from the seals every six to nine weeks and made various measurements of immune system function. Almost immediately after the experiment began, vitamin A levels dropped 20 to 40 percent in the blood of seals fed fish from the [more polluted] Baltic and remained low throughout the 2-year experiment. Vitamin A is associated with disease resistance; lower vitamin A levels in the blood correspond to greater vulnerability to disease.
>
> Seals fed Baltic fish showed another important change: the level of NK cells in the blood remained 20 to 50 percent below normal throughout the study. NK cells are "natural killer" cells that attack foreign bodies in the blood, thus providing important immune protection.
>
> Other key components of the immune system were compromised in the Baltic-fed seals. In a healthy immune system, B-cells produce antibodies and T-cells orchestrate the immune response to foreign invaders. In the Baltic-fed seals, the T-cell response to a standard set of antigens dropped 25 to 60 percent, compared to the Atlantic-fed seals.[55]

It is important to remember that both groups of seals, those fed the heavily contaminated fish and those fed the less contaminated fish, were eating fish that were destined for, and considered perfectly fit for, human consumption. It may thus be expected that the immune systems of other mammals, including humans, might be similarly affected by exposure to such foodborne organochlorines.

We might be wise to recall Chief Sealth's[56] dictum: "Whatever happens to the beasts soon happens to man. All things are connected."[57]

Another series of immune system studies examined the impact of organochlorines on human beings, specifically Inuit natives in northern Quebec. These studies found that "organochlorine contamination of the food chain (including many pesticides) leads to a buildup of these toxic substances in breast-fed Inuit babies."[58] One consequence of the resulting damage to these infants' immune systems is that sometimes "they cannot be vaccinated against disease because their immune systems cannot produce the needed antibodies."[59]

This kind of damage to the immune system from organochlorine compounds in the environment does not bode well for the future control of epidemic infectious diseases.

These health consequences, naturally, are not limited to seals and Inuit natives. Human breast milk, we are discovering, often contains high levels of these lipophilic toxins. John Wargo tells us, in his superb study of the checkered history of pesticide control legislation, that DDT, DDE, and other organochlorines have often been found in high concentrations in human breast milk.

> Because the human breast is largely adipose tissue, fat-soluble compounds such as DDT or DDE tend to concentrate there. The high lipid content of human breast milk (3–5 percent) thus explains the relatively high levels of DDT found in it.[60]

Other chlorinated pesticides have also been found in breast milk.[61] Nor is this new knowledge. Rachel Carson pointed this out to us four decades ago in *Silent Spring*.[62] She summarized the situation thus:

> Insecticide residues have been recovered from human milk in samples tested by Food and Drug Administration scientists.... In experimental animals the chlorinated hydrocarbon [i.e., organochlorine] insecticides freely cross the barrier of the placenta, the traditional protective shield between the embryo and harmful substances in the mother's body. While the [absolute] quantities so received by human infants would normally be small, they are not unimportant because children are more susceptible to poisoning than adults. This situation also means that today the average individual almost certainly starts life with the first deposit of a growing load of chemicals his body will be required to carry henceforth.[63]

This should all have been predictable, we can now see in hindsight, because the mammalian mother draws on her fat resources in order to produce fat-rich milk. As Theo Colburn explains,

> While nursing, a mammalian mother (including humans) draws down her fat stores, dumping not only the fat but also the persistent toxic

chemicals she has accumulated in her body fat over the years into her milk. In this way, a load of contaminants that it has taken the mother decades to accumulate is passed on to her baby in a very short time. By the time a baby beluga [whale] stops nursing at two years of age, it will have acquired a toxic load that, relative to its size, far exceeds that of its mother.[64]

[Furthermore,] according to various studies of breast milk contamination, nursing babies take in the highest doses of contaminants they will experience in their entire lives—levels ten to forty times greater than the daily exposure of an adult.[65]

Breast feeding, therefore, may likely result in some level of impact on the infant immune system, perhaps on the endocrine system, and perhaps on development of the infant's other organ systems. Levels of these chlorinated pesticides found in human milk do vary somewhat, depending (probably) primarily on the amount of pesticide to which the mother herself has been exposed. Some women living in areas (such as parts of sub–Saharan Africa) where the incidence of malaria is high, and hence where the use of organochlorine insecticides (to control mosquito vectors) has been heavy, do show evidence of some of the highest milk levels of these chemicals anywhere in the world.[66] In the United States in recent decades, however, where the use of many organochlorine pesticides has been banned for over a decade, the levels of these chemicals in breast milk seems to be diminishing somewhat.[67]

(It should be noted that none of this is intended to argue that women should stop breast feeding their infants. While it is true that nursing probably results in a certain level of exposure of the infant to these toxins, this potentially adverse impact of breast feeding must also be balanced against the long-recognized positive effects that breast feeding has, among other things, on the nursing infant's ability to resist disease by the passing on of maternal antibodies. The question of the impact of breast feeding on infants born to mothers who may have suffered high exposures to lipophilic toxins, however, certainly deserves more research.)

In any case, one thing seems clear: exposure to certain environmental toxicants, particularly insecticides and herbicides, and most particularly chlorinated compounds of any sort, does sometimes have an adverse impact on the human immune system. Given the importance of the immune system in protecting us from infectious disease (as well as from some cancers), anything which compromises immune function must be taken very seriously.

Thus, when policymakers are assessing the risks and benefits associated with the use and dispersal of environmental toxicants to which a large percentage of the community will eventually be exposed, the costs that could result from large numbers of people suffering compromised immune function must clearly be factored into the risk assessment equation. If increased incidence of some cancers and some opportunistic infections is a likely consequence of impaired immune function, then the social costs (both direct and indirect) of immune system damaging toxicants will also need to be taken into consideration when policy is being formulated.

Peter Montague, a long-time analyst of government environmental policy, is not confident that the U.S. government is presently capable of successfully dealing with this challenge. He writes:

> To prevent damage to the immune system would require strong action to curb the release of immunotoxic chemicals into the environment. This would require a government that is independent of, and stronger than, the corporations releasing the chemicals. At present we do not have anything close to that kind of government.[68]

Whether or not Montague is correct in this assessment remains to be seen. What we can say, at the least, is that it should be incumbent on legislators and policymakers to closely examine and seriously consider all possible means of reducing the load of immunotoxic contaminants in the air, water, soil, and food supplies.

One reason for the need to control immunotoxic contaminants, after all, is that an increase in the number of people with compromised immune systems might also be expected to lead to an increase in the incidence of infectious diseases.

5. Increased Incidence of Infectious Diseases

Widespread compromise of the human immune system may result in a higher incidence of infectious diseases in the general population. After all, if it is true that: "A competent immune system is essential for health"[69]; and if it is also true that "certain synthetic chemicals affect the immune system (e.g., aromatic hydrocarbons; carbamates; heavy metals; organohalogens [such as organochlorines]; organophosphates; organotins; oxidant air pollutants, such as ozone and nitrogen dioxide"[70]; and if it is further true (as it is) that these immune system alterations are more likely to affect the very young, whose immune systems and detoxification systems are not yet fully developed; and finally, if it is true that these "Alterations in the developing and mature immune systems may not be [clinically] recognized as an adverse health effect until long after the exposure"[71]—then we may conclude that "The potential exists for widespread immunotoxicity in humans and wildlife species because of the worldwide lack of appropriate protective standards."[72]

One consequence we could expect to see of this increasing compromising of human immune system function is a decrease in the ability of human immune systems to adequately protect against infectious diseases and cancers. We might, as a corollary, expect to see an overall increase in the incidence of infectious diseases, and perhaps an increase in the incidence of cancers.[73]

Recent data indicate that this is in fact the case. We have already discussed the increase in cancer rates. What is now becoming evident is that there has also been, in recent decades, an increase in infectious diseases. "Between 1980 and 1992 in the U.S., the death rate due to infectious diseases as the underlying cause of death increased 58 percent, from 41 to 65 deaths per 100,000 population, according to the *Journal of the American Medical Association*."[74]

AIDS first appeared in 1981 in the United States, so some of that increase can be accounted for by the emergence of HIV infection and AIDS. However, as Peter Montague points out:

> Deaths from infectious diseases *not* related to AIDS [also] increased substantially during the period. For example, the death rate for respiratory infections increased 20 percent, from 25 to 30 deaths per 100,000, and the rate of death from septicemia (a blood infection) increased 83 percent, from 4.2 to 7.7 per 100,000.[75]

If it is true that the incidence of infectious diseases is increasing, then this is significant and is something policymakers would want to be aware of. This too, after all, can be expected to take its toll on society and on the ability of society to do its necessary work. When it comes time to tally up the true costs of toxicants and toxicant induced disorders, those costs should include losses due to an increase in the incidence of infectious diseases and cancers resulting from toxicant-compromised immune systems.

6. The Blood-Brain Barrier

Under certain conditions, the Blood-Brain Barrier (BBB) can also be severely compromised, sometimes enough to allow toxicants direct access to the brain.

Just as the immune system is one of the body's primary ways of protecting against the threat of disease-causing organisms, so the BBB is one of the brain's primary defenses against internal exposure to neurotoxic chemicals that could cause it damage. (The BBB consists of the formation of extremely tight junctions between the cells in vessels that serve the brain. These tight junctions are able to prevent molecules of a certain size from passing between these cells, and thus moving out of the bloodstream and directly into brain tissues.) Without the BBB, our highly sensitive mammalian brains would be exposed to potential damage from all the toxins, endogenous and exogenous, that may be circulating in our bloodstream at any given moment.

Israeli researchers have found, though, that under certain conditions of high stress, either physical or psychological, the integrity of the blood-brain barrier can be compromised to such an extent that it no longer adequately protects the brain from toxins.[76] Their studies show that, under certain stressful conditions, xenobiotic toxins which would ordinarily have virtually no access to brain tissues can sometimes have relatively free access.[77] If this early work is corroborated with further studies, it may offer a plausible explanation for how the already documented injuries to the central nervous system could occur.

The Israeli researchers specifically examined the hypothesis that high stress significantly compromises the effectiveness of the blood-brain barrier. During the Gulf War, many soldiers were given pyridostigmine bromide (PB) as a sort of preventive "vaccine" against neurologic damage that could result from exposure to enemy chemical weapons. Little thought seems to have been given to the possibility that the PB itself may also have had neurotoxic effects, or that it may at least have added to soldiers' total body load of contaminants, and thus may have potentially made them even more vulnerable to neurotoxicity.

In any case, these researchers had epidemiologic data showing that soldiers who were given the PB in wartime had a much higher percentage of adverse neurologic side effects (almost 25 percent suffered neurologic abnormalities) than soldiers who were given PB in peacetime (when only 8 percent experienced adverse effects).[78] The researchers hypothesized that stress may have been one factor that significantly differentiated the two groups.

To test their hypothesis, they injected PB into mice which had been put under stress (by being forced to swim for several minutes; something mice would normally avoid if possible). Then they injected it into mice (the control group) which had not been stressed. "The researchers found that it took over 100 times more pyridostigmine to penetrate the brains of the unstressed mice as the brains of stressed mice. Tests using a larger molecule, a blue dye, showed a similar effect."[79] Photographs accompany the published study and show images of the blue dye in both the stressed and unstressed mouse brains, and the difference is striking.

This study suggests that experiencing high levels of stress may predispose some persons to be more susceptible to the neurotoxic effects of ambient chemicals in the air, water, and food supply.

(Future studies should perhaps approach the concept of "stress" with somewhat more conceptual subtlety than this study did and try to distinguish between what some psychologists have called eustress and dystress.[80] According to this distinction, eustress is the kind of stress that is invigorating and enlivening, perhaps partly because it is freely chosen and is stoppable—in other words, it is under the subject's control. Physical exercise, mountain climbing, skiing and bungee jumping may create eustress, since a person may choose to do these activities or not, and usually may stop them when they wish. Dystress is not invigorating but debilitating, is highly unpleasant, and is out of one's control. Thus, the stresses of war and combat—or the mouse's stress of being placed into a tub of water with no means of escape—may count as dystress; But the stress of race car driving, watching scary movies, and playing competitive sports would probably be experienced as eustress. In any case, future studies on the effects of stress on the BBB may need to take this distinction, or one similar to it, into account.)

In conclusion, it should come as no great surprise that high levels of stress can weaken a body's immune system, its Blood-Brain Barrier, and perhaps other of its protective mechanisms as well, and thus render it much more vulnerable to assault from both microorganisms and environmental toxicants.

7. Sleep Abnormalities

A recent study[81] has found objective evidence of measurable sleep disturbances in persons who report even just mild levels of sensitivity to environmental chemicals. It found that

> [I]nsomnia and other sleep disturbances are typical problems that multiple chemical sensitivity (MCS) patients report in association with low level chemical exposure.... Objective evidence of biologically disturbed sleep patterns (as assessed by polysomnography) was found in this study of primarily healthy elderly people who subjectively report chemical odor intolerance.[82]

The study found that, compared to controls, these subjects with mild chemical sensitivities "had significantly less total sleep time, lower total rapid eye movement (REM) sleep, more wakefulness, and a trend toward longer latency between sleep onset and REM sleep. These findings are significant because they corroborate what people with MCS, CFIDS and other toxicant induced illnesses have reported for some time: their sleep patterns have been compromised and their sleep is much less restful and restorative. Interestingly, the findings in this study emerged despite the fact that none of these subjects were consciously aware of having any problematic sleep disturbances. Furthermore, none of them had chemical sensitivities severe enough to have received a physician's diagnosis of MCS, chronic fatigue, or multiple food intolerances. They had no expectations of finding disturbed sleep patterns. The only characteristic that distinguished subjects from controls in this study was that the subjects reported moderate illness from exposure to low levels of chemicals such as perfumes, pesticides, paint products, new carpeting and diesel exhaust, while the controls did not.

If further studies confirm what chemically sensitive people already know from personal experience—that they sometimes do experience disturbed sleep patterns when exposed to low levels of environmental chemicals—this would be a significant finding.

Moreover, if all the research on the healing and restorative powers of sleep is valid, then those whose sleep patterns are disturbed would seem to be at increased risk of biologic harm due to lack of sufficient recuperative rest. Their various body systems would not be as effectively restored as those of other people.

8. *Intellectual Function*

Exposure to low levels of environmental toxicants can result in compromised intellectual function, including compromised learning abilities and measurable deficits in short-term memory. According to Ashford and Miller, this may be a result of the fact that "the human nervous system, because it is so highly evolved, may be most susceptible to environmental agents."[83]

A recent study published in the *New England Journal of Medicine*[84] confirms that "children exposed to low levels of polychlorinated biphenyls (PCBs) in the womb grow up with low IQs, poor reading comprehension, difficulty paying attention, and memory problems."[85] The study examined 242 children of mothers who had eaten an average of two to three meals per month of salmon or lake trout from Lake Michigan for at least six years prior to giving birth. This is not an unusually large quantity of those fish to have eaten. It is probable that a significant percentage of the several million people who live on the shores and in the vicinity of Lake Michigan have regularly consumed at least this quantity of the lake's fish. The reason the study focused on the larger species of fish is because they, due to biomagnification of toxicants up the food chain, have been found to contain higher levels of PCBs.

In this study, the greatest mental deficits occurred in the children whose mothers ate the most fish, thus establishing a clear dose-response relationship. Objective determination of the fetuses' PCB exposure was obtained by measuring PCB levels in the blood of the babies' umbilical cords, which is probably a relatively accurate measure of actual intrauterine exposure. These PCB measurements also correlated well with the mothers' self-reports of their own fish consumption.

The 242 infant subjects were compared with 71 infant controls, i.e., babies whose mothers had not eaten Lake Michigan fish.

At birth, the subject babies were clearly different from the controls. They had abnormally weak reflexes, they were less responsive to stimuli, they were more jerky and unbalanced, and they were more easily startled.

Mental capacity of these child subjects was then assessed at age seven months (using the Fagan Test of Infant Intelligence), again at age four, and most recently at age 11. According to *Rachel's Environment and Health Weekly*, the study found that

At age 11, maternal exposure to PCBs was correlated with lower over-all IQ and lower verbal IQ score. The 11 percent of the children whose mothers had the highest exposures now have IQs 6.2 points lower than average. In these 11-year-olds, prenatal exposure to PCBs was linked to poor word comprehension and poor reading ability. The highest-exposed children were twice as likely to be at least two years behind their peers in word comprehension. The Jacobsons summarize: "Our IQ results indicate deficits in general intellectual ability, short-term and long-term memory, and focused and sustained attention." They spec-ulate that PCBs interfere with thyroid hormones, which are essential for development of the brain.[86]

The researchers were able to determine that it is not just the PCBs passed *post partum* to children during breast feeding that are responsible for reduced intelligence. The significant factor in this study was the intrauterine PCB exposure. But the fish the mothers had eaten *during* the nine months of pregnancy was not the only problem, the *Rachel's* article went on to point out.

It was not the mothers' fish-eating habits [only] during pregnancy that was important—it was the mothers' *cumulative lifetime exposure* to PCBs that lowered their children's IQs. In other words, exposure of females to PCBs at any time in their lives before they bear children may eventually translate into mental deficits for their offspring. This has profound implications for regulatory agencies. *Lifetime* exposure [particularly for females] must be regulated.[87]

PCBs, commercialized by Monsanto in 1929, are highly persis-tent chlorinated compounds, and their use was banned in the United States in 1976. It is still legal, however, to manufacture PCBs in the U.S. Twenty-two million pounds per year were manufactured throughout the world between 1984 and 1989, much of that in the U.S. Where are these PCBs now? Apparently, more than 30 percent of them are still in use, another 30 percent or so can be found in landfills, in storage, or in the sediments of lakes, rivers and estuar-ies, and another 30 percent (roughly one billion pounds) is com-pletely unaccounted for.[88] It is estimated that "about one-third of the world's total production of PCBs [has] ... escaped into the gen-eral environment."[89] As Steingraber says in *Living Downstream*:

Like thousands of tiny bombs exploding in slow motion, pieces of discarded equipment containing the oily fluid—electrical transform-ers, television sets, old french friers—leak their contents drop by drop into soil and water. From here, PCB molecules rise into the atmosphere, circulate with the wind, and are redeposited all over the globe. They then enter the food chain. The fatty tissues of nearly all Americans are believed to contain PCB molecules.... In rodent assays, PCBs cause liver cancer, pituitary tumors, leukemia, lymphoma, and intestinal cancers.[90]

And as we have just seen, exposure to PCBs can have many more adverse health effects in addition to their carcinogenicity, including immune system damage, endocrine system dysregulation, and damage to the central nervous system.

The study (discussed above) of the effects of PCBs on childhood development is only the latest to reach similar conclusions. "Four previous studies of children had reported similar problems from PCB exposures, ranging from small size at birth to developmental disorders."[91] Animal studies have confirmed these findings as well.

Another recent study has found environmental factors to be significant in the development of IQ. This study found that, contrary to what we have thought in the past, genetic influences on individual IQ may be weaker, and chemotoxic environmental influences greater, than previously assumed.[92] According to the publication *Nature*,

> [This study] supports the view that the main environmental influences on IQ occur early in life [and this] improved cognitive functioning might be an unexpected benefit of public health initiatives aimed at improving maternal nutrition and reducing pre-natal exposure to toxins.[93]

This study, therefore, clearly supports "the increasingly dominant view that the major toxicant-related environmental influences on IQ occur in the first few years of life, as well as *in utero*, and do directly affect the development of the brain.[94]

If further studies continue to corroborate what these studies have shown—that certain persistent chemical compounds (particularly chlorinated compounds) do adversely affect the mental capacities of human (and other mammalian) offspring—then societies must decide whether they want their future generations to struggle with the burden of measurable intelligence deficits.

9. Endocrine System Dysregulation

Long-term exposure to low levels of environmental toxicants may also result in endocrine system dysregulation. A substantial amount of recent research is providing convincing evidence that many ambient environmental toxicants can have serious dysregulating effects on the endocrine and reproductive systems of a variety of animals, including humans and other mammals.[95] "The evidence that has accumulated in the scientific literature is compelling that the endocrine systems of certain fish and wildlife have indeed been disturbed by chemicals that contaminate their habitats."[96] For example, "Female molluscs (snails, mussels, etc.) have turned into males as a result of exposure to endocrine-disrupting chemicals (a condition called imposex),"[97] and "hermaphroditism has been observed in fish (a single fish having both male and female sex organs)."[98] Phenomena such as these have given rise to the popular term "gender benders" to designate xenobiotic hormone disrupters.

Furthermore, "these chemicals that affect fish and wildlife in their natural habitat have been shown to [also] cause similar adverse effects in laboratory test animals."[99] For instance, "Rats exposed to PCBs prior to birth have disturbed thyroid hormones."[100] There is also evidence, according to Peter Montague, that

> permanent exposure to low levels of dioxin can cause endometriosis in monkeys. Endometriosis is a painful disease of the tissues lining the uterus, which often results in sterility; it presently afflicts an estimated 5 to 9 million American women.[101]

Moreover, he continues, exposing rodents to endocrine-disrupting chemicals

> can cause them to undergo puberty at an early age and can cause persistent estrus (meaning, being "in heat" for an abnormal, prolonged time).[102] In addition, male rodents "can be born with hypospadias (a birth defect of the penis) and cryptorchidism (undescended testicles).... The Weybridge Report [from the European Environment Agency] specifically associates these effects (in rodents) with exposure to Vinclozolin, a powerful anti-androgenic pesticide. (In the U.S. today, Vinclozolin is legal for use on cucumbers, grapes, lettuce, onions, bell peppers, raspberries, strawberries, tomatoes, and Belgian endive. U.S. Environmental Protection Agency has no published plans for banning Vinclozolin.)[103]

These endocrine disrupting effects, among others, have been observed in both wildlife and laboratory animals, and most "evidence supports the idea that if a chemical is estrogenic in one species, it will be in all others."[104]

What this research is discovering is that certain chemical agents that are currently ambient in the air, water, and food supply do sometimes act as endocrine disrupters, sometimes actually binding to, or blocking, the same cell sites that were originally intended to be receptors for the body's own endogenous hormones. Molecules of DDT, chlordane, PCBs and other chlorinated compounds, for example, when circulating in the bloodstream, seem to have enough surface similarity to circulating endogenous estrogen molecules, that they can bind to, or in other ways directly affect, the identical cell site receptors to which natural estrogens would normally bind. Sometimes endocrine disruption can occur via other biochemical mechanisms as well. "Some chemicals imitate the hormone directly, while others interfere with the various systems that regulate the body's production and metabolism of natural estrogens. Still others seem to work by blocking the receptor sites for male hormones [androgens]."[105] Thus, endocrine disruption can occur and work its pathogenic effects by a variety of different mechanisms.

An endocrine disrupter may be described as "an exogenous substance or mixture that alters the function of the endocrine system and consequently causes adverse health effects in an intact organism or its progeny or subpopulations."[106] Researchers are suggesting that endocrine disruption may well be responsible for some of the reproductive changes that have been noted in recent studies, such as earlier puberty and menstruation in human females and the "significant decline in sperm density" in human males.[107]

These endocrine mimics, moreover, can be found in the most common places. An article in the May 1997 issue of *Endocrinology*,[108] for example, reports that bisphenol A, a key ingredient in polycarbonate plastics—drinking water, juices, soft drinks, and other consumable fluids are commonly stored in bottles made of polycarbonate plastics—mimics the female hormone estrogen in some rats. Whether it acts this way in humans has not yet been determined (because it has not yet been studied). Some estrogen mimics, notably those in certain pesticide compounds, have deliberately been synthesized "to function intentionally as hormone/growth regulators to control pest populations."[109] Whether these specific compounds adversely affect the human endocrine system as well has not yet been scientifically determined, but it would probably not come as any great surprise if we found that they did.

What exactly is the endocrine system? The endocrine system is, like the nervous system, one of our key integrating and regulating systems. It allows the body's billions of cells to stay in communication with each other.[110] Major glands in the endocrine system include the thyroid, pituitary, pancreas, adrenal, pineal, testes and ovaries. These finely tuned ductless glands secrete minuscule quantities of natural hormones directly into the bloodstream. These hormones "travel in the blood in very small concentrations [parts per trillion] and bind to specific cell sites called receptors in the distant target tissues and organs, where they exert their effects on development, growth, and reproduction in addition to other bodily functions."[111] Hormones, therefore, have the highly important function of signaling all the various specialized cells in the body to behave in specific ways; and when these signal systems are disrupted by exogenous synthetic endocrine mimics, effects on body function and development can be significant.

Exogenous endocrine system disrupters have been more precisely defined by Crisp, Clegg and Cooper in their *Special Report on Environmental Endocrine Disruption*:

> An environmental endocrine disruptor is defined as an exogenous [originating outside the body] agent that interferes with the synthesis, secretion, transport, binding, action, or elimination of natural hormones in the body that are responsible for homeostasis, reproduction, development, and/or behavior.[112]

Endocrine disrupters have the potential to effect changes in a wide variety of bodily organs and systems that might otherwise have been considered relatively independent of each other. This unfortunate fact, it has been suggested, has sometimes made the process of clinical diagnosis quite challenging.

Many old school diagnosticians expect to see their patients with clinically evident symptoms in one or two body systems. When they see a patient who describes symptoms relating to a multiplicity of systems (e.g., headache, some nausea, paraesthesias, dermatitis, memory loss, difficulty concentrating, and asthma-like symptoms), they are not sure how to proceed. A little principle that has been commonly taught (or at least commonly learned) in many medical schools is that the more symptoms a patient has and the more body systems about which they have complaints, the more likely it is that the patient's problem is psychosomatic.[113] This *petitio principium* has turned out to be the bane of many people who suffer toxicant induced illnesses such as MCS. Some of their physicians believe it is "all in their heads," largely because of the inscrutability of a condition that often manifests itself in such a multiplicity of body systems.

Actually, however, because the body's multiplicity of constantly interacting systems are so integrated, it should come as no great surprise to discover that dysfunction in one system might well lead to dysfunction in others. If a person's gastrointestinal tract, for example, is unable to effectively absorb and process nutrients well, then it is little wonder that other body systems may suffer adverse effects from a lack of cellular nutrition. In the same way, if the integrating and regulatory functions of the endocrine system have been disrupted by exogenous chemicals, we should perhaps be surprised if we did *not* find symptoms developing in various organs and systems.

In addition to the simple endocrine disrupting effects that appear to result from exposure to certain environmental toxicants, some recent research has shown that the effects of exposure to *mixtures* of toxicants may sometimes be multiplicative and synergistic rather than merely additive. This should perhaps come as no great surprise to us. Synergistic effects of chemical mixtures have been recognized as long as there have been chemicals. Chemical synergisms are well known in the pharmaceutical world. For example, "The combination of aspirin and opioids is more analgesic than the summed effect of each drug given separately."[114] Effects of chemical mixtures, in other words, can be much more potent than the summed effects of the individual chemicals in the mixture.

What this means, unfortunately, is that ambient environmental toxicants may actually be even more toxic in the real world than they are in laboratory tests, because in the real world people are normally exposed to mixtures of toxicants, and not just to one chemical at a time as laboratory rodents are. For instance, a study published not long ago in *Science* suggested that synergistic multiplicative effects of such mixtures, particularly of organochlorines, can be very potent indeed:

> Tests on four pesticides believed to be only very weakly estrogenic—the pesticides dieldrin, endosulfan, toxaphene, and chlordane—yielded little or no response, as expected. When the chemicals were paired, however, the activity shot up by a factor of 160 to 1600.[115]

So these endocrine disrupters may be even more potent in combination than singly. While these findings have been considered controversial (and pressures were exerted on the authors to rescind their article), more recent studies continue to provide evidence of the multiplicative effects of chemical synergisms. Thus, it should be of concern to us that the more chemicals that are released into the environment, and the more varieties that are released (particularly of the chlorinated compounds), the greater may be our risk of doing increasingly significant damage to human (and other animal) biological systems.[116]

A report from the U.S. Environmental Protection Agency, released in February 1997, indicates that the risk of endocrine disruption may actually be greater than had heretofore been appreciated.[117] This preliminary report was issued by "a technical panel of EPA scientists assembled by the Agency's Risk Assessment Forum," which had looked at "nearly 300 peer-reviewed studies that examine the effects of a number of chemicals on the endocrine systems of humans, laboratory animals and wildlife."[118] According to Robert Huggett, EPA Assistant Administrator for the Office of Research and Development,

> The studies we reviewed demonstrate that exposure to certain endocrine disrupting chemicals can lead to disturbing health effects in animals, including cancer, sterility ... [and] developmental problems.[119]

Since the endocrine system is so integral to the functioning of a wide variety of profoundly interconnected body systems, the consequences of endocrine disruption can be enormous, both for those who have themselves been directly exposed to endocrine disrupting toxicants in their environment, and potentially for their offspring as well.

10. Detoxification Pathways

Just as one primary function of the immune system is to help protect the body from attack by bacteria, viruses, parasites, and other such pathogens and carcinogens, so likewise our detoxification systems are designed to help our bodies break down and metabolize both the toxins that originate within our bodies from normal metabolic processes and those xenobiotic toxicants that are introduced from without.

There are two basic processes by which the body eliminates toxins. One is to use enzymes to break them down into molecules that are less toxic, and then excrete them via the urine, sweat and feces.

The other is to conjoin them with other molecules—the conjugation process—so that those new larger molecules can then be excreted via the urine and feces.

Both these processes require the employment of certain nutrients at the cellular level. When a person has been exposed to a quantity of toxicants large enough that it temporarily depletes the nutrients necessary for breaking down (or conjugating) and excreting them, those toxicants can remain in the body and are able to do more physical damage (as we have seen in previous pages) than they might normally be able to do. This damage may then eventually become serious enough that it results in measurable deficits in CNS function, a weakening of the immune system, endocrine system dysregulation, and so on. It may also include the kind of central nervous system damage that can sometimes result in behavioral disorders.

11. Behavioral Disorders

Exposure to low levels of toxicants may sometimes result in various behavioral disorders, perhaps including such abnormalities as attention deficit hyperactivity disorder (ADHD).

One recent study, for example, has attempted to explore a possible link between violent crime and exposure to neurotoxic agents.[120] Roger Masters, the principal author of this study, has developed what he terms the neurotoxicity hypothesis of violent crime.

> According to this hypothesis, toxic pollutants—specifically the toxic metals lead and manganese—cause learning disabilities, an increase in aggressive behavior, and—most importantly—loss of control over impulsive behavior. These traits combine with poverty, social stress, alcohol and drug abuse, individual character, and other social factors to produce individuals who commit violent crimes.[121]

Masters argues that in order for this hypothesis to be taken seriously it must meet five requirements. It must

1. [show] that individuals who engage in criminal behavior are more likely to have absorbed toxic chemicals than a comparable control population....
2. be able to predict future violent behavior of young people exposed to toxins....

3. [show that there is] a biological basis for believing that lead, manganese and other toxic metals could cause a person to lose control over impulsive and aggressive behavior....

4. [show that] individuals ... receive doses of toxic metals sufficient to be associated with violent behavior....

5. [show that] measures of environmental pollution ... correlate with higher rates of violent crime.[122]

Masters believes that his data support and meet these five tests.

Clearly, this study is preliminary. It is, however, suggestive of a possible connection between long-term exposure to certain kinds of environmental pollutants and the later acting out in violent behaviors. This possible connection, it would seem, deserves more research.

Evidence of increased acting out behavior in school children exposed to toxics has been documented by Environmental Medicine physician Doris Rapp.[123] Her preliminary evidence too deserves further exploration.

Finally, some increased incidence of suicide among those with toxicant induced illnesses may partially result from the psychoneurotoxic effects of certain toxicants on the limbic system of the midbrain and thus on the emotions. Other suicides, of course, may simply be caused by the great sense of personal and social loss many with toxicant induced illnesses experience.

12. MCS

Multiple Chemical Sensitivity is an acquired condition characterized by more or less severe symptomatic reactions in a wide variety of organ systems, to low levels of common ambient toxicants. In people with MCS, these symptoms can be triggered by exposure to doses of chemicals—such as ambient pesticides, solvents in artificial fragrances, industrial toxicants and formaldehyde—at levels to which most people do not normally react. Some people with MCS may react also to residues of commonly used herbicides and persistent insecticides that are in their drinking water[124] and shower water, as well as to the pesticide residues commonly found on and in supermarket foods.

Reactions can range from symptoms as mild as sudden fatigue, a sharp metallic taste in the mouth or other unusual paraesthesias, to more serious symptoms such as nausea, severe skin rashes, headaches and brain fog, and even to very dramatic symptoms such as intense migraines, disabling cerebral dysfunction, loss of consciousness, and life-threatening asthma.

MCS is an acquired condition. People are not normally born with it. Many people with the condition can clearly identify the time and place when it began. Most people with MCS live healthy, productive and normal lives up to the time their condition is initiated, either by one large exposure or by a long accumulation of lesser exposures to chemicals which, at some point, simply reach a critical mass in their tissues.

The condition is considered controversial by some practicing physicians and by virtually all executives in the employ of the chemical manufacturing corporations. Some less knowledgeable physicians have wanted to dismiss the condition as psychosomatic simply because they are not aware of other options readily available to them in the normal repertoire of diagnoses. In addition, most chemical manufacturers would like to see MCS dismissed as psychogenic. They are concerned about sullying the public image of their chemical products; they are concerned about the possibility of toxic torts litigation; and they are deeply concerned about the potential impact on corporate profits that might result from a public recognition that chemicals can be pathogenic.

On the other hand, eight states[125] now officially recognize MCS for workers' compensation claims, and "19 federal and 22 state agencies, other than workers' compensation departments, recognize the condition as a legitimate illness."[126] Research studies in the 1990s were finally validating and corroborating what people with MCS have known for years: their bodies have been dramatically impacted by exposure to chemicals.

Estimates of MCS prevalence vary from 4 percent to 34 percent of the general population.[127] Slightly more than 4 percent of the population has been formally diagnosed with MCS by an MD, whereas 30 to 40 percent (depending on the study) report that they are often made sick in some way from exposure to chemicals such as pesticides, diesel exhaust and artificial fragrances. (Most artificial fragrance products contain more than one hundred chemicals and solvents; the perfume Red by Giorgio, for example, includes over 600 ingredients.[128])

The most successful treatment option for people stricken with MCS is to minimize further exposure to toxicants. In this way, they can diminish the risk of experiencing their sometimes disabling symptoms. In today's world, though, avoiding exposure to these toxicants is virtually impossible, or is at least a Herculean task. Fortunately, at least five states in the U.S. (New Mexico, Missouri, North Carolina, Connecticut and Washington) have recently established MCS Awareness Weeks as a way of raising public understanding of the formidable challenges faced by sufferers of the disorder.[129]

Ashford and Miller, in their classic text *Chemical Exposures: Low Levels, High Stakes* (a work which won the World Health Organization's Macedo award in public health), sum up MCS thus: "chemical sensitivity is a debilitating condition and a serious public health concern, but one that can be addressed by aggressive, coordinated public and private sector efforts."[130]

13. Pesticides

Pesticides are a unique class of toxicants, and therefore need to be considered separately. They are special for several reasons:

Any product which is deliberately designed to be biocidal—intentionally manufactured in such a way as to kill living things, to be toxic to neural tissue, to disrupt the endocrinologic regulation of growth processes (as some herbicides are designed to do), or to interrupt other vital life processes necessary for healthy function in living organisms—should clearly be treated separately from toxicants which produce their adverse effects as accidental or unintended side effects. Public policy should be designed in ways that would allow people who need or wish to protect themselves (as well as their children and families) from exposure to such agents to be able to do so. Increasing scientific evidence continues to support the claim that some pesticides may be responsible for a wide variety of adverse health effects including, as we have seen, cancers, respiratory disorders, neural damage (as in Parkinson's Disease and other CNS disorders), immune system damage, and endocrine system dysregulation both in those who have been directly exposed and in their offspring.[131]

Furthermore, pesticides are so widely used outdoors and indoors—"researchers estimate that pesticides are used in 90% of U.S. homes"[132]—in agriculture, on golf courses, in schools, public buildings, private office buildings, storage warehouses, city, county and state parks, apartment buildings, restaurants, grocery stores, in neighborhoods, along roadways, in bedding, and in clothing, that it is virtually impossible to avoid exposure to them. Pesticide residues are found in our air, water, and food, on the surfaces on which we and our families walk, sit, play, work and sleep, and even on the surfaces of baby's toys.[133] Researchers have found that "household toys, pillows, bedding, furniture, and other sorbent objects in homes readily absorb and hold pesticides that volatilize from indoor applications."[134] This can be a special problem for children, of course, since they are more biologically susceptible to these agents, and because of the almost constant hand-to-mouth activity in which infants engage. In addition, opportunity for skin absorption is greater in children who regularly crawl and play on carpets and other sorbent surfaces. Moreover, researchers have found that "washing with soap and water does not completely remove pesticides because they bind to the skin. [Therefore] ... 'this incomplete removal of the pesticide from hands may allow pesticides to persist for days after [initial] exposure....'"[135] And pesticides in clothes can be in continuous contact with the skin and absorbed into the body.

It is not necessary to have pesticides sprayed inside the home for these exposures to occur. "Households can pull pesticides offgassing from neighboring lawns and agricultural fields into the indoor environment through outdoor air exchange systems or open windows."[136] And pesticide drift often occurs over hundreds and sometimes thousands of miles. "Pesticides primarily used in the southern U.S. states have been found in remote formerly pristine regions in Canada."[137] Pesticide drift residues are also found in both polar icecaps.

The ubiquity of pesticide applications and residues, therefore, means that it is virtually impossible for any given person to effectively avoid exposure to them. Pesticides are used in such enormous quantities that no agency anywhere in the world[138] even monitors, let alone regulates, the quantity of pesticides purchased and used in the U.S. or in any other nation. "The EPA does not know who is using what pesticides in what quantities on which crops in which locations. There is simply no record of pesticide use in this country (except for a state program in California), and the new law [the Food Quality Protection Act of 1996] does not change that fact.[139] Furthermore, "After more than 20 years of effort, EPA remains astonishingly ignorant about the health effects of pesticides."[140]

And yet a certain percentage of people do suffer quite severe physical reactions to these agents,[141] as we have seen above. This should be entirely unsurprising and understandable, since pesticides are intended and designed to be toxic to living tissues. And yet all our public policy to date, including a large body of relatively ineffective pesticide legislation,[142] has provided no effective protection for people from exposures to pesticides.

It is ironic that, as matters stand now, in order to purchase or use many pharmaceutical products (i.e., products which are designed to heal) it is necessary to have a prescription from a physician who has been educated in the effects of that medication; and yet no such prescription or certification is required for the purchase of pesticides which are designed to kill. Even worse, those who buy these deadly chemicals are not even required to be able to read the label on the containers.

Future generations and future civilizations may well look back on us—as we look back on the faults and weaknesses of the decaying Roman Empire—and wonder what kind of thinking allowed us to knowingly poison ourselves, our children, our pets, wildlife, and environment through the virtually indiscriminate use of herbicides, insecticides, rodenticides, fungicides and microbicides. Will those peoples in the future be astonished that we did not stop the wholesale damage to our planet and its multiplicity of life forms, even when we knew the damage might be irreperable?

Rachel Carson made this point quite starkly: "All this is not to say that there is no insect problem and no need of control. I am saying, rather, that ... the methods employed must be such that they do not destroy us along with the insects."[143]

What Carson said about insects can be applied to the whole variety of pests and scourges that human beings deal with, including fungi, weeds, rodents, and microbes. There really are pests in the world[144] and they sometimes really do need to be controlled, but chemical interventions need not always be the first or primary method. There are plenty of less toxic alternatives that can be deployed before turning to chemicals.[145]

14. Life Disruption

The lives of many people with chemical sensitivity disorders and other toxicant induced illnesses have often been dramatically and severely disrupted. One rather typical example will illustrate some of the key themes. A person with MCS describes her situation in this manner:

> My husband and I were poisoned by chronic low levels of organophosphate and carbamate pesticides over a period of ten months. We did

not know we were being exposed to them because they leached into our house from an adjoining wall in the next building. We both worked and lived in our house.

The people next door did not live there and were hardly ever there because of the nature of their business. They had a pesticide service do a "crack and crevice spray" every two weeks. We felt ill within weeks of moving there, and had no idea what was wrong. As the months passed we began to feel as though we had a terminal illness. Strange thing was that the symptoms were exactly the same as Gulf War Syndrome, although we had never been there.

When we finally discovered what the trigger was it was too late. Even six years later we experience severe symptoms when exposed to neurotoxins. And believe me, they are very, very prevalent. It is hard to go anywhere without being exposed.

We can't even use polyester clothing because pesticides and other petrochemical contaminants cling to the fibers and bond molecularly with them. Polyester is also a petrochemical product and it is next to impossible to wash out other petrochemicals that cling to [it].

Six years after we moved from our house we are improved only because we have taken extraordinary steps to protect ourselves ... mainly, through avoidance of neurotoxins. When we come in contact with them, we [still] suffer many of the same symptoms ... in this approximate order: difficulty concentrating, tight band pressure around head, headache, joint pain, cramping in legs and feet, gastrointestinal problems, urgency to urinate, bowel movements like clay, pain in kidneys, pain in liver, bleeding from nose, chest pressure, pain in mitral valve area of heart, pain in left arm, testicular pain (husband, of course), mood swings, and many other symptoms.

It is important to know that we lived a wonderful lifestyle before this happened. We had two homes, we owned our own business, we traveled around the world and we both had a 4.0 grade average at the University. We had it made.

When we became ill we did not know what to do because very few doctors are trained in recognition and management of pesticide poisoning.

It took us years to search existing medical literature to figure out what had happened to our nervous systems. Unfortunately, [by the time we had learned of chemical sensitivity and how to deal with it] we had lost over $500,000 and were living in our van because it was the only place where we didn't get ill. We had to dump about 99% of our belongings because they were so contaminated.

We think about Gulf War Veterans a lot, and about how they sent and brought their toxic belongings home to their families. The issues of cross contaminations are not well understood by the general population, and certainly not by our vets. But we know how sick we get even six years later when we go into the shed where we still have a few of our belongings such as photographs. We get ill after being inside that shed for only a few minutes.[146]

Several key themes emerge from this account, many of which are tragically common to people who have contracted toxicant induced illnesses such as MCS.

1. Ordinary people in the ordinary course of their regular lives, not doing anything unusual, can be made sick by toxicants that are present in their environment.

2. They can be made sick by toxicants to which they were unknowingly exposed in the normal course of their life and work.

3. They may learn of the cause of their ill health only long after the damage has been irretrievably done and the situation can no longer be remedied.

4. They can experience a wide variety of symptoms in multiple organs and body systems, and the symptoms seem to them to be similar to those reported by soldiers who returned from the Gulf with Gulf War Syndrome.

5. Their regular physicians are seldom able to recognize the nature of their condition, largely because the physicians have had no training in either recognizing the condition or even in asking their patients about past exposures to environmental toxicants. "Most physicians do not obtain occupational or environmental histories from their patients."[147]

6. It was largely by their own efforts that they were able to search the medical literature and learn about the condition themselves, and it was largely by their own efforts that they have dealt with the new life challenges caused by their condition.[148]

7. Their sensitivity to ambient toxicants persists for years, probably for the rest of their lives.

8. They find it virtually impossible to avoid exposure to ambient toxicants except by taking extraordinary (and sometimes extreme) measures.

9. Their daily life, work, home, possessions, and literally every dimension of their lives have been dramatically (and negatively) impacted by their new physical condition.

10. They have often spent themselves into poverty in the attempt to understand and deal with their chemical sensitivity disorder, and are now reduced to living in severely distressed circumstances.

11. They eventually come to realize that there are enormous forces arrayed against the formal recognition of toxicant induced disorders.

Many forces want to deny "that there are *any* long-term effects from such exposure," says this MCS sufferer. She adds:

> The petrochemical industry has enormous influence and spends a lot of money funding chairs and research at various universities including the medical schools. When doctors and scientists try to pursue an avenue of inquiry regarding chemical injury, they often find themselves without their next grant, or out of a job, or discredited ... and [under] many other pressures that take their toll ... and create a complicity of silence. It was not until the Gulf War and the vets becoming ill that doctors and scientists began speaking out. There is a long list of brave men and women who have lost their positions because of speaking out.[149]

Tragic as this couple's personal experience is, and dramatic as the impact on their lives has been, their story is unfortunately all too common. In addition, in more cases than not, contracting a chemical sensitivity disorder will turn out to have devastating consequences for the personal relationships in the lives of people with MCS, and many marriages, friendships, and family relationships eventually break under the strain. The well people in these relationships have difficulty believing that their partners, friends or family members are actually sick since they sometimes do not appear to be sick. The well people may also have difficulty believing that the environment in which they themselves live and work, and which had previously been comfortable and acceptable for everyone, now suddenly makes the MCS sufferer sick. And all with no tangible cause. It often seems implausible to the well person. They may begin to feel that their partner, friend or family member is simply malingering or looking for attention. The newly ill person, on the other hand, is suddenly feeling very sick much of the time, their emotional states and cognitive processes are sometimes dramatically affected by exposure to chemicals in their environment, and the lack of understanding by the well people can eventually take a significant toll on the relationship.

The impact on health, on productivity, on the ability to work, and on virtually every aspect of a sufferer's life, is often dramatic.[150] Although there have as yet been no studies directly assessing the frequency of suicide among those with toxicant induced disorders (especially among those with MCS and CFIDs), estimates are that the rate is higher than the societal norm.

Fortunately, personal accounts of how devastated individual lives have been by toxicant induced illnesses, and of how devastated the lives of their families have been as well, have begun to be published, albeit slowly.[151] When personal stories began to be published about the horror of AIDS created in the lives of those suffering from it, public awareness of the newly discovered disease increased. At that point policymakers, legislators, and the public at large started to take the disease seriously. In the case of toxicant induced disorders such as MCS and CFIDs, the personal impact of them is still mostly hidden and not commonly recognized. But as more accounts of these diseases are published, and as they become better known and understood, we will see them too taken more and more seriously.

15. Actual Costs

In addition to impacting individual lives, the effects of toxicant induced illnesses may impact society in a wide variety of ways as well, including that of lessened productivity.

Any increased incidence of morbidity, particularly morbidity that is as disabling as that experienced by many people with MCS, asthma, Chronic Fatigue Syndrome, Reactive Airway Disease Syndrome, and other toxicant induced disorders, can have significant economic impact on a community. Unfortunately, no thorough studies have yet been done which effectively examine the actual and potential economic impact of chemical injury diseases and chemical sensitivity disorders on a community. However, WHO has called for studies to be done which will determine "the true personal and financial costs of human disease due to environmental chemical allergies."[152]

According to the World Health Organization,

> The need to assess the problem and to develop preventive measures became evident with the increase in the amount of chemical substances to which a large number of people are exposed.
> During the past 10 years [i.e., 1985–1995], about 10,000 new substances have been marketed in the European Region, and the prevalence and severity of respiratory hypersensitivity have increased. Asthma mortality worldwide has also increased. In 11 of the 14 countries, the death rate from asthma was higher in the 1980s than in the 1970s. In six countries, the increase in asthma mortality was over 20%.[153]

If it is true that the morbidity and mortality associated with increased exposure to the growing quantities of environmental toxicants are higher now than in past decades—asthma alone has increased 40 percent in the past decade and "it is now the number one cause of absenteeism for American schoolchildren"[154]—then there is little doubt that the economic impact will eventually need to be tallied so that it can be properly factored in to policy decisions.

16. How Many People Are Affected?

At this point in our study it would be perfectly reasonable to ask: if these toxicants are so pathogenic, then why aren't more people made obviously sick by them? The question is an important one and deserves an answer, but any adequate answer will have to have many parts and include several different elements. Before we turn to those elements, let us look briefly (by way of illustration) at some of the disease processes known to be caused by smoking tobacco products.

We are already aware that both human epidemiological data and animal research data clearly indicate that tobacco use is pathogenic. Tobacco use has been clearly shown to be associated with increased incidence of cancer, especially lung cancer, as well as with increased incidence of emphysema, cardiovascular disease and erectile dysfunction. And yet not everyone who uses tobacco products contracts cancer or cardiovascular disease. Why not? There are probably several factors that explain this. Some smokers die of other causes before they are diagnosed with or die of tobacco-related causes, so they would not be counted in any statistics about tobacco's pathogenicity. Genetic variability is probably also responsible for some people being more, and others being less, at risk than others. Length of time smoking may account for some differences in morbidity and mortality, and there may be other factors as well. The point is that, even when there is clear and virtually irrefutable evidence that a substance is pathogenic, still, not everyone exposed to that substance always develops a clinically evident disease.

In the case of the ubiquitous toxicants that seem to have been such a large part of life in the last third of the 20th century and in the beginning of this, if they are indeed as pathogenic as the evidence indicates, then the question inevitably arises: why aren't there more people suffering from symptoms attributable to toxicant exposures?

Several elements of the explanation, none of them mutually exclusive, deserve mention.

It is likely that different people have varying degrees of genetic susceptibility to these pathogens just as they do to many other kinds of pathogens, including bacteria and viruses. This genetic variability may account for the fact that lower doses of certain toxicants make some people sicker than others. This variability may explain why some people are made sick by certain *combinations* of toxicants, while others are not made sick by them at all. Thus, genetic variability may be a factor in some people being more susceptible than others to the pathogenic effects of ambient toxicants.

A higher or lower total life-to-date exposure to toxicants may be another factor that accounts for some people having developed pathologies while others have not. Different lifestyles may contribute to higher toxicant exposures as well. Urban or rural living may affect levels of exposure. Living in agricultural or nonagricultural areas may contribute to different levels of exposure to pesticides. A history of using various lawn and household chemicals, solvents, and cleaning agents may contribute to higher levels of exposure. Living or working in certain kinds of "tight" buildings may contribute to higher levels of indoor contaminant exposure. Certain kinds of employment may contribute to more exposures. In other words, there are probably a wide variety of factors that contribute to the total quantity of life-to-date exposures.

In addition, the length of time a person has been living and absorbing toxicants—their simple biological age—may be a factor. The era during which they have lived may also be a factor. The later in the 20th century a person was born, or if they were born in the 21st, will probably be a factor in the total quantity of toxicants to which they have been exposed, if only because synthetic chemical production and use steadily escalated as the last century progressed.

Data illustrates the difference in total life-to-date toxicant exposure between a person born in the early 1940s, who probably experienced a smaller total toxicant exposure in the first decade or so of life, and persons born in subsequent decades, who are likely to experience significantly higher total life-to-date exposures during their lifetimes. It also illustrates how those born later in the 20th century, after the development and widespread use of pesticides, artificial fragrances, and the burgeoning emergence of so many household, office, industrial and other chemical compounds and byproducts, may be at notably higher risk of being exposed to much higher levels of synthetic toxicants than those born earlier. Furthermore, persons born later in the last century or in this one will have been exposed to these pollutants at a much earlier period in their lives when many of their organ systems were still developing, and consequently when they were more susceptible to toxicant damage. They may therefore be at higher risk of developing toxicant induced pathologies.

Data suggests that persons born later in the 20th century or in the 21st may be at greater risk of contracting toxicant induced pathologies than those born earlier, even though these pathologies may not become clinically evident in some cases until the third or fourth decade of life, or later. This means that national and international public health agencies (such as the U.S. Centers for Disease Control and Prevention, and the World Health Organization) should seriously consider monitoring those generations born later in the last century and in this for the possible increased incidence of toxicant induced pathologies. Only in this way will they have a chance of detecting any emerging patterns soon enough to take nationwide preventive measures.

People born earlier in the 20th century may be at somewhat lower risk of developing toxicant induced pathologies since they have (as a group) had lower total life-to-date exposures. They will probably also have had far less toxicant exposure in their early developing years.

The period of life during which a person is exposed to pollutants may be a third factor in the likelihood of developing adverse health effects. When young children, for example, are exposed to certain toxicants, that exposure will affect them much more dramatically than it will adults.

There are actually several reasons why children are so much more likely than adults to be harmed by exposure to toxicants. One reason is that children's bodies are smaller, so a dose of toxicants that may not seriously affect a 70 kilogram male,[155] could seriously affect the much smaller child because of the higher dose per body weight. In addition, children respire much more frequently than adults, and thus are exposed to larger doses of inhalants than adults. They also eat much more food and drink more water than adults (in proportion to their body size), so they are exposed to proportionately much larger doses of toxicants in food and water. In addition, children's organ systems (including all the detoxification pathways) are not yet fully matured and are not able to perform their functions as effectively as those same systems in adults. For these reasons, small children are much more likely to be adversely affected by exposure to toxicants (such as ambient pesticide residues, for example, or the solvents and chemicals in artificial fragrances) than adults would be.

Thus, another factor that may put some people more at risk for developing toxicant induced pathologies is the time of life at which they have endured certain exposures.

"If these chemicals are so toxic, why aren't more people sick?" In answer to our question, we have so far suggested genetic variability, varying levels of total life-to-date exposures, and the time of life at which those exposures occurred as possible factors that may affect the likelihood of developing pathology. There may be another factor as well.

It is probable that more people than realize it are actually affected by, and have already developed symptoms related to, toxicants in their environment. The increase in asthma and other respiratory disorders in recent decades, for instance, may well be a form of increased illness due to higher levels of exposure to toxicants. Epidemiological evidence of increased incidence and prevalence of infectious diseases[156] may also be suggestive that ambient toxicants have had compromising effects on the immune system. The increased incidence of breast cancer[157] and childhood cancers may also be a consequence of increased exposure to environmental toxicants.[158] Thus many more people than realize it may already be suffering the effects of overexposure to environmental toxicants.

Furthermore, it may be that some diseases which so far are poorly understood by traditional medicine (some autoimmune disorders, for example, including systemic lupus erythematosus,[159] and perhaps other rheumatoid and neurologic conditions) may actually turn out to be consequences of increased exposure to environmental pollutants. If this is true, then even more people may actually be adversely affected by toxicants than presently realize it.

We know that most practicing physicians today do not commonly ask their patients about, or even consider the possibility of, long-term low dose exposures to common toxicants. They do not ask about exposure to the toxicants that may be found in their patients' newly constructed homes or in mobile homes, or in new furniture and new carpeting. They do not commonly ask about exposure to lawn care products, to local pesticide spraying (in parks and cemeteries, on golf courses, private timberlands, lawns, streets and roadways), or exposure to artificial fragrances such as may be found in laundry detergents and other household cleaning products. So it may well be that some poorly understood clinical conditions have an environmental component that plays a significant role in their etiology.[160]

Thus it may be that more people are made noticeably and clinically sick by environmental toxicants than presently realize it, because they themselves have not yet associated their symptoms and conditions with exposure to toxicants. Even the initial exposure event which brings about a loss of tolerance to toxicants and sensitizes a person to future low level exposures may sometimes "go unnoticed entirely or may not [consciously] be connected causally with onset of illness by patient or physician."[161] In the journal *Toxicology*, Dr. Claudia Miller writes:

> For example, an illness that develops following routine household extermination [of insects] or administration of a general anesthetic may be attributed to some other cause. If several residents of a home recently treated with pesticides develop flu-like symptoms at the same time, an infectious cause may be assumed erroneously.[162]

For these reasons, Miller refers to chemical sensitivity, or TILT, as a kind of "cryptotoxicity" (from the Greek *crypto*, meaning "hidden").[163] That is, the sensitizing effects of the original exposure may sometimes not be immediately evident; it may be only in retrospect that a person is able to identify an original sensitizing exposure. And then, following that initiating exposure, according to the model of toxicant induced loss of tolerance, sensitized persons will begin to experience physical reactions to low levels of other ambient toxicants, some of which may be chemically related to the original sensitizing agent and some of which may be entirely unrelated.

Proving a causal relationship between the clinical symptoms and the offending toxicants may, of course, be scientifically challenging. It will probably ultimately require use of the hospital Environmental Medical Units developed by Randolph,[164] Rea,[165] and others,[166] along with double blind toxicant challenge testing. (For more details regarding the design of such trials, see section one in Chapter Three below.)

One piece of evidence which may indicate an increased incidence of toxicant induced illnesses is the rise in recent decades, in the number of people turning to alternative medical practitioners for help. It may be that many people are experiencing symptoms and disabilities for which they find little understanding or help among traditional medicinal practitioners. Some people with toxicant induced pathologies may find sympathetic understanding among naturopaths, chiropractors, and acupuncturists when they have not been taken seriously by traditional clinicians. Most medical schools today simply do not teach students about pathologies that result from long-term exposure to low doses of environmental toxicants. When these students graduate and begin medical practice, they seldom think in terms of toxicant induced pathologies (except perhaps for their patients in some occupational settings), and they especially are not likely to think in terms of long-term, low dose exposure to toxicants. It is not hard to see that people experiencing symptoms that are little understood by traditional medicine may feel they are a better off with alternative medical practitioners.

Finally, it may be that a significant number of people are perhaps being adversely affected by toxicants, but the effects are still developing and have not yet emerged into a clinically visible form. Cancers can, of course, take 20 to 40 years post exposure to become clinically evident.[167] Reproductive disorders that have resulted from *in utero* or early childhood exposures to toxicants may not become clinically evident until a child reaches puberty, or even later. Endocrine system disorders too can sometimes show up many years post exposure, and can sometimes show up only later in the offspring of mothers who were exposed to endocrine disrupters. Furthermore, many of these toxicants are lipophilic, and are thus able to pass through various barriers and membrane systems[168] and bioaccumulate in tissues over time (because they are not fully metabolized and excreted, and instead build up and magnify). As a result, it may only be that a sufficiently critical quantity of these toxicants has not yet accumulated in some people to cause manifest clinical symptoms.

If this is the case, then many more people than are presently symptomatic may actually be accumulating levels of these toxins in their tissues which will lead to toxicant induced illnesses. These people, then, would be analogous to those who have been infected with HIV but who have not yet developed any clinically evident symptoms of AIDS. One could look at these asymptomatic HIV positive people and mistakenly claim, since they have no symptoms of disease and since they appear to be perfectly healthy and do not have AIDS, that therefore HIV is not a cause of AIDS. This postulation would be just as faulty as the suggestion that environmental toxicants are not pathogenic because they have not yet caused clinically evident disease in everyone. What must be realized is that it may take years from the time a person is first infected with HIV before enough virus builds up in the body to produce symptoms,[169] and in a similar way it may take years before the toxicant load in a person's cells reaches a level high enough to cause clinically evident disease.

As exposure of populations to ambient synthetic chemical products and byproducts continues to increase, therefore, an ever larger number of people may well over time, develop adverse health effects attributable to environmental toxicants.

All these reasons taken together explain why the connection between toxicants and the illnesses they cause has not been commonly recognized.

17. Mechanisms

Several plausible biological mechanisms by which low level toxicants may cause adverse health effects have been proposed. Before outlining those mechanisms, however, it needs to be remembered that the human organism is in reality an integrated whole, and has only been artificially divided into "systems" (such as respiratory, circulatory, neurologic, etc.) for purposes of formal study. Interactions between these various body systems are necessarily much more complex than the simplified heuristic separation into single, separable systems might imply. Toxicant induced illnesses, which seem often to manifest symptoms in a multiplicity of body systems, could well affect interaction of one system with another. It may well be that these illnesses " involve the entire neuroimmunoendocrine axis. Teasing out the subtle biochemical interactions involved in adaptation to the plethora of substances in the environment may be extremely difficult."[170] The deeply integrated character of the mammalian organism must be kept in mind as we look at the various hypotheses that suggest mechanisms to explain toxicant induced illnesses.[171]

IMMUNE SYSTEM

One plausible mechanism by which environmental toxicants may cause physical injury is by compromising the immune system. Although we usually think of the immune system as having the primary function of dealing with the invasion of organisms that can cause infectious diseases, evidence is beginning to accumulate which indicates that the immune system probably has much broader functions than that alone. Ashford and Miller explain:

> In truth, the immune system may have evolved to help control the body's [entire] internal milieu. Thus, its purpose is not simply to ward

off infections but also to carry out precise regulatory interactions between the immune system, endocrine system, and nervous system.[172]

If this is true, then any toxicant damage to the immune system may impair its internal regulatory functions as well and thereby impact a variety of other body systems.

Laboratory findings in persons with chemical sensitivity disorders often do show evidence of immune system dysregulation, such as altered T cell counts, altered T4/T8 ratios, lower natural killer cell counts, and sometimes evidence of antibodies to some of the host's own tissues.[173]

One intriguing study even suggested that exposure to *lower* doses of toxicants (in this case, residues of the herbicide aldicarb in drinking water) seemed to suppress immune function significantly more dramatically than did exposure to *higher* doses. This experiment "was carried out several times with two different mouse strains and two sources of aldicarb, with the same results."[174] How might this counterintuitive finding be explained? Ashford and Miller hypothesize that "lower levels of toxic substances could be more damaging than higher levels, perhaps because damage from the former is so slight that usual cell repair mechanisms are not triggered and the damage becomes permanent."[175]

In any case, however toxicant induced damage to the immune system might be caused, compromised immune function may account for some of the variety of clinical symptoms experienced by people with chemical sensitivity disorders.

Central Nervous System Mechanisms

A second proposed mechanism of injury by toxicants may be direct mechanical damage to the neural tissues of the central or peripheral nervous systems, or both.

As for direct toxic injury to the brain, researchers have described two potential routes of entry. One is passage of molecules from the nasal surfaces, along the olfactory nerve trunk, and directly into the midbrain, particularly into the limbic system of the midbrain.[176] This route would explain the almost instantaneous reactions that many with chemical sensitivity disorders experience in the presence of neurotoxins.

A second possible route of access of toxicants to the brain would be by crossing a compromised Blood-Brain Barrier. As noted earlier, researchers have found that, under certain conditions of high stress, the integrity of the BBB can be compromised to such an extent that xenobiotic toxicants which would ordinarily have virtually no access to the brain can have relatively free access via the bloodstream.[177]

The hypothesis that toxicants may have direct access to the limbic system is an intriguing and a promising one. The limbic system is one of the most primitive elements of the early brain, and it serves a wide variety of functions. Some of its various elements are involved in the laying down of memories, in learning, and in the regulation of "feelings and activities related to self-preservation, such as searching for food, feeding, fighting, and self-protection."[178] Ashford and Miller write:

> The most vital component of the limbic system, the hypothalamus, governs: (1) body temperature via vasoconstriction, shivering, vasodilation, sweating, fever, and behaviors such as moving to a cooler or warmer environment or putting on or taking off clothing; (2) reproductive physiology and behavior; (3) feeding, drinking, digestive, and metabolic activities, including water balance, addictive eating leading to obesity, and complete refusal of food and water leading to death; (4) aggressive behavior, including such physical manifestations of emotion as increased heart rate, elevated blood pressure, dry mouth, and gastrointestinal responses. The hypothalamus is also the locus at which sympathetic and parasympathetic nervous systems converge.[179]

Another author, Corwin, suggests a promising metaphor to help make clear the complexity and significance of the functions served by the hypothalamus.

> Imagine, if you will, a chemical laboratory set up to monitor a stream of fluid continuously. This laboratory is equipped to perform analyses for simple substances such as acids, bases, and salts, ions such as sodium, potassium, calcium, and chloride, and more complex substances such as glucose and cholesterol, simple hormones such as adrenaline and thyroxine, more complex hormones such as the peptide hormones. This laboratory has a built-in computer which evaluates the balance between all these substances and controls this balance so that in case one is formed in excess, the valves can be tightened electrically to decrease the production or to generate an antagonist. In addition, this laboratory has the means for the synthesis of organic chemicals which can be released into the flowing stream of fluid at appropriate points to alter the action of the way stations producing the desired or undesired materials.... The human body has its analytical laboratory, computer controller, and hormone factory compressed into a few grams of hypothalamus, a true marvel of microminiaturization.[180]

Chemical injury to a system so intimately involved in all the regulatory subsystems of human physiology and behavior could certainly explain the variety of symptoms that are expressed in toxicant induced illnesses.[181]

VASCULAR MECHANISMS

A third proposed mechanism of chemical injury is xenobiotic toxicants compromising peripheral blood flow. The SPECT scans[182] of the brains of people with chemical sensitivities often show clear visual evidence of decreased blood flow to certain areas of the brain during exposure to toxicants. The SPECT scans also show evidence of *increased* blood flow to these areas after several weeks of participating in a medical detoxification treatment program.[183] This evidence suggests that the presence of xenobiotic toxicants in the body may indeed have a direct compromising effect on cerebral blood flow—and perhaps on blood flow to other organ systems. Toxicants in the bloodstream may cause inflammation or tissue damage to vessels, potentially leading to either vasoconstriction or vessel leakage, perhaps both. The consequent decreased blood flow to various organ systems could result in compromised organ function which may account for some of the multiple system complaints reported by people with toxicant induced illnesses. Dr. William Rea, Director of the Environmental Health Center in Dallas, Texas, is one of the proponents of this explanation. He suggests that

> particular complaints may simply mirror the site and size of affected blood vessels. Spasms in large-caliber arteries, either acutely or chronically, could reduce blood supply to an organ or limb and result in dysfunction, pain, or even necrosis. Chemical injury to the fragile walls of smaller vessels, however, would be more likely to cause hemorrhage (resulting in petechiae and bruises) or edema.[184]

Further research will be needed, of course, to test this vascular damage hypothesis. But preliminary evidence is quite promising.

AN ENDOCRINE SYSTEM MECHANISM

A fourth plausible mechanism, as we have seen above, is direct action of toxicants on the endocrine system.[185] The endocrine system and the hormones it produces are central to the body's billions of cells staying in communication with each other, and when these signal systems become disrupted by endocrine mimics, effects on the functioning of multiple body systems be significant.

A BIOCHEMICAL MECHANISM

Our biological detoxification systems require the presence of various enzymes to help the body metabolize and eliminate both endogenous and exogenous toxins. Most of these enzymes are synthesized by the body from molecules absorbed from various nutrients. Nutritional deficiencies or depletion of cellular nutrient stores (or even genetically weaker detoxification pathways) may severely compromise these detoxification processes, thereby allowing for a buildup of toxins at the cellular level. As evidence supporting this hypothesis, Dr William Rea "has noted that many of his chemically sensitive patients [at the Environmental Health Center] have decreased levels of detoxifying enzymes, such as glutathione peroxidase."[186] If these detoxification pathways become compromised and are unable to adequately break down and eliminate toxins, these toxins may build up and cause direct adverse effects on any number of body systems. This could also account for the wide variety of symptoms reported by those with toxicant induced illnesses.

STOCHASTIC RESONANCE

This final hypothesis for explaining some of the phenomena typically found in chemical sensitivity disorders is inspired by an issue of *Chaos: An Interdisciplinary Journal of Nonlinear Science*, a journal sponsored by the American Institute of Physics. The September 1998 issue was devoted entirely to principles of stochastic resonance (a concept to be explained briefly below), and several of the articles were devoted to the function of stochastic resonance in biological systems. Some of the articles relating to biological systems discussed studies on subjects such as "Detection of weak electric fields by sharks, rays, and skates," "Stochastic resonance in mammalian neuronal networks," and "Noise sustained waves in subexcitable media: From chemical waves to brain waves."

People with chemical sensitivity disorders find that they have become hypersensitized to the presence of very low levels of toxicants in their environment; that is, they find that their bodies develop physical reactions to levels of environmental toxicants that most people are not even aware are present. The phenomenon of stochastic resonance may provide one possible explanation for why these reactions develop.

Stochastic resonance is the name for the intriguing physical phenomenon whereby the detectability of a signal is sometimes actually *enhanced* by the presence of small amounts of noise around the signal. We usually think of noise as an obstacle which impedes the ability of a signal to be detected. But as is pointed out in these articles, "in nonlinear systems that display stochastic resonance, the presence of noise *enhances* the detection of weak signals."[187]

> Stochastic resonance is now firmly established as a common phenomenon which appears in a wide variety of physical systems. Interest in the subject has now crossed disciplinary boundaries, as researchers ask whether it may be relevant to problems in sensory biology.[188]

Stated a bit more technically: "Stochastic resonance (SR) is a phenomenon wherein the response of a nonlinear system to a weak input signal is optimized by the presence of a particular, nonzero level of noise."[189] Too much noise, of course, drowns out the signal, but at some optimal "nonzero" level of noise, the signal's detectability is actually strengthened.

This phenomenon holds true in systems as diverse as radio receivers, detection of pressure signals on the skin, and the passage of electrochemical signals along nerve pathways.[190] It may operate at the cellular level of organisms as well (according to articles in this issue of *Chaos*), and perhaps even at the subcellular level. In any case, there is little doubt that the phenomenon of stochastic resonance applies as much to biological systems as to other nonlinear physical systems.[191]

The hypothesis suggested here is that stochastic resonance may be functioning in the neural tissues of some people with MCS. It may be that the presence of accumulated toxins, particularly in the lipid tissues of the myelin sheaths that cover the surface of neurons, operates as a kind of chemical "noise" along those neurons. If neurons function largely as vehicles for electrochemical signal transmission, then it may be that some nerve "signals" are in effect intensified by the presence of chemical "noise," following the principles of stochastic resonance. Too much chemical noise, according to this hypothesis, would not produce the same effect,[192] but low levels of noise would.

This hypothesis may help explain at least three of the phenomena associated with chemical sensitivity disorders. Firstly, it may partially account for the fact that even very low levels of environmental toxicants seem to cause physical reactions. It may also account for an "enhanced" or "hyperreactive" sensitivity to certain neural signals (either afferent or efferent), leading to experiences of sensory overload, various paraesthesias, and perhaps even some of the sensations associated with fibromyalgia. Thirdly, this hypothesis may help account for the wide variety of multisystem complaints that so dramatically affect people with MCS.

Finally, according to the principles of stochastic resonance, the presence of accumulated chemical "noise," even at the cellular level, may in some ways affect the signals emitted by, and received by, individual cells and clusters of cells. This could lead to significant alterations in the cellular communications that are so necessary for normal biological functioning.

While it may be difficult to design research studies to determine whether SR is functioning at these levels, the hypothesis should at least not be immediately dismissed. It may turn out to be yet one more piece in the difficult and complex puzzle that faces those who are trying to understand the underlying physiology of chemical hypersensitivity disorders.

These six possible mechanisms may partially explain the variety of physical symptoms suffered by those with toxicant induced disorders. Except for SR, enough substantial preliminary research has been conducted to render these mechanisms at least plausible, perhaps even likely, and to strongly suggest the need for additional corroborating (or disproving) research.

As a cautionary note, however, it should be remembered that when searching for plausible biomedical mechanisms, the concept of plausibility is largely a function of whatever the current medical paradigm understands about physiologic processes. Explanatory mechanisms that do not appear plausible one year may well be accepted as plausible the next.

We saw a major shift like this happen within the span of just a few months in early 1995 when one very powerful piece of research changed our understanding of how HIV interacts with the human immune system. It explained the long delay between infection with HIV and the onset of AIDS-like symptoms.[193] We had earlier believed that this delay was explained by the "latency" phenomenon and that HIV somehow "went dormant" for a period of months or years until an unknown factor somehow stimulated it to reemerge and become active again. This explanatory mechanism fit the model of other infectious agents that we already knew behaved in a similar manner, so we found this "latency" model of HIV's behavior to be entirely plausible. However, when David Ho's research came out in January of 1995, we discovered that what we had considered to be plausible was in fact empirically quite wrong, and that an entirely different mechanism of action more accurately explained the long lapse of time between HIV infection and the onset of AIDS-like symptoms. Ho discovered that during those symptom-free years HIV was anything but dormant: it was in fact replicating by the billions of particles every day. The only reason the infected person was free of symptoms was because his or her immune system was able to wage such an energetic and largely successful battle against the virus. This model of an ongoing pitched battle between virus and immune system became our new explanatory paradigm for understanding the symptom-free period.

So while dormancy had been accepted for over a decade as the reason for the symptom-free period, it was, in fact, entirely wrong. Dormancy had been considered plausible only because it fit the then current medical paradigm.

This is not an uncommon occurrence in the history of medicine. Often an accepted explanation for a certain phenomenon, while it was indeed quite plausible at the time, turned out, with increased knowledge, to be absolutely mistaken.[194]

When the four humors were the dominant medical paradigm, for example, plausible disease mechanisms needed to have been couched in terms of humors. When 19th century scientific medicine developed the germ theory of disease causation, plausible explanations of disease processes needed to be couched in terms of bacterial infection. Later in the century, viruses and viral infection became part of the germ theory paradigm. Currently, a full century later, prions are slowly becoming recognized as a kind of quasi-infectious agent, probably responsible for certain diseases such as bovine spongiform encephalopathy (BSE), and a human form of the disease, Creutzfeldt-Jakob Disease (CJD). Prions may eventually be considered to fit, or perhaps not to fit, the germ model of disease. As yet, there is simply too little understood about how they work to know whether they will fit or not.

Plausibility, therefore, must be clearly recognized as a function of whatever the current ruling medical thinking is. As Dr. Claudia Miller says, "What is [considered] plausible depends on the biological knowledge of the time."[195] This historical realization should perhaps temper our intellectual hubris and our uncritical assumption that the currently dominant medical paradigm will always be able to explain virtually all disease manifestations. It should especially cause both medical researchers and clinicians to remember the primacy of empirical data and to listen very carefully to what their patients tell them. Empirical data, including that derived from taking medical histories, must be given a certain privilege of place in diagnosis, even if there is as yet no adequately plausible model for explaining that data. This should be particularly so in areas of newly emerging medical knowledge.

Indeed, until the mid 1990s, although we all had clear empirical data indicating that insects were indeed capable of flight—i.e., we could watch them fly—we did not yet understand the actual aerodynamic mechanisms of that flight.[196]

In the same way, even though it would be preferable to have plausible explanations for how toxic chemicals cause adverse health effects, it may be that we will not discover any adequate model until more research has been completed. In fact, as Miller's work suggests, Toxicant-Induced Loss of Tolerance (TILT) may itself be the operating mechanism in chemical sensitivity disorders,[197] and we may be dealing with a mechanism of disease causality that is entirely new and has not yet been adequately characterized by contemporary conventional medicine. Her work, fortunately, does nicely outline several clear research protocols for testing the TILT theory of disease causation[198] (protocols which will be described below in the first section of Chapter Three).

In the meantime, until definitive explanatory models have been fully worked out, medical practitioners may be forced to choose between holding tightly to their current models of medical plausibility on the one hand, and on the other hand recognizing the reality of the empirical givens in their patients' experience. It may well be the case, after all, that toxicants do, even in relatively low doses, actually cause serious adverse chronic health effects in some people, even though we may not as yet have a proven and plausible explanation for precisely how that process occurs.

Nor should it be forgotten that, even in the absence of proven mechanisms of action, it is still possible to take measures to prevent the spread of diseases. John Snow, for example, was able to prevent the continued spread of cholera by removing the handle from the Broad Street pump even though he had no understanding at all of the physiological processes which led to the symptoms of cholera. As Ashford and Miller explain,

> Although knowledge of the mechanism of a disease may be useful for
> developing better therapies, such knowledge is not a prerequisite for

intervention. Preventing the development of multiple chemical sensitivities in those not yet afflicted may be possible by controlling environmental exposures that cause the initial sensitization.[199]

And yet, understanding the mechanism of action in a disease
process can be extremely valuable, and as we have seen above, some
plausible mechanisms have already been suggested.[200] Nor should it
be forgotten that environmental toxicants may cause adverse health
effects by more than one mechanism.

18. Controversy

The data presented in this chapter are well supported by solid
scientific findings, and are thus, in all likelihood, valid. However, one
may wish to argue that some of the postulations have not yet been
adequately supported by scientific evidence.

It should be remembered, though, that sometimes even true
claims can be made to *appear* unproven, especially by parties with
a financial interest in the matter. The Tobacco Institute, for example, still holds that the Surgeon General's claims of tobacco's carcinogenicity are unproven, that claims of tobacco's addictiveness are
unproven, and that there is inadequate scientific data linking tobacco
use to cardiovascular disease. They repeat the refrain, "More
research is needed," as a way of perpetuating the position that
tobacco's pathogenicity is controversial. In fact, it is not controversial at all except to those who have a reason for refusing to see that
tobacco use does cause increased risk of disease.

The same may well be true of environmental toxicants. It should
not come as any surprise to learn that synthetic chemical pollutants
can make people sick. Nor should it come as a surprise to learn that
chronic exposure to increasing quantities of these pollutants can
make even more people even sicker.

The more appropriate question might be to ask what steps societies should take when they have strong scientific data which con-
vincingly support, though they may not conclusively prove, a clear
association between increased exposure to toxicants and increased
incidence of certain kinds of disease. This, of course, is a policy question, and thus concerns the primary focus of this book. It will therefore be taken up in Chapter Three where some clear policy recommendations will be advanced.

Before we can discuss policy recommendations, though, we must

examine some of the fundamental working principles by which policymaking should be guided. We turn to this now in Chapter Two.

Notes

1. J.G. Vos, M. Younes and F. Smith, eds., *Allergic Hypersensitivities
Induced by Chemicals: Recommendations for Prevention* (London: CRC
Press (on behalf of the World Health Organization Regional Office for
Europe), 1996) 348. p. 3.

2. From S. Lester and L. Gibbs. *A Citizen's Guide to Risk Studies.* Citizens' Clearinghouse for Hazardous Waste, 1988, as quoted in S. Kroll-
Smith and H.H. Floyd. *Bodies in Protest: Environmental Illness and the
Struggle Over Medical Knowledge* (New York : New York University Press,
1997) 223+xiv. p. 195

3. The April 8, 1997, issue of the journal *Pediatrics* published a study
by Marcia Herman-Giddens of the University of North Carolina, Chapel
Hill, reporting that the age of puberty for U.S. girls seems to be younger
than previously thought. "[T]he authors speculate that something new may
be going on: perhaps higher exposures to estrogens [estrogen mimics, actu-
ally] in plastics, insecticides and even hair products." "Puberty Signs Evident in 7- and 8-Year-Old Girls," *USA Today*, 8 April 1997. 1A.

4. T. Colburn, D. Dumanoski and J.P. Myers. *Our Stolen Future: Are
We Threatening Our Fertility, Intelligence and Survival?—A Scientific Detective Story* (New York: Penguin Books USA, 1996) 306+xii.

5. C. Duehring, "Gulf Vets' Injuries Echo MCS," *Medical and Legal
Briefs*, 2, #6 (May/June 1997) 5–6. p. 5.

6. Chloracne is a skin condition that seems to occur most commonly in
persons exposed to chlorine compounds. One author's description sounds
distressingly unpleasant. She says that it often manifests as "an eruption of
the skin of the neck, back, and chest into a mass of ulcerations, comedones,
cysts and pustules. Chloracne has been repeatedly described by the chemical industry as 'only a slight skin rash.' Their euphemistic description does
not indicate other more serious symptoms of the disease, including urinary
disturbances, liver damage, leg cramps, shortness of breath, intolerance to
cold, loss of sensation in extremities, demyelination of peripheral nerves,
fatigue, nervousness, irritability, insomnia, loss of libido, and vertigo. The
condition can persist or recur for many years. Chloracne has been known
since 1899 in factories producing chlorine by hydrolysis. It was a common
affliction during World War II among workers in plants producing chlorinated naphthalenes. In 1936, over three hundred workers in Mississippi
contracted severe cases of chloracne after treating lumber with a Dowicide
formulation of tetrachloraphenol, used as a wood preservative. In Dow's
own plant in Midland, Michigan, in 1937, twenty-one workers suffered
from the disease." C. Van Strum, *A Bitter Fog: Herbicides and Human
Rights* (San Francisco: Sierra Club Books, 1983) 288+x. p. 69–70.

7. Many of these disorders are listed on a U.S. Air Force document reproduced in *ibid.*, Appendix A. As we learn more about some of these conditions, we may discover them to be rather closely related to each other. See, for example, D. Buchwald and D. Garrity, "Comparison of Patients with Chronic Fatigue Syndrome, Fibromyalgia, and Multiple Chemical Sensitivities," *Archives of Internal Medicine*, 154 (September 26, 1994) 2049–53.

8. This study found "a gradient of increasing exposure" between non-Hodgkins lymphoma and length of exposure to chlorophenate wood preservatives. C. Hertzman, et al., "Mortality and Cancer Incidence Among Sawmill workers Exposed to Chlorophenate Wood Preservatives," *American Journal of Public Health*, 87, No. 1 (January 1997) 71–9. p. 77.

9. For somewhat more detailed overviews of some of these disorders, see the remaining sections here in Chapter One, as well as the sources cited in those sections.

10. R. Repetto and S.S. Baliga, *Pesticides and the Immune System* (Washington, DC: World Resources Institute, 1996) 100. See also P. Montague, "Infectious disease and pollution," *Rachel's Environment and Health Weekly*, #528 (January 9, 1997).

11. See P. Montague, "Toxics affect behavior," *Rachel's Environment and Health Weekly*, #529 (January 16, 1997) D.J. Rapp, *Is This Your Child? Discovering and Treating Unrecognized Allergies in Children and Adults* (New York: William Morrow, 1991) 626+. D.J. Rapp, *Is This Your Child's World? How You Can Fix the Schools and Homes That Are Making Your Children Sick* (New York: Bantam, 1996) 635+xix.

12. P. Montague, "Toxics affect behavior."

13. W. Rea, MD, *Chemical Sensitivity*, 4 (Boca Raton, FL: Lewis Publishers, and CRC Press, 1992–97) 2924.

14. See, for example, N. Ashford and C.S. Miller, *Chemical Exposures: Low Levels, High Stakes*. First ed. (New York: Van Nostrand Reinhold, 1991) 214. See also W. Rea, MD, *Chemical Sensitivity*, 4 (Boca Raton, FL: Lewis Publishers, and CRC Press, 1992–97) 2924.

15. C. Duehring, "The global problem of MCS part one: overview of investigative reports' findings," *Medical and Legal Briefs*, 2, Number 5. March/April (1997) 1–5. p. 1.

16. *Ibid.*

17. *Ibid.*, p. 2.

18. *Ibid.*

19. "According to the World Health Organization in 1964, 80 percent of cancers are caused by human-produced carcinogens." J. Brady, "The Goose and the Golden Egg," *One in Three: Women with Cancer Confront an Epidemic*, ed. J. Brady (San Francisco and Pittsburgh: Cleis Press, 1991) 13–35. p. 14. The citation provided in Brady is from Environmental Defense Fund and Robert H. Boyle, *Malignant Neglect* (New York: Vintage Books, 1980). p. 5. See also P. Montague, "Living downstream," *Rachel's Environment and Health Weekly*, 565 (September 25, 1997).

20. D. Fagin and M. Lavelle, *Toxic Deception: How the Chemical*

Industry Manipulates Science, Bends the Law, and Endangers Your Health (Seacaucus, NJ: Carol Publishing Group, 1997) 294+xxvi. p. 7.

21. J. Brady, "The Goose and the Golden Egg," *One in Three: Women with Cancer Confront an Epidemic*, ed. J. Brady (San Francisco and Pittsburgh: Cleis Press, 1991) 13–35. p. 34.

22. *Ibid.*, p. 30.

23. A. Lorde. *The Cancer Journals* (San Francisco: Aunt Lute Books, 1980) 77. p. 73.

24. Mostly because of the fact that several executives from chemical manufacturing corporations have traditionally sat on the board of directors of the NCI.

25. Cancer at the Crossroads: A Report to Congress for the Nation, Cancer Advisory Board, September 1994. Quoted in J. Stauber and S. Rampton, *Toxic Sludge Is Good for You: Lies, Damn Lies, and the Public Relations Industry* (Monroe, ME: Common Courage Press, 1995) 236+iv. p. 192.

26. C. Sellers, "Discovering Environmental Cancer: Wilhelm Hueper, Post-World War II Epidemiology, and the Vanishing Clinician's Eye," *American Journal of Public Health*, 87, #11 (November 1997) 1824–35.

27. S. Steingraber. *Living Downstream: An Ecologist Looks at Cancer and the Environment* (Reading, MA: Addison-Wesley Publishing Co., Inc. 1997) 357+vi. p. 40.

28. The chapter is titled "One in Four." R. Carson, *Silent Spring* (Boston: Houghton Mifflin Co., 1962, 1994) 368+xxvi.

29. S. Steingraber, p. 40.

30. *Ibid.*, p. 45.

31. J.H. Cushman, Jr., "U.S. Reshaping Cancer Strategy As Incidence in Children Rises," *New York Times*, September 29, 1997. A1 & A13.

32. *Ibid.*, p. A1.

33. *Ibid.*, p. A13.

34. *Ibid.*

35. *Ibid.*

36. S. Steingraber, *op. cit.*, p. 45. Davis' statistics are restricted to Caucasians only because the statistics for these groups have been somewhat more reliable. One might well suppose that the increased incidence of many cancers may be even more dramatic in some more marginalized social groups.

37. The National Cancer Institute (NCI) of the U.S. Department of Health and Human Services, which is a department of the National Institutes of Health, takes the position that "There is no adequate evidence that there is a safe level of exposure for any carcinogen." C. Duehring, "Nat'l Cancer Institute Statements Counteract Junk Science," *Medical and Legal Briefs*, 2, No. 4 (January/February 1997) 10. NCI cites evidence such as those "family members of asbestos workers who have brought the particles home on their clothes," who were thus exposed to very low levels of this carcinogen, and yet who nonetheless developed cancers. This principle, viz., that there is no safe level of exposure for any carcinogenic toxicant, would

mean that once a substance is determined to be carcinogenic, no amount of it should be considered acceptable for human exposure. This would be particularly true for toxic exposures which individuals are unable to avoid by their own actions, but which policymakers could render avoidable by means of policy decisions and legislative actions.

38. D. Fagin and M. Lavelle, *Toxic Deception: How the Chemical Industry Manipulates Science, Bends the Law, and Endangers Your Health* (Seacaucus, NJ: Carol Publishing, 1997) 294+xxvi. p. 9.

39. M.A. Kiettles, et al., "Triazine Herbicide Exposure and Breast Cancer Incidence: An Ecologic Study of Kentucky Counties," *Environmental Health Perspectives*, 105, Number 11 (November 1997) 1222–27.

40. J.M. Pogoda and S. Preston-Martin, "Household Pesticides and Risk of Pediatric Brain Tumors," *Environmental Health Perspectives*, 105, Number 11 (November 1997) 1214–20.

41. S. Steingraber, *op. cit.* p. 126.

42. *Ibid.*, p. 127.

43. *Ibid.*, p. 131.

44. There is too much work in this connection to cite here, but for a few examples see *ibid.*, *passim*; R.N. Proctor, *Cancer Wars: How Politics Shapes What We Know and Don't Know About Cancer* (New York: Basic Books, 1995) 356+xii; C. Van Strum, *op. cit.*, *passim*; C. Sellers, "Discovering Environmental Cancer: Wilhelm Hueper, Post-World War II Epidemiology, and the Vanishing Clinician's Eye," *American Journal of Public Health*, 87, #11 (November 1997) 1824–35.

45. N. Ashford and C.S. Miller, *Chemical Exposures: Low Levels, High Stakes*, 2nd ed. (New York: Van Nostrand Reinhold / John Wiley & Sons, 1998) 440+xxiii. p. 9.

46. *Ibid.*

47. Quoted in J.B. Berkson, *A Canary's Tale: The Final Battle, Politics, Poisons, and Pollution vs. the Environment and the Public Health* (Hagerstown, MD: self-published, 1996) 452+siii. p. 140.

48. P. Montague, "Immune system toxins," *Rachel's Environment and Health Weekly*, #536 (March 6, 1997).

49. R. Repetto and S.S. Baliga, *op. cit.*

50. S. Steingraber, *op. cit.*, p. 112.

51. *Ibid.*, p. 114.

52. One recent story in *USA Today* (October 2, 1998, p. B3), for example, reported that the FDA and the Navy were trying to determine how chlordane had gotten into a grease trap at the Chief Petty Officers' Club at Little Creek Naval Amphibious Base in Virginia Beach. This was a puzzle for them because chlordane had been banned for use in the U.S. (though *not* banned for manufacture in the U.S.) since 1988.

53. P. Montague, "Infectious disease and pollution."

54. *Ibid.*

55. *Ibid.*

56. The city of Seattle is named after Chief Sealth.

57. Suquamish Tribe, 1788–1866.

58. P. Montague, "Infectious disease and pollution."

59. *Ibid.*

60. J. Wargo, *Our Children's Toxic Legacy: How Science and Law Fail to Protect Us from Pesticides* (New Haven: Yale University Press, 1996) 380+xvi. p. 169.

61. *Ibid.* See also K. Hooper, et al., "Analysis of Breast Milk to Assess Exposure to Chlorinated Contaminants in Kazakhstan: PCBs and Organochlorine Pesticides in Southern Kazakhstan," *Environmental Health Perspectives*, 105, Number 11 (November 1997) 1250–54.

62. R. Carson, *Silent Spring* (Boston: Houghton Mifflin Co., 1962, 1994) 368+xxvi.

63. Quoted in J. Wargo.

64. T. Colburn, D. Dumanoski and J.P. Myers, *Our Stolen Future: Are We Threatening Our Fertility, Intelligence and Survival?—A Scientific Detective Story* (New York: Penguin Books USA Inc., 1996) 306+xii. 145–6.

65. T. Colburn, D. Dumanoski and J.P. Myers, *op. cit.* p. 215. Colburn concludes: "It is indeed tragic that breast-feeding is the only efficient way to remove these persistent chemicals from the human body." Many of the synthetic chemical toxicants that are pathogenic for human beings are lipophilic, and hence bioaccumulate in fatty tissues throughout the body. So one possible reason for the finding that a large percentage (75–80 percent) of those who suffer from chemical sensitivities and other environmental illnesses are women is that women have, as a rule, a larger percentage of body fat than males, and hence may have accumulated a greater quantity (per unit of weight) of these toxicants. One possible methodology for treating chemical sensitivities and other environmental illnesses is to detoxify the body as much as possible, via sauna sweating, colonics, and so on. But given that "wet nurses" have been able, throughout history, to induce lactation without the prior necessity of first becoming pregnant and giving birth, and modern medicine has methods for inducing lactation, would it not be possible to use the process of lactation to bring about some amount of detoxification? That is, might it not be possible, as a method of detoxification of accumulated synthetic lipophilic toxicants, to induce lactation in women suffering from symptoms of chemical sensitivities and other environmental illnesses, and then use a breast pump for some period of time to withdraw the milk? It is true that the contaminants in such breast milk are so high, then it would probably be best to not use that milk for infant nourishment. There may be questions other than strictly medical about using lactation as a method of detoxification. Some women, for example, may find the idea objectionable or offensive. To think of one's breast milk as toxic may well offend some people's feelings about the special intimacy of breast feeding. Or some might feel that such a practice would violate the intended purpose of lactation, and hence be viewed as unethical. Others may feel the procedure to be too uncomfortable, or may have other objections.

66. J. Wargo, *op. cit.*, p. 170.

67. *Ibid.*, p. 171. The levels of xenobiotic chemicals in human fat stores may not be diminishing in developing nations, however. One recent study

reports that, "In the late 1980s, worldwide total DDT (in human fat samples) averaged 1,000 ng/g fat, with levels in developing countries 10–100 times higher," K. Hooper, et al., *op. cit.*, p. 1253.

68. P. Montague, "Immune system toxins."

69. P. Montague, "Statement on immune toxins," *Rachel's Environment and Health Weekly*, #544 (May 1, 1997).

70. *Ibid.*

71. *Ibid.*

72. *Ibid.*

73. "The World Health Organization's annual report, Conquering Suffering, Enriching Humanity, says the number of cancer cases is expected to at least double in most countries during the next 25 years." "WHO says chronic and infectious diseases are increasing worldwide," *The Nation's Health*, 27, #5 (May/June 1997) 11.

74. P. Montague, "Infectious disease and pollution."

75. *Ibid.* Emphasis mine.

76. I. Hanin, "GWS: Expanding knowledge on permeability of Blood-Brain Barrier," *Our Toxic Times*, 8, Number 4 (April 1997) 1–4.

77. D. Vergano, "Stress may weaken the blood-brain barrier," *Science News*, 150 (December 14, 1996) 375.

78. *Ibid.*

79. *Ibid.*

80. I first encountered this distinction 30 years ago in a book (long since lost) titled *Why Men Seek Stress*.

81. I.R. Bell, R.R. Bootzin et al., "A Polysomnographic Study of Sleep Disturbance in Community Elderly with Self-reported Environmental Chemical Odor Intolerance," *Biology Psychiatry*, 40 (1996) 123–33.

82. C. Duehring, "Objective Sleep Abnormalities Found Even with Mild Chemical Sensitivities," *Medical and Legal Briefs*, 2, No. 4 (January/February 1997) 6–7. p. 6.

83. Ashford and C.S. Miller, *Chemical Exposures: Low Levels, High Stakes*, 2nd ed.

84. J.L. Jacobson and S.W. Jacobson, "Intellectual Impairment in Children Exposed to Polychlorinated Biphenyls in Utero," *New England Journal of Medicine*, 335, No. 11 (September 12, 1996) 435–45.

85. Montague, "PCB exposure linked to low IQ," Rachel's Environment and Health Weekly, #512 (September 19, 1996).

86. *Ibid.*

87. *Ibid.* Emphasis in original (except for *Lifetime*).

88. *Ibid.*

89. S. Steingraber, *op. cit.*, p. 126.

90. *Ibid.*

91. P. Montague, "PCB exposure linked to low IQ."

92. M. McGue, "The democracy of genes," *Nature*, 388 (July 31, 1997) 417–18. p. 417. See also B. Devlin, M. Daniels and K. Raeder, "The democracy of genes," *Nature*, 388 (July 31, 1997) 468–74.

93. M. McGue, *ibid., passim.*

94. *Ibid.*

95. Much of that research is summarized in T. Colburn, D. Dumanoski and J.P. Myers, *op. cit.* "Scientists estimate that at least 50 different chemicals, many of which are discharged into the environment, exhibit estrogenic activity." "Estrogens in the Environment," *Environmental Health Perspectives*, 105, Number 9 (September 1997) 910.

96. T. M. Crisp, E.D. Clegg and R.L. Cooper, *Special Report on Environmental Endocrine Disruption: An Effects Assessment and Analysis.* U.S. Environmental Protection Agency (February 1997). p. 81.

97. P. Montague, "The Weybridge Report," *Rachel's Environment and Health Weekly*, #547 (May 22, 1997).

98. *Ibid.*

99. T.M. Crisp, E.D. Clegg and R.L. Cooper.

100. P. Montague, "The Weybridge Report." Other studies are suggesting a strong association between PCBs and both estrogenic and anti-estrogenic activity. M.R. Fielden, et al., "Examination of the Estrogenicity of 2,4,6,2',6'-Pentachlorobiphenyl (PCB 104), Its Hydroxylated Metabolite 2,4,5,2',6'-Pentachloro-4-Biphenylol (HO-PCB 104), and a Further Chlorinated Derivative, 2,4,6,2',4',6'-Hexachlorobiphenyl (PCB 155)," *Environmental Health Perspectives*, 105, Number 11 (November 1997) 1238–48.

101. P. Montague, "The Weybridge Report."

102. *Ibid.*

103. *Ibid.*

104. P. Montague, "Fish Sex Hormones," *Rachel's Environment and Health Weekly*, #545 (May 8, 1997).

105. S. Steingraber, *op. cit.*, p. 109.

106. "The state of the science on endocrine disruptors," *Environmental Health Perspectives*, 106, #7 (July 1998) A319–20.

107. S.H. Swan, E.P. Elkin and L. Fenster, "Have Sperm Densities Declined? A Reanalysis of Global Trend Data," *Environmental Health Perspectives*, 105, #11 (November 1997) 1228–32. This article does a critical analysis of 61 studies on sperm density and concludes that sperm density has indeed declined, at least in the United States and Western Europe. See also C. Duehring, "Sperm Density Decline Confirmed," *Medical and Legal Briefs*, 3, No. 6 (May/June 1998) 6.

108. Quoted in the *Washington Post*, April 2, 1997, p. A2.

109. T.M. Crisp, E.D. Clegg and R.L. Cooper, *op. cit.*, p. 82.

110. *Ibid.*, p. 2.

111. *Ibid.*

112. *Ibid.*, p. 1.

113. "Some of the physicians we interviewed recalled being told as medical students that the more symptoms a patient complained of, the less validity any of them had." N. Ashford and C.S. Miller, *Chemical Exposures: Low Levels, High Stakes*, 2nd ed., p. 74.

114. J.T. Williams, "The painless synergism of aspirin and opium," *Nature*, 390 (December 11, 1997) 557–58. p. 557.

115. J. Kaiser, "New Yeast Study Finds Strength in Numbers," *Science*,

272 (June 7, 1996) 1418. Also: S.F. Arnold, et al., "Synergistic Activation of Estrogen Receptor with Combinations of Environmental Chemicals," *Science*, 272 (June 7, 1996) 1489–92. It should be noted that these findings have been considered controversial, as noted in a letter to *Nature* by researchers at Zeneca Central Toxicology Laboratory in Cheshire, UK, and at Brunel University in Uxbridge, UK. See J. Ashby, et al., "Synergy between synthetic oestrogens?" *Nature*, 385 (February 6, 1997) 494. The lead author of the original study has stated: "Whatever merit this publication contained, and despite the enthusiasm it generated, it is clear that any conclusions drawn from this paper must be suspended until such time, if ever, the data can be substantiated." Meanwhile, their laboratory "will continue to aggressively conduct research on environmental endocrinology," because they believe "there are important and verifiable discoveries to be made." Quoted in C. Duehring, "Synergy Findings Withdrawn Re: Environmental Estrogens," *Medical and Legal Briefs*, 3, #2 (1997) 7. For results from another study that also supports the claim that mixtures are more powerful than single chemicals, see P. Montague, "Fish Sex Hormones."

116. "There clearly is a need to expand our thinking about ... how best to address possible human health risk associated with exposure to chemical mixtures with potential for hormone mimetic chemical interactions." J.D. McKinney, "Interactive Hormonal Activity of Chemical Mixtures," *Environmental Health Perspectives*, 105, Number 9 (September 1997) 896.

117. T.M. Crisp, E.D. Clegg and R.L. Cooper, *op cit., passim.*

118. A.P., "Hormone disruptors require additional study, EPA says," *New York Times.* March 14, 1997. A26.

119. *Ibid.*

120. R.D. Masters, B. Hone and A. Doshi, "Environmental Pollution, Neurotoxicity, and Criminal Violence," *Environmental Toxicology*, ed. J. Rose (London and New York: Gordon and Breach Publishers, 1997).

121. P. Montague, "Toxics and Violent Crime," *Rachel's Environment and Health Weekly*, #551 (June 19, 1997).

122. *Ibid.*

123. D.J. Rapp, *Is This Your Child's World?* See also her earlier book: D.J. Rapp, *Is This Your Child?*

124. According to a story in *USA Today*, Oct. 2, 1998, p6A, a local water company in Zelienople, PA warned that pregnant women, nursing mothers, and children under six months of age should not drink the local tap water due to high nitrate levels.

125. Alaska, Connecticut, Delaware, Maryland, Massachusetts, New Mexico, New York and Ohio. D.M. Blank, "A Growing Sensitivity to What's in the Air," *New York Times*, February 11, 1998. BU 11.

126. D.M. Blank, *ibid.*

127. N. Ashford and C.S. Miller, *Chemical Exposures: Low Levels, High Stakes*, 2nd ed., p. 332–33.

128. C. Duehring, "Perfume Toxicity, Sensitivity, Accommodation and Disability—Part One: Evidence of Health Hazards," *Medical and Legal Briefs*, 4, Number 1 (July/August 1998) 1–6. p. 3. Later in the same article,

after detailing some of the cerebral and pulmonary inadequacies that can result, even in nonsensitized people, from exposure to artificial fragrances, the author notes that "the U.S. Food and Drug Administration (FDA) lacks authority to require toxicity testing and premarket testing of cosmetics." p. 5.

129. Most of these states have issued declarations worded almost identically to the declaration issued by Washington State. It read: MCS awareness week in Washington. **The State of Washington.** Proclamation. WHEREAS, people of all ages in Washington have developed a condition known as Multiple Chemical Sensitivity as a result of a single massive exposure or repeated low level exposures to toxic chemicals and other irritants in the environment; and WHEREAS, MCS is a chronic condition for which there is no known cure and which symptoms include chronic fatigue, muscle and joint pain, rashes, asthma, short term memory loss, headaches and other respiratory and neurological problems; and WHEREAS, MCS can cause major financial, employment, housing, health and social consequences for people who have this disability; and WHEREAS, the health of the general population is at risk from chemical exposures that can lead to illnesses that may be preventable through reduction or avoidance of chemicals in the air, water and food in both the indoor and outdoor environments; and WHEREAS, MCS is recognized by the Americans with Disabilities Act, Social Security Administration, U.S. Department of Housing and Urban Development, Environmental Protection Agency, as well as other state and national government agencies and commissions which have supported the health and welfare of the chemically injured; and WHEREAS, reasonable accommodations, information about and recognition of MCS can provide opportunities for people with this disability to enjoy access to work, schooling, public facilities and other settings where they can continue to contribute their skills, ideas, creativity, abilities and knowledge; and WHEREAS, people with MCS need the support and understanding of family, friends, co-workers and society as they struggle with their illness and adapt to new life styles; NOW THEREFORE, I, Gary Locke, Governor of the state of Washington, do hereby proclaim July 13-17, 1998, as Multiple Chemical Sensitivity Awareness Week in Washington State and urge all citizens to support increased understanding, education and research of MCS. Signed this 30th day of June, 1998. Gary Locke, Governor

130. N. Ashford and C.S. Miller, *Chemical Exposures: Low Levels, High Stakes,* 2nd ed., p. 343.

131. For a summary of some of these studies, see T. Colburn, D. Dumanoski and J.P. Myers, *op. cit.*

132. C. Duehring, "Overexposure from legal pesticiding: a generation at risk," *Medical and Legal Briefs*, 3, No. 6 (May/June 1998) 1–4. p. 1.

133. "It has been established for the first time that a semivolatile pesticide will accumulate on and in toys and other sorbent surfaces in a home via a two phase physical process that continues for at least 2 weeks postapplication.... Estimates of a child's nondietary exposure to chlorpyrifos associated with toys and other sorbent surfaces for a period of 1 week following application appear to be of public health concern." S. Gurunathan, et al., "Accumulation of Chlorpyrifos on Residential Surfaces and Toys

Accessible to Children," *Environmental Health Perspectives*, 106, Number 1 (January 1998) 9–16.

134. C. Duehring, "Overexposure from legal pesticiding: a generation at risk." p. 1.

135. *Ibid.*, p. 2.

136. *Ibid.*, *passim.*

137. *Ibid.*, p. 2. One researcher explains: "When it's warm down south and cold up north, it pulls the airstream up and causes these materials to be carried on the air until they hit a cold region where they deposit out. In this manner, pesticides can be transported literally thousands of miles." *Ibid*. Moreover, Dr. Sheldon Wagner, a physician and professor of clinical toxicology at Oregon State University, "noted that with typical applications on calm days (winds under six mph), one can generally anticipate drift within five to six miles, with the major portion drifting within 100 meters of the source." Thus, largely because of the problem of pesticide drift, "in general, less that 0.1 percent of pesticides to crops reaches the target pest for which it was intended. The rest goes wherever the wind carries it." *Ibid.*

138. With the exception of a small program in California.

139. P. Montague, "1997 Snapshots—Part 2," *Rachel's Environment and Health Weekly*, #579 (January 1, 1998).

140. *Ibid.*

141. For some direct accounts of poisoning due to exposure to locally sprayed herbicides such as 2,4-D and 2,45-T, see C. Van Strum, *op. cit.*, *passim.*

142. As clearly documented in J. Wargo, *op. cit.*, *passim.*

143. Quoted in M.L. Winston, *Nature Wars: People vs. Pests* (Cambridge, MA: Harvard University Press, 1997) 210+x. p. 1.

144. These pests, of course, are seen as pests only when looked at from the point of view of another competing species, such as human beings.

145. For alternatives to chemical pesticide solutions, two organizations provide superb information: the Northwest Coalition for Alternatives to Pesticides (NCAP) in Eugene, Oregon, and the National Coalition Against the Misuse of Pesticides (NCAMP).

146. Personal communication.

147. N. Ashford and C.S. Miller, *Chemical Exposures: Low Levels, High Stakes,* 2nd ed., p. 208.

148. P.R. Gibson, J. Cheavens and M.L. Warren, "Social Support in Persons with Self-Reported Sensitivity to Chemicals," *Research in Nursing and Health*, 21 (1998) 103–105.

149. Personal communication.

150. For more details on life impact, see P.R. Gibson, "Environmental Illness/Multiple Chemical Sensitivities: Invisible Disabilities," *Women and Therapy*, 14, Number 3/4 (1993) 171–85.

151. See, for example, T. Svoboda, "Every Breath She Takes," *Utne Reader* (March-April 1987) 59–63. See also J. Harr. *A Civil Action* (New York: Random House, 1995) 500. L. Lawson, *Staying Well in a Toxic World*

(Chicago: Noble Press, 1993) 488. E. Royte, "Where the Skies Are Not Toxic All Day," *Outside* (May 1996) 45–55. H. Millar and M. Millar, *The Toxic Labyrinth* (Vancouver, British Columbia: NICO Professional Services Ltd. 1995) 301. C. Van Strum, *op. cit.* J. B. Berkson, *op. cit.* R. Jerome and M. Nelson, "Toxic Avenger," *People*, February 9, 1998; 113–15.

152. J.G. Vos, M. Younes and E. Smith, eds., *loc. cit.*

153. *Ibid.*, p. 4.

154. S. Steingraber, *op. cit.*, p. 187.

155. The usual standard for toxicology testing is the 70 kilogram adult Caucasian male.

156. P. Montague, "Infectious disease and pollution."

157. I mention breast cancer only because so many environmental toxicants are lipophilic and gravitate toward fatty tissues in the body, and it is now widely accepted that residues of many of these toxicants do accumulate in breast tissues.

158. "Symptoms developed from prolonged low-level exposure to organochlorine pesticides may be gradual in onset and may not necessarily be [consciously] associated with chemical insults." Quoted in C. Duehring, "Organochlorines linked with CFS and chemical sensitivities," *Medical and Legal Briefs*, 4, Number 1 (July/August 1998) 7.

159. "Lupus is a multisystem inflammatory disorder characterized by activation of the B-lymphocytes of the immune system and autoantibodies which attack the body's own cell components and tissues." C. Duehring, "Lupus Linked to Industrial Pollution," *Medical and Legal Briefs*, 3, Number 3 (November/December 1997) 5. A Recent study assessing the association between exposure to industrial pollutants and the development of lupus argues that "The hypothesis that environmental toxins may induce lupus is consistent with the known ability of certain medications to do the same." The data in the study argue that "long standing exposure to industrial emissions may be associated with an increased risk of lupus." T. Kardestuncer and H. Frumkin, "Systemic Lupus Erythematosus in Relation to Environmental Pollution: An Investigation in an African-American Community in North Georgia," *Archives of Environmental Health*, 52, Number 2 (March/April 1997) 85–90.

160. One case of acute hepatitis, for example, was found in a golfer who routinely cleaned his golf balls by licking them. This practice had not ever caused any problem for the 65 year old man until the golf course at which he golfed daily began to use the common herbicide 2,4-D. See C. Duehring, "'Golf ball liver' caused by herbicides," *Medical and Legal Briefs*, 4, Number 1 (July/August 1998) 6.

161. C.S. Miller, "Chemical Sensitivity: symptom, syndrome or mechanism for disease?" *Toxicology*, 111 (1996) 69–86, 81.

162. *Ibid.*

163. *Ibid.*

164. T.G. Randolph and R.W. Moss. *An Alternative Approach to Allergies,* rev. ed. (New York: Harper & Row, 1980, 1989) 337+viii.

165. W. Rea, MD, *op. cit.*

166. See N. Ashford and C.S. Miller, *Chemical Exposures: Low Levels, High Stakes*, first ed., 305ff. See also C.S. Miller, et al., "Empirical Approaches for the Investigation of Toxicant-induced Loss of Tolerance," *Environmental Health Perspectives*, 105, Supplement 2 (March 1997) 515–19.

167. "Cancers can take forty years to develop." L. Gayle, "Mother's Milk—as Safe as Apple Pie?" *One in Three: Women with Cancer Confront an Epidemic*, ed. J. Brady, p. 83.

168. C. Duehring, "Plasticizers and Diesel Particulates Impair Sperm Motility," *Medical and Legal Briefs*, 3, Number 3 (November/December 1997) 6.

169. D.D. Ho, et al., "Rapid turnover of plasma virions and DC4 lymphocytes in HIV-1 infection," *Nature*, 373 (January 1995) 123ff.

170. N. Ashford and C.S. Miller, *Chemical Exposures: Low Levels, High Stakes*, 2nd ed., p. 89. "Therefore, the endocrine, immune, and nervous systems, once perceived as separate compartments, are increasingly recognized as interconnected. The hypothalamus (part of the limbic system) has attracted considerable attention because it is the focal point in the brain where the immune nervouse, and endocrine systems interact." *Ibid.*, p. 91.

171. See especially the following lengthy and thorough examination of this hypothesis, S.C. Rowat, "Integrated defense system overlaps as a disease model: with examples for Multiple Chemical Sensitivity," *Environmental Health Perspectives*, 106, Supplement I (February 1998) 85–106.

172. N. Ashford and C.S. Miller. *Chemical Exposures: Low Levels, High Stakes*, 2nd ed., p. 98.

173. *Ibid.*, p. 98–107.

174. *Ibid.*, p. 106–7.

175. *Ibid.*, p. 107. Another possible explanation may involve the physical principles of stochastic resonance. See the final section in this chapter on mechanisms of action.

176. "A direct pathway from the oropharynx to the brain and hypothalamic and limbic region has been demonstrated in rats. Substances placed in the oropharynx migrated to the brain in minutes [seconds?] via a pathway other than the blood stream and in higher concentrations than if administered via the gastrointestinal tract, suggesting a direct route from mouth (or nose) to brain." *Ibid.*, p. 91.

177. Vergano, 1996.

178. N. Ashford and C.S. Miller, *Chemical Exposures: Low Levels, High Stakes*, 2nd ed., p. 92.

179. *Ibid.*, p. 93–4.

180. A. Corwin, as quoted *ibid.*, p. 95.

181. These themes are laid out much more fully *ibid.*, p. 91–8 and p. 257–61.

182. Single Photon Emission Computed Tomography.

183. See the work of Gerald Roxx, MD, at the Environmental Health Center, Dallas, Texas.

184. Referenced in N. Ashford and C.S. Miller, *Chemical Exposures: Low Levels, High Stakes*, 2nd ed., p. 110.

185. Much of the relevant research can be found summarized in Colburn, 1996.

186. N. Ashford and C.S. Miller, *Chemical Exposures: Low Levels, High Stakes*, 2nd ed., p. 107.

187. K. Wiesenfeld and F. Jaramillo, "Minireview of stochastic resonance," *Chaos*, 8, Number 3 (September 1998) 539–48. p. 539. Emphasis mine.

188. Wiesenfeld, 1998, p. 539.

189. K.A. Richardson, et al., "Using electrical noise to enhance the ability of humans to detect subthreshold mechanical cutaneous stimuli," *Chaos*, 8, Number 3 (September 1998) 599–603. p. 599.

190. ...the ability of an individual to detect a subthreshold mechanical cutaneous stimulus can be significantly enhanced by introducing a particular level of mechanical noise.... These results suggested that a mechanical noise-based technique could be used to improve tactile sensation in humans. *Ibid.*, p. 600.

191. The suggestion that SR might play a role in biological systems was discussed at least as early as 1991. K. Wiesenfeld and F. Jaramillo, *op. cit.*, p. 544.

192. Large quantities of accumulated toxics may, of course, produce the symptoms associated with classical toxicology.

193. Ho, 1995.

194. Another historical illustration of this phenomenon occurred when Edward Jenner, in 1796, was trying to explain how it happened that inoculation with cowpox could prevent infection with smallpox. His explanation—that no two sytemic diseases could co-exist in the same body at the same time—was perfectly plausible at the time and in fact was endorsed by Sir John Hunter, perhaps the most prominent physician of the time. Yet, with increasing knowledge, this plausible explanation turned out to be quite wrong. See Kerns, 1997.

195. C.S. Miller, "Toxicant-induced Loss of Tolerance—An Emerging Theory of Disease?" *Environmental Health Perspectives*, 105, Supplement 2 (March 1997) 445–53. p. 452.

196. In fact, we have actually been plagued with just such ignorance in our understanding of the aerodynamics of insect flight. Only very recent research has offered what may well turn out to be a plausible explanation of the aerodynamics of insect flight. Fortunately, scientists in this field were not so foolish as to declare that insects were incapable of flight simply because they has as yet no plausible aerodynamic mechanism to explain it. See C.P. Ellington, et al., "Leading-edge vortices in insect flight," *Nature*, 384 (December 19/26, 1996) 626–30.

197. C.S. Miller, "Chemical Sensitivity: symptom, syndrome or mechanism for disease?"

198. C.S. Miller, "Toxicant-induced Loss of Tolerance—An Emerging Theory of Disease?" *Passim*. See also C.S. Miller, et al., "Empirical Approaches for the Investigation of Toxicant-induced Loss of Tolerance." See also N. Ashford and C.S. Miller, *Chemical Exposures: Low Levels, High Stakes*, second ed., *passim*.

199. N. Ashford and C.S. Miller, *ibid.*, p. 90.

200. Several other more detailed possible mechanisms, such as Iris Bell's "kindling" and neurogenic inflammation mechanisms, have also offered important explanatory potential.

Two

──── Principles ────

Wise action and good public policy must be based on three things: good information, well-grounded ethical principles, and wise judgment about how best to put those principles into action. In Chapter One we offered an overview of some of the information related to the health effects of long-term, low dose exposures to ubiquitous environmental toxicants. Here in Chapter Two we will lay out some of the main ethical principles that ought to guide wise policy-making. In Chapter Three, then, we will make some modest policy recommendations, and in Chapter Four we will detail some of the obstacles and challenges that will need to be met and dealt with in the process of implementing those recommendations.

To begin: our first principle, that preventing a problem is usually a better idea than having to solve that problem after it has developed, is simply one of the standard principles of wise and healthy living, a principle readily to be found in most of the wisdom traditions around the world. To that simple principle we now turn our attention.

1. Prevention

One of the lessons that the U.S. Centers for Disease Control and Prevention (CDC) learned in the first 50 years of its existence (the fiftieth anniversary was celebrated during 1996) is that prevention modalities are almost always both more effective and less expensive than treatment modalities. Prevention is obviously more effective than treatment when it successfully reduces the sum total of potential human suffering and increases the overall health and well-being of people and communities. But, in addition, it is also more cost effective to prevent diseases than to wait for them to occur and then try to treat them. Prevention, says the CDC, is literally "the best investment we can make in health."[1]

In the arena of infectious diseases alone, for example, according D. Satcher in the American Journal of Public Health,

> $21 is saved for every dollar spent immunizing children against measles, mumps, and rubella. For diphtheria/pertussis/tetanus, the savings are $29 for every dollar, and for polio, $6.
>   It cost $32 million to eradicate smallpox globally. Now more than that amount is saved every 26 days as a result of that eradication and the elimination of immunizations and quarantine programs no longer required.... With the introduction of the HiB[2] conjugate vaccine in the late 1980s, invasive HiB disease has been virtually eliminated, with savings estimated at $350 million annually.[3]

In addition to savings that result from preventive immunization programs, significant savings have also resulted from prevention programs based on behavioral interventions. One clear example of savings that resulted from preventing a disease by relying on behavioral modalities involved Byssinosis, or "brown lung" disease, "a disabling and potentially fatal lung disease caused by breathing cotton dust."[4] This condition affected 20 percent of textile workers in 1978. Satcher wrote:

> Following CDC research and recommendations, the Department of Labor established a national health standard to reduce cotton dust exposure through the textile industry. Consequently, in the United States today, the 1978 prevalence of 40,000 cases has been reduced to fewer than 1000. The direct cost savings of this success in medical care [i.e., not counting all the indirect costs] are estimated at over $365 million *annually*.[5]

What the CDC has thus learned is that prevention is indeed a much more cost-effective way for society to maintain its health and productivity than is treatment. Prevention is also, *a fortiori*, an effective way for society to reduce the indirect costs that result from sickness and disabilities. Indirect costs can include loss of productivity due to sick time, increased accidents due to impaired employees, high costs of treatment for conditions that have resulted from inadequate prevention, long-term disability insurance payouts, total years of productive life lost, and so on.

While chemical corporation executives, some elected officials, and others with relatively short-term financial interests may wish to avoid spending monies today, the CDC's long term calculations clearly indicate that funds spent on prevention today can lead to enormous economic savings in the long term. As Benjamin Franklin's Poor Richard reminded us, "a stitch in time saves nine."

Unfortunately, newly developed treatments to cure or ameliorate disease processes that are already under way are usually much more visible and sensational than the somewhat less spectacular public health interventions which are designed to prevent disease. This is reflected even in the fact that many of the nation's leading medical schools are highly visible to the public (the task of medicine being to *treat* diseases), whereas the leading schools of public health (the task of public health being more focused on *preventing* diseases), "often in the same universities, are relatively unknown."[6] Nonetheless, it has long been accepted that the most significant improvements in overall health in this century, as well as "the major increases in life expectancy ... are mainly the result of improvements in [preventive] public health [measures] rather than improvements in the treatment of disease."[7] Although prevention modalities, while much less dramatic and less visible than treatment modalities, do seem to be ultimately much more effective in controlling diseases, in the years since 1970, "the U.S. has spent 98% of its health dollars trying to cure diseases, and only 2% trying to prevent them."[8]

Moreover, it is not even entirely necessary to have a full scientific understanding of the mechanisms of disease causality before a community can begin to institute effective measures to prevent increased incidence of a disease. It was possible, for example, for Ignaz Semmelweis[9] to know that handwashing by physicians at Vienna's Lying-in hospital in 1846 diminished the incidence of "childbed fever," even though he did not know the full microbial explanation for why it did. And Edward Jenner knew that vaccination with cowpox pus effectively prevented subsequent infection with smallpox, even though he had no understanding at all of the microbial nature of infection or of the immunologic nature of protection.

It is, therefore, as we see in these historical examples, entirely possible to know what preventive measures should be taken to diminish the incidence of a disease even before there is a complete understanding of what the mechanisms are that cause that disease. This fact will become particularly important in Chapter Three in our discussion of measures for the prevention of toxicant induced illnesses.

The importance of the concept of prevention in the world of public health is hardly new. But, "Public health officials often bemoan, quite appropriately, the lack of political commitment to and public interest in prevention, even after its economic and humane benefits have been abundantly demonstrated."[10] And yet, particularly with diseases that cannot yet be effectively treated (as is the case with many toxicant induced illnesses), the imperative to prevent them becomes even more critical.

A four-year study, in which 14 nations participated, was coordinated some years ago by the Hastings Center, a center for the study of ethical and policy issues in clinical medicine and biomedical research. The final report of the study was titled *The Goals of Medicine: Setting New Priorities*. One of the key (and rather unsurprising) recommendations urged by this international study was that national priorities need to be "shifted toward public health strategies to prevent disease."[11] And *Healthy People 2010*, the study prepared by Office of Disease Prevention and Health Promotion of the U.S. Department of Health and Human Services (in its version released for public comment in the fall of 1998) states clearly that, "Efficient programs to improve environmental health must be based on primary prevention."[12]

In other words, the more we learn about the health of the world's communities, the more we come to realize the importance of prevention.

Therefore, any prevention measures that can be implemented sooner are likely to do much toward saving money later, toward reducing acute and chronic human suffering both now and later, and toward reducing the impact (economic and otherwise) that toxicant induced illnesses will continue to have on society.

The implications of this prevention principle for toxicant induced illnesses will become more evident in the policy recommendations outlined in Chapter Three.

2. Risk-Benefit Assessment

A PRELIMINARY EXCURSUS ON METAETHICAL METHODS

In the study of philosophical ethics, at least in the history of the West, a wide variety of methods have been devised for assessing right and wrong actions, i.e., for determining what the right, or best, course of action is in a given situation. These many methods, however, have been more or less distilled into two primary classes of methods[13]: 1. Those that are primarily teleological, consequentialist, or utilitarian-based, and 2. those that are primarily deontological, or duty-based methods. The practice of risk assessment belongs to the first class of methods, and human rights documents belong to the second class. We will turn first (in this section) to an analysis of risk assessment methods, and then in the next sections to a study of some relevant human rights documents.

We turn now to the method of thinking currently used in virtually all matters involving toxics policy, viz., the method of risk assessment. We will consider risk assessment under four headings: what it is; a recent attempt at improving the guidelines that should govern risk assessment practices; what is fundamentally wrong with risk assessment; and a proposed counterbalance to risk assessment.

What Risk Assessment Is

It was a philosopher-economist (Jeremy Bentham, 1748–1832) who first articulated, and a philosopher-ethicist (John Stuart Mill, 1806–1873[14]) who best articulated the cost-benefit method of decisionmaking. Mill's teleological principle for guiding the making of ethical decisions was simply to consider which actions would lead to the *greatest total benefit* and the *least total cost* for the largest number of persons over the longest period of time, and which actions would lead to the opposite. This method of decisionmaking is based on trying to accurately estimate the likely future outcomes of any given course of action, both its total future costs[15] and its total future benefits,[16] and then choosing the action with the lowest costs and highest benefits. Today's practice of environmental health risk assessment is a relatively young stepchild[17] of Bentham's and Mill's consequentialist method of decisionmaking.

One or two preliminary definitions: a risk is a potential for any future adverse event. In our context, a risk is a potential for any future adverse health or environmental effect. Risk has two dimensions, each of which must be taken seriously. One dimension of risk is the perceived severity of the adverse event, i.e., its degree of badness, since some events are clearly more serious, more tragic, and less remediable than others. This might be termed the value dimension of risk. The other dimension of risk is the probability or likelihood of that adverse event actually coming to pass. This might be termed the probability dimension of risk. Thus, some potential future adverse health effects may not be considered very serious, but may be fairly likely to occur, whereas other adverse health effects may be much more serious or irreversible, but not very likely to occur. Others may be both serious and likely. The same two dimensions, value and likelihood, apply equally well to potential future benefits.

Environmental health risk assessment, then, is the practice of attempting to assess these likely future costs to community health and the environment that would result from any given environmental policy decision, and then weighing them against the potential future benefits. Good risk assessment practices should require that all potential costs and benefits be evaluated in both the value and probability dimensions.

After this the risk *management* process takes place. It consists of the policy decisions and regulations which are undertaken as a result of the data gathered and the judgments made in the risk assessment portion of the process.

Because the practice of environmental risk assessment has sometimes been so heavily criticized, a U.S. Presidential/Congressional Commission on Risk Assessment and Risk Management was convened in May 1994 to develop a new set of guiding principles for environmental health risk assessment and management. This commission, as we will see below, made several recommendations which, if they were followed and implemented, could represent some level of improvement over past environmental risk assessment practices.

An Attempt at Improvement

The presidential commission completed its work and issued its final report in January 1997. Titled *Framework for Environmental Health Risk Management*, it makes several recommendations for improvements in the health risk assessment and risk management processes.

In the first place, the *Framework* defines the process of risk assessment and management as the process of identifying, evaluating, selecting, and implementing actions to reduce risk to human health and to ecosystems. The goal of risk management is scientifically sound, cost-effective, integrated actions that reduce or prevent risks while taking into account social, cultural, ethical, political, and legal considerations.[18]

The document does at least give verbal mention to those values listed in that last line above, and this in itself represents something of an improvement over past risk assessment standards which did not even mention most of those values. Whether this brief mention will turn out to be window dressing only, or a set of actual guiding principles that will shape and determine public policymaking still remains to be seen. It may be wise to not expect great changes.

One of the more significant recommendations of the new guidelines is that the risk assessment process should include a full mix of relevant "stakeholders." A stakeholder, says this document, is anyone who has a "stake," or interest, in a risk management decision.

> Stakeholders typically include groups that are affected or potentially affected by the risk, the risk managers, and groups that will be affected by any efforts to manage the source of the risk.... In the case of an application for a pesticide reregistration [for example], stakeholders would include the pesticide manufacturer, owners of the farms where the pesticide is used, laborers who apply the pesticide, consumers who may be exposed to pesticide residues in foods, scientist who seek further pesticide research funding, trade associations like the Grocery Manufacturers' Association, those who speak on behalf of ecological considerations, and those with regulatory responsibility.[19]

The document's list of possible stakeholders does not, unfortunately, include any mention of representatives from the public health community. More specifically it does not include any mention of representatives of those with pesticide intolerances or with chemical sensitivities (who comprise, at minimum, 5 percent—probably more—of the population, as we have seen above), who have already been made highly reactive to pesticides, artificial fragrances, industrial byproducts, and other contaminants. These people can certainly be expected to suffer significant (and almost immediate) adverse health effects from exposure to pesticide drift and environmental residues of other contaminants. They should, therefore, clearly be included as stakeholders, since there is no doubt that their bodies will be very directly "affected or potentially affected by the risk." Not only does this new framework not mention them as stakeholders or as parties with an interest in the policies being considered, it does not even include a category of stakeholders who could represent their interests.

Nevertheless, in this newly proposed risk assessment framework, the participant stakeholders are clearly all interested parties. Most, if not all, of the stakeholders will probably be directly affected, most of them financially, by the risk management decisions that will be made based on their assessments. They are thus clearly not impartial observers.

In this context, therefore, it would stand to reason that a full disclosure of each stakeholder's interests in the issue should also be required so that the entire process of deliberation is fully transparent and aboveboard. But the *Framework* does not suggest this requirement. I think it should have. Full disclosure of each stakeholder's interests should be made readily available to everyone.

While involving those with direct financial and personal interests in the outcome may appear to compromise the objectivity of the risk assessment process, there are some sound reasons for doing so. The *Framework* itself lists seven benefits that might accrue from including stakeholders in the process:

1. Supports democratic decision-making.
2. Ensures that [some] public values are considered.
3. Develops the understanding needed to make better decisions.
4. Improves the knowledge base for decision-making.
5. Can reduce the overall time and expense involved in decision-making.
6. May improve the credibility of agencies responsible for managing risks.
7. Should generate better accepted, more readily implemented risk management decisions.[20]

These benefits may eventually accrue from a process that includes a wide variety of stakeholders, but they will accrue only if *all* interested groups are included. If some stakeholders are intentionally excluded—for example, if the public health constituency, or those whose health would be directly impacted, are excluded—then the process is much less likely to be properly democratic, and the outcomes are less likely to be fair and just. Thus, public health advocates and people whose physical health may be immediately or eventually affected by the outcome of the deliberations should be given a strong voice in the risk assessment process. Though these stake-holders and representatives from the public health community are not specifically mentioned in the *Framework*, a generously benevolent interpretation of the document would hope that it does at least leave room for them to be recognized as stakeholders and participants.

Although the *Framework* does not mention this following point at all, we would hope that policymakers will, when it comes time to make the difficult risk management decisions that follow from the risk assessment process, have the good sense to insure that some voices and some considerations will be weighed somewhat more heavily than others. The public health voices, for example, if they eventually get included in the process, should perhaps be given more weight than the voices of those with a direct, near-term financial interest in the outcome of the process. Theodore Roosevelt said it most clearly: "Public rights come first, and private interests second."

Furthermore, it would also be important to insure that all stake-holders be given access to the same level of resources during the deliberation process. That is, the process should insure that corporate stakeholders, who will doubtless have enormous financial and legal resources available to them, do not overwhelm those stake-holders who have far fewer resources. In addition, it will be important to insure an equal voice not only to those who suffer from environmentally related disorders that will cause them to be directly and immediately affected by risk management decisions (those with asthma and chemical sensitivity disorders, for example), but also to representatives of those stakeholders who live in poverty, and to stakeholders who are members of ethnic minorities or indigenous populations, and to those who live in neighborhoods and regions that may be more directly affected by risk management decisions. If these much less affluent stakeholders are not provided with an equivalent level of resources to help them in the deliberation process, then their voices will almost certainly not be adequately heard. The failure to deal with this problem is a special weakness in the proposed *Framework*.

In another recommended improvement to the process, the *Framework* finally recognizes for the first time that it is no longer sufficient to consider the toxicity of single chemicals only. The process must now ask: "Do other pollutants from the same source pose additional risks to the population of concern? Do the pollutants interact? Are their effects cumulative?"[21] This recommendation, if it were to be implemented, would represent a large step forward in the risk assessment process, because almost never in the real world do people encounter chemicals one at a time. In the real world, people encounter chemicals in multiple combinations and a wide range of mixes, and it may well be that certain combinations of chemicals have significantly different health effects than any of the chemicals singly.

This improvement would seem to represent a significant step forward in improving the risk assessment process. To what extent risk assessment teams will actually follow this recommendation is another question, however, especially since it would be very difficult indeed to actually test the health effects of all the possible chemical combinations that people are likely to encounter in their environment. The possible parametric combinations of 80,000 chemicals is an astronomically large number, and there would not be time to test them all before the end of this century. If these tests were to be done, however, they would provide the kind of information that risk managers, according to this new document, ought to be looking for.

Nor is it any longer adequate, says the *Framework*, simply to examine the health effects of exposures to a given toxicant which comes from only one source, or via only one pathway. The process must now also ask: "Is the population exposed to the same pollutant from other sources? ... Is exposure to the pollutant also occurring from other environmental media?"[22] This information too will be important in assessing the potential additive human health effects of toxicants.

In another recommended improvement, the risk assessment process should now be expected to consider how a given pollutant, or combination of pollutants, may interact with other public health factors, such as a high rate of local poverty, or certain ethnic or cultural factors, or the presence in a community of certain infectious diseases such as HIV/AIDS or tuberculosis, as well as other factors. This recommendation, if actually implemented, would also constitute a significant improvement in the process.

These new guidelines also recommend that the process now consider a much wider variety of potential adverse health effects from exposure to toxicants. Instead of focusing primarily (or even, as in the past, sometimes exclusively) on the carcinogenicity of toxicants, it is now recommended that the process consider adverse health outcomes other than cancer. Potential adverse effects on the reproductive system, on the respiratory system, possible neurotoxic effects, immune system dysregulation, and endocrine disruption are some of the other health effects that the risk assessment process should now also be expected to consider.

In addition, although the *Framework* nowhere makes any recommendations regarding "environmental justice," it does at least mention the term here and there. The concept of environmental justice is never defined, but it presumably includes issues such as equitable distribution of costs and benefits across regions, neighborhoods, and ethnic and socioeconomic groups.[23] The mention of this concept, however, while left entirely general, undefined and vague in the document, does at least represent some improvement over past risk assessment documents which failed to mention the concept of environmental justice at all. The *Framework* could have, in this regard, taken some lessons from the relevant human rights documents which we will be examining below,[24] but unfortunately it did not.

Finally, the *Framework* also recommends that the entire risk assessment be peer reviewed by independent (and disinterested) third parties. This would mean that the process might be somewhat more open than it is now, and this requirement would, it seems to me, if it were actually followed, have some potential for keeping the process much more honest and somewhat more objective.

What's Wrong with Risk Assessment?

One of the difficulties with any version of utilitarian thinking, including this one of environmental risk assessment, is that the process can be so broadly flexible, and judgments about the estimated future outcomes so unfounded and so widely variable, that the process inherently has an enormous amount of "slop," or "give," or "wiggle room" in it. As John Wargo has said, in referring to the conceptual looseness of the risk assessment process, "risk estimates may be easily manipulated to trivialize or exaggerate hazards."[25]

Utilitarian thinking of this sort can readily be used to justify a very wide range of possible risk management decisions, ranging from those that may be healthy and wise to those that may be self-serving, nefarious or corrupt.

There is evidence,[26] for example, that some Nazi doctors attempted to justify some of their horrendous medical experiments on prisoners in the concentration camps by using just such utilitarian justifications. We know that a number of them did in fact say that, "Yes, it may be unfortunate that some prisoners will suffer during our biological experiments, but their suffering will at least work for the greater good of society, and for the good of many thousands of other human beings who will benefit from our work and their suffering. The benefits to be gained from these experiments by a large number of people will far outweigh the costs in physical suffering to a small number of individual camp prisoners."[27] Other approaches to ethical decisionmaking will find this kind of thinking morally unacceptable.

One of the fundamental problems with much utilitarian thinking, including that of environmental risk assessment, is that, at root, it requires decision-makers to assess and make judgments about the future; and it is well known that "futurology" can be a highly inexact science at best. We all know that the future will be affected by an enormously wide variety of interconnected variables, and that in fact there are no guarantees at all that the future will be very much like we have experienced the past to be. People often see in the future only what they want to see—i.e., it can often serve as a kind of giant Rorschach inkblot—and thus their judgments about it can be highly influenced by their biases. Therefore, any thinking that relies primarily on our ability to assess the future—and which is based on no other ethical principles at all (such as principles of justice, moral obligation, and human rights)—runs the risk of being highly flexible and self-serving indeed.

In order for any consequentialist method of decisionmaking to have a good chance of working well and leading to ethical and just decisions, those who use the method must remember to be guided by at least the following five principles:

1. They must, in their deliberations, consider the likely future consequences of *all* feasible alternative courses of action, or at least of a very broad spectrum of possible actions, and not just of one or a few.
2. They must judiciously weigh *both* the costs and the benefits, i.e., not consider only the costs or only the benefits.
3. They must examine the likely future consequences *from the point of view of those persons most likely to suffer or enjoy those consequences*, and not just from their own personal or corporate point of view.
4. They must make every effort to examine *the sum total of all the likely consequences*, even the interactions, conflicts, and synergies of those consequences, and not focus on only one or a few consequences.

5. And finally, they must insure, when it comes time to make recommendations for managing the risk, that it is approximately the same community of persons which both suffers the costs and enjoys the benefits; i.e., they must insure that it will not be the case that one group suffers almost all the costs while a different group enjoys almost all the benefits.

If these five principles are not brought fully to mind during, and thoroughly applied to, the risk assessment process—in other words, if the cost-benefit analysis of the actions under consideration is not complete—then the deliberations are not likely to result either in an adequately democratic assessment process, or in appropriately ethical risk management decisions.

How does the current practice of environmental risk assessment measure up against these five principles? Let us look briefly at each principle.

Does today's practice of risk assessment consider a wide variety of possible feasible courses of action, and not just one or a few of them?

Perhaps theoretically today's risk assessment process could consider all (or at least many) possible courses of action, but in actuality it seems not to. In practice it seems that environmental risk assessment is usually asked to evaluate only one, or at best a very few, proposed courses of action, and not a broad spectrum of possible actions. For example, a risk assessment process might be asked to analyze and assess the likely risks associated with applying a certain brand of commercial herbicide to the grounds in local city parks. The risk assessment process would then examine only the issues surrounding use of that herbicide (or perhaps one or two others) in its city parks, considering the costs and benefits of only that single action. It would then attempt to assess potential economic impact, potential ecological impact, and (in the best case) the potential public health impact, i.e., how much morbidity or mortality is likely to result from such herbicide use, which populations are more likely to be exposed to that herbicide if it is used,[28] and what specific health effects might be likely to result for them.[29] The process may even explore which specific herbicides are likely to be safer or more effective at weed-killing.

What we should notice here, though, is that the risk assessment process in this hypothetical case was asked to consider only one course of action, or perhaps a few courses of action. It was not asked to consider a wide imaginative range of other possible courses of action, such as perhaps designating some city parks as herbicide free, for instance, or allowing the entire community to vote on herbicide use issues, or using alternative methods of weed control (such as boiling-water applicators and hand pulling), or even simply allowing some weeds to grow in some city parks.[30] Each of these other courses of action is, naturally, accompanied by certain costs and benefits which could also then be weighed and assessed. But unfortunately the process is not usually asked to consider a variety of alternative courses of action like these. I believe it should be. The risk assessment process should, as a rule, consider a wide range of creative options, perhaps arriving at alternatives that can satisfy those with public health interests, those with horticultural interests (in the example of the city parks), and those with primarily economic interests.

Mary O'Brien, an environmental writer and activist, proposes a process she terms "alternatives assessment" in place of the current practice of risk assessment. She offers an analogy to illustrate the value of her alternatives assessment approach.

> A woman is standing by an icy river. There are four risk assessors behind her. The toxicologist says the woman should wade across the river because it is not even toxic; it is only icy. The cardiologist says that the woman does not look old, or hypothermic, so she should wade across the river. The hydrologist says he has seen other rivers like this, and this river probably doesn't have whirlpools, and probably isn't deeper than four feet, so she should wade across. Finally a U.S. Environmental Protection Agency comparative risk analyst notes that the risk to the woman of wading across is nothing compared to the risks of global warming or the loss of biological diversity.
>
> The woman refuses to wade across.
>
> The risk assessors show her their numbers and formulas. They explain to her that her chance of dying as a result of wading across the river is one in 40 million.
>
> She refuses to cross.
>
> Exasperated, they ask her why she won't wade across.
>
> She points upstream. "Because there's a bridge," she says.[31]

O'Brien's alternatives assessment approach also urges that a wise assessment procedure should examine the costs and benefits of a wide variety of alternative courses of action, and not just the one or two courses of action that have been formally presented to it.

Does risk assessment weigh both the costs and the benefits?

The risk assessment process, almost by definition, seems to focus primarily on assessing the costs, and not the benefits. So focused is the process on managing risks, that it is almost unable to conceive of benefits except in terms of reducing risks. At one point, in fact, the *Framework* even says that, "The most obvious benefit from risk management is risk reduction or elimination."[32] One of the most glaring weaknesses in the new *Framework* despite its numerous improvements over the older risk assessment guidelines, is that it does not focus on the anticipated benefits which would be the whole *raison d'être* for undertaking any policy or course of action. Even the new guidelines seem not to require risk assessors to weigh and assess the anticipated benefits of any proposed course of action. And yet, we must wonder how any wise or just decisions could ever be adequately made without a full analysis of both the cost side and the benefit side of the equation.

Philosophers and psychologists have long recognized that people usually undertake an action because they expect some benefit to accrue from undertaking that action. How could policymakers justly deliberate about a course of action without some adequate understanding of the benefits that are anticipated to accrue from that action? In order for the risk assessment process to be fair, adequate, and equitable, such benefits should be analyzed and articulated just as fully and assiduously as are the risks.

Policymakers may believe that the benefits are clear to them and to everyone involved in the process and therefore that they do not need to be as fully articulated as the risks are. Others may just as foolishly believe that the risks are so obvious as not to need full articulation. The health and well-being of the public, however, would ultimately be better served by a full analysis, outline, and disclosure of both the expected future costs and the expected future benefits of any given course of action. These formal analyses of both costs and benefits would, furthermore, have the added value of articulating a clear rationale and justification for the proposed action, and of leaving a complete record of deliberations to document the thinking behind the policy decisions that will eventually be made. Moreover, it would seem that peer reviewers of the process would not be able to adequately follow and understand the process of deliberation and the reasons for the decision outcomes unless both the costs and the benefits had been fully articulated and analyzed.

Obviously, one of the most common expected benefits will be the opportunity for accrual of profits by the corporate developers, manufacturers, and distributors of the products which will be affected by the course of action under consideration. Profit is, of course, an entirely legitimate benefit, but it should be clearly articulated and analyzed just as fully as the risks are, and then should be weighed properly into the risk management decision.

Furthermore, in weighing the various goods that may accrue from a given course of action, it will be important for policymakers to have some sense of which goods should be taken to count more heavily than others. In weighing the interests of the parties involved, risk managers are called on to choose those options that best suit the community (including perhaps the global community) as a whole. In a letter to the *Wall Street Journal* on January 3, 1997, Nancy Krieger of the Harvard School of Public Health wrote, "Public welfare must be placed before corporate welfare and social equality before unrestricted freedom of the economic market.... Social Justice is the foundation of public health."[33]

While it may be argued that a strong economic market is important to the public welfare, it is even more true that an unhealthy working population will be much less useful to the economy, and may in fact turn out to be a serious economic impediment. The physical health of the community, in other words, will need to take precedence in the decisions of policymakers, even over the pressing near-term financial interests of corporate managers.

Does the risk assessment process examine the likely consequences of the policies being considered *from the point of view of those persons most likely to suffer or enjoy those consequences?*

In considering any questions of cost and risk, it is important to keep in mind the wise little proverb: "The burdens that appear easiest to bear are those that are borne by others." This is particularly important to remember because those who suffer the risks of a given policy may be in groups other than those which include the stakeholders and policymakers who are considering the policy decision, and hence they may be perceived by those decisionmakers as "other." It may well be that these policymakers would find certain risks acceptable for other people to bear, even though they themselves might not wish to bear them.

Mrs. Eva Mozes-Kor and her twin sister were, in their childhood, research subjects in some of the horrible medical experiments performed by Dr. Josef Mengele at Birkenau in the early 1940s. She says:

> To look back at my childhood is to remember my experiences as a human guinea pig in the Birkenau laboratory of Dr. Josef Mengele.

To recount such painful memories is to relive the horrors of human experimentation, where people were used as merely objects or means to a scientific end.... Every time scientists are involved in human experimentation, they should try to put themselves in the place of the subject and see how they would feel. The scientists of the world must remember that the research is being done for the sake of mankind and not for the sake of science; scientists must never detach themselves from the humans they serve.[34]

In a similar manner, policymakers must remember that the policies about which they are deliberating are being made for the sake of the community, not merely for the sake of industrial or commercial interests. Hence, if Mrs. Mozes-Kor is right, policymakers must never emotionally detach themselves from the individual human beings who make up the community they serve, but must instead examine the likely consequences of the proposed policy from the viewpoint of those who are most likely to bear them.

Does the risk assessment process currently do this? It certainly does not appear so, given that the groups who will often bear those costs are often not even represented on the risk assessment team. With the improved *Framework* recommendations, within which each set of stakeholders will be looking out primarily for their own interests, we could hope that those most likely to bear the brunt of the policy will be given a voice at least as loud as those of the participants who stand to profit economically.

Does the risk assessment process make every effort to examine the sum total of all the likely consequences, even the possible additive and multiplicative effects, as well as the possible interactions, conflicts, and synergies between those consequences, and not to simply focus on only the few more readily apparent individual consequences?

In principle, the new risk assessment guidelines do urge that the full range of potential consequences be analyzed. But in practice to analyze such a broad range of potential effects, health and otherwise, would be almost impossible. In addition, most analyses tend to focus more on near-term consequences since longer term consequences are so much more difficult to assess. (It is the longer-term consequences, after all, which require so much more far-seeing judgment, and hence which also have that much more potential for wandering from actuality.) Potential additive effects, multiplicative effects, and synergies among all the likely consequences are even more difficult to assess. Any given policy is likely to lead to consequences that are multifactorial, that are highly dynamic, and that will interact with other parts of the environment and culture in ways that will also be extremely difficult to assess.

For example, in the case of exposures to ambient toxicants in the environment, most studies examining the health effects of these chemicals have, in the past, focused on the health effects of only one chemical at a time and via only one environmental medium at a time (e.g., air, or water, or food). They have not considered the potential toxicity of the breakdown products and metabolites of environmental chemicals. In the real world, people are almost never exposed to just one chemical at a time; nor are they exposed to a given chemical through only one medium. Instead, they are exposed to a complex mixture of chemicals as well as to the breakdown products and metabolites of those mixtures, and they are exposed to them through a wide variety of environmental media.

In one sense, as noted above, the new *Framework* does attempt to rectify this problem. It recommends that risk assessors analyze the risks that communities face on a chemical by chemical basis, and not just via a single environmental medium, and that they examine the risks posed by the mixture of multiple agents via different environmental media. This, of course, would be good advice for risk assessment teams to follow.

In actuality, though, to perform such testing of chemical mixtures would be an enormously time consuming and expensive task, and would almost certainly take many decades to accomplish. According to an article in *Rachel's Environment and Health Weekly,*

> [To] test just the commonest 1000 toxic chemicals in unique combinations of 3 would require at least 166 million different experiments (and this disregards the need to study varying doses given to animals at varying times during their lives).[35] If we wanted to conduct the 166 million experiments in just 20 years, we would have to complete 8.3 million tests each year. The U.S. presently has the capacity to conduct only a few hundred such tests each year.[36]

The author adds that, "Just training sufficient personnel to conduct 8.3 million animal tests each year is [currently] beyond our national capacity."[37] And 20 years, of course, is quite a long time to wait for research to tell us what damage a given mixture of chemicals may be doing to human bodies.

With the results of such research currently unavailable to us, the question we should instead be asking is: in the absence of adequate data, what position should society take with respect to allowing untested chemicals to be dispersed into the environment? It would seem that, even given the assumptions in this new *Framework*, it would be best for policymakers to err on the side of caution and to take steps which would lead to the minimizing of risk to the public health. (For a further development of this question, see section 5 below, "The Precautionary Principle.")

If risk assessors actually did follow these new recommendations conscientiously, and if they were actually able to develop this potential data about likely adverse health effects, it could represent a significant improvement over traditional risk assessment methods. It seems unlikely, however, that chemical manufacturing interests will find these recommendations appealing.

Finally, do risk managers try to insure, when it comes time to make recommendations for managing the risk, that it is approximately the same community of persons who will both suffer the costs and enjoy the benefits? That is, do policymakers try to insure that their chosen policies will not result in one group suffering virtually all the costs of the policy, while a different group enjoys virtually all the benefits? Such an outcome would violate most accepted norms of social justice. To date, however, environmental risk assessors and managers have paid little attention to social justice concerns of this sort. Whether this will improve in the future remains to be seen.

Conflicts of Interest

There is one additional element that would help insure that a risk assessment and management process is undertaken in an ethically proper manner. This would be to require the absolute avoidance of any potential (or even seeming) conflicts of interest on the part of those who will—after all the assessing has been completed—ultimately be making the final decisions regarding environmental risk management practices. At least a full public disclosure and full investigation of any potential apparent conflicts of interest should be required by the process.

Apples and Oranges

And finally, it bears mentioning that one of the almost inescapable difficulties inherent in the process of risk assessment is that the process is asked to compare apples and oranges. A given risk assessment panel, for example, may be asked to weigh the costs associated with a certain number of people being made sick or killed by aerial herbicide spraying of private timberland (with 2,4-D, for example), against the economic benefits of increased timber yields that may result from that spraying.[38] These two entirely different kinds of values—human life and health vs. increased timber yields—are virtually impossible to compare, and to attempt to weigh them in the same scale is a difficult, if not impossible (and therefore potentially misleading), task.

Furthermore, one of the consequences of such herbicide spraying—people being made sick—could happen fairly soon after the spraying and may affect those sick people and their families for the rest of their lives. The other consequences—a potential for increased timber yields—may not come to pass for decades, and may even then be a relatively short-lived benefit. Or in another situation the profits may be almost immediate, and the health effects may not become evident for two or three decades. To compare these two kinds of consequences clearly involves an attempt to compare very different *kinds* of values.

And yet these are the sorts of judgments that risk assessors are asked to make every day, and it constitutes one of the central weaknesses of the risk assessment process.

A COUNTERBALANCE

We see that environmental risk assessment and risk management are such open ended, highly flexible, and indeterminate processes because of the ultimate unpredictability of the future, because of the kinds of comparisons and judgments that it requires risk assessors and managers to make, and because of the highly complex (and almost impossible to acquire) scientific data which must be available to risk assessors. Risk assessment and management, therefore, because they are such open ended processes, often leave an enormous amount of room for the effects of personal bias and self interest. We know, for instance, that chemical corporations have been able to manipulate these processes largely for their own benefit, and this is due to the highly flexible nature of the risk assessment process itself.

Because of these inherent weaknesses in the risk assessment process—indeed in any utilitarian or consequentialist approach to decisionmaking—it will be important to have as a counterbalance, a quite different method of assessing how society ought to make decisions about these matters. That counterbalancing method lies in the public recognition, the explicit official affirmation, and the effective legislative implementation of certain basic, fundamental human rights.

3. Human Rights:
An Ethical Counterbalance

Deontological methods of determining ethical obligation, i.e., methods grounded in moral rights and obligations, are *not* based on, as the risk assessment method is based on, estimating possible and probable future outcomes of a given course of action and then weighing the expected negative consequences against the expected beneficial consequences. The central problem with teleological methods, as we have seen, is that they are far too susceptible to the influence of personal biases, self-serving distortions, miscalculations, and simple bad judgments, all of which can be so easily shaped by the desires, hopes, and intentions of those fallible persons doing the assessing.

What is needed instead is an ethical decision-making methodology that is more solidly grounded in fundamental principles of moral rights and duties, and is thus less susceptible to such stakeholder biases and misjudgments. Fortunately, the concept of human rights offers just such an alternative.

Alexis de Tocqueville, in 1840, said of the concept of rights: "After the general idea of virtue, I know no higher principle than that of right; or rather these two ideas are united in one. The idea of right is simply that of virtue introduced into the political world."[39] More recently, a long and highly respected tradition of well-founded codes of human rights has helped clarify ethical thinking, particularly in matters of health and biomedical research, for a much longer period of history than has the relatively recent practice of risk assessment.

It is true, moreover, that we are presently experiencing an unprecedented moment in human history when the efforts of the human rights movement and the efforts of the public health movement are just beginning to meet and learn from each other. Dr. Jonathan Mann, the first Director of the World Health Organization's Global Programme on AIDS, and later Professor of Health and Human Rights and Professor of Epidemiology and International Health at the Harvard School of Public Health, has said that we are witnessing "an extraordinary moment in social history—the emergence of a health and human rights movement."

> Stimulated in the first instance by pressures within each field, both public health and human rights are undergoing major transformations, so that the linkages between them and the outcomes of their association have now become dynamic and even more challenging

than may have been evident just a few years ago. Fortunately, as the tectonic plates are shifting in the domains of both public health and human rights, interest in health and human rights has intensified.[40]

The perspectives expressed in this book fall within this emerging paradigm of a confluence of human rights and public health traditions, particularly in the book's insistence on the need for a heavy counterbalance to the risk assessment approach to policymaking regarding toxics.

In this section we will examine some of the key documents in this human rights tradition and some of their implications for control of environmental toxicants, for maintaining the health of the environment, and for reducing the incidence of toxicant induced human pathologies. We will examine these issues in four brief segments, corresponding to four (actually five) readily available human rights documents: 1. the *Universal Declaration of Human Rights*, one of the earliest foundational statements of human rights in the world; 2. the 1994 *Draft Declaration of Human Rights and the Environment*; 3. the *Charter on Industrial Hazards and Human Rights*; and 4. the *Nuremberg Code* and the WHO/CIOMS *International Ethical Guidelines*, (both of which focus on ethical guidelines for biomedical research involving human subjects.)

THE UNIVERSAL DECLARATION OF HUMAN RIGHTS

The *Universal Declaration of Human Rights* was written at the United Nations in 1948 based on the realization that "disregard and contempt for human rights have resulted in barbarous acts which have outraged the conscience of mankind," and from the belief that every member of the human family deserved to be free of fear.[41] The document was based on the tenet that "it is essential, if man is not to be compelled to have recourse, as a last resort, to rebellion against tyranny and oppression, that human rights should be protected by the rule of law." For these reasons and others, "Member States ... pledged themselves to achieve ... the promotion of universal respect for and observance of human rights...."[42] The Preamble recognizes that when people and communities feel that their basic rights have been ignored and violated they may be more likely to instigate rebellion. The document emphasizes that it is thus in the self-interest of governments and societies to insure that certain basic human rights are respected within their national boundaries.

The *Universal Declaration* intends itself to be "a common

standard of achievement for all peoples and all nations, to the end that every individual and every organ of society ... shall strive by teaching and education to promote respect for these rights."[43]

In addition to some of the more general rights articulated in the *Universal Declaration*, four key rights which have a bearing on matters of environmental health are clearly enunciated:

Article 3. Everyone has the right to life, liberty and security of person.

People who have been made sick or disabled by nonconsensual exposure to insecticides, herbicides, industrial pollutants, and other ambient environmental toxicants in their air and water, may well feel that their fundamental right to security of person has been violated.

Article 12. No one shall be subjected to arbitrary interference with his [or her] privacy, family, [or] home.

People whose homes or property have been contaminated, perhaps by industrial byproducts or by pesticide application or drift, and whose families have been made sick by pesticides and other environmental toxicants in their common air and water, may well feel that this right has been violated. Families, such as the one we heard from in Chapter One, who have been forced to leave their homes because of pesticide poisoning, could justly feel that this right (as well as the next one) had been violated.

Article 17. No one shall be arbitrarily deprived of his [or her] property.

Numerous people (some of whom I know personally) have been forced to leave their homes and abandon all their belongings due solely to nonconsensual exposure to highly toxic pesticides and other environmental contaminants.[44] They may well feel that they have been arbitrarily, and for no just cause, deprived of their property.

Article 25. Motherhood and childhood are entitled to special care and assistance.

While motherhood and childhood are entitled to special care and assistance according to the *Universal Declaration*, we have seen in Chapter One that they have in fact been given no special care at all in matters related to exposures to toxics. Mothers, fetuses, and children, despite their much greater vulnerability to environmental toxicants, have been granted no special exemptions or protections from such exposures. Despite their unique physical vulnerabilities, they enjoy no more protections than the much less vulnerable 70 kilogram adult Caucasian male[45] whose body has come to represent the standard for most research involving the health effects of toxics on humans. If their unique status, vulnerabilities, and importance to the community entitle them to special care, as the *Universal Declaration* affirms, then we may well conclude that their rights have not been properly protected in this regard at all.

In fact, anyone who has been physically injured by pesticide residues, for example, or whose children have been injured by the application of pesticides in their schools, knows that they have been subjected to a violation of the security of their persons. Anyone who has been injured by sick buildings, or by industrial byproducts in their air or water, or by any number of other potentially toxic chemical agents, knows that industrial interests have arbitrarily interfered with their privacy and family.[46] Anyone who has been forced from their home, and anyone who has been forced to abandon or discard their possessions due to nonconsensual contamination with toxic chemical agents,[47] may rightly feel that they too have been arbitrarily deprived of their home and property.

As another recent human rights draft document clearly states, "Human beings deserve the maximal protection under the law from non-consensual exposure to toxic substances."[48]

These principles will be important to bear in mind when we consider, in Chapter Three, what policy changes will be necessary in order that these basic human rights are adequately complied with.

The 1994 Draft Declaration of Human Rights and the Environment

The genesis of this document was the convening in May 1994 of a group of human rights and environmental protection experts at the United Nations headquarters in Geneva. The group had been assembled at the invitation of the Sierra Club Legal Defense Fund, the Association Mondiale pour l'École Instrument de Paix, and the Societé Suisse pour la Protection de l'Environnement. The group met under the aegis of the United Nations Sub-Commission on Prevention of Discrimination and Protection of Minorities. The Draft Declaration was presented to this Sub-Commission in 1994.

In its preamble, the *Declaration* clearly acknowledges its foundations and roots in previous human rights documents, such as the *Universal Declaration of Human Rights*, the United Nations *Charter*, and the *International Covenant on Civil and Political Rights*, as well as in previous environmental documents such as the *Stockholm Declaration* of the United Nations Conference on the Human Environment, the *World Charter on Nature*, and others. It is also guided by many of the principles embodied in international humanitarian law.[49]

The preamble notes that "the potential irreversibility of environmental harm gives rise to special responsibility to prevent such harm." It is therefore incumbent on governments, according to the document, to recognize their special responsibility to prevent such irreparable harm to human beings and their environment.

Though this particular document is focused on protecting the environment, it states that because of the seamless interconnections between human beings and their environment, human health can be expected to be adversely effected by any degradation in the health of the environment. The *Declaration* affirms that

> All persons have the right to freedom from pollution, environmental degradation and activities that adversely affect the environment, threaten life, health, livelihood, well-being or sustainable development within, across or outside national boundaries.[50]

Furthermore, "All persons have the right to the highest attainable standard of health free from environmental [hazards]."[51] They have the right to "a secure, healthy, and ecologically sound environment."[52] And in order to protect and promote a state of health, "All persons have a right to safe and healthy food and water adequate to their well-being."[53]

Indigenous peoples in particular have a special right to be protected against environmental degradation.

> Indigenous peoples have the right to protection against any action or course of conduct that may result in the destruction or degradation of their territories, including land, air, water, sea-ice, wildlife or other resources.[54]

In addition, "special attention shall be given to [other] vulnerable persons and groups."[55]

Several articles of the *Declaration* also affirm the right of individuals and communities to ready availability of information about potential environmental contaminants, the right to widely disseminate that information to all potentially interested parties and groups, and the right to participate in decisionmaking about the dispersal of toxicants into the environment. In accord with the principle of informed consent, the *Declaration* clearly affirms that

> All persons have the right to information concerning the environment. This includes information, howsoever compiled, on actions and courses of conduct that may affect the environment and information necessary to enable effective public participation in environmental decision-making. The information shall be timely, clear, understandable and available without undue financial burden to the applicant.[56]

Thus, the *Declaration* clearly affirms the right of individuals and communities to live healthy lives free of endangerment by nonconsensual exposure to environmental toxicants. It affirms the right of individuals and communities to be given full information about the use and dispersal, and especially about the *proposed* use and dispersal, of environmental toxicants. *The Charter on Industrial Hazards and Human Rights*, to which we now turn, affirms these rights even more explicitly, and with much more emphasis on the human health effects of synthetic chemical compounds.

The Charter on Industrial Hazards and Human Rights

Perhaps the most intriguing and promising of the human rights documents relevant to issues of toxicant exposures and their effects on human health is the 1996 *Charter on Industrial Hazards and Human Rights*. This charter was nearly five years in the making, and arose, as did *The Nuremberg Code*, from the immediate experience of human tragedy. While the *Nuremberg Code* emerged out of the horribly tragic human medical experiments conducted in the Nazi concentration camps during World War II, the charter originated in the wake of the tragic industrial devastations that resulted from two catastrophic environmental tragedies: 1) the explosion (and subsequent massive release of feedstock chemicals) at the Union Carbide pesticide factory in Bhopal, India in 1984, where over 2,000 people were killed and over 100,000 were injured[57]; and 2) the devastation to human health which resulted two years later from the nuclear power plant explosion at Chernobyl, Ukraine in 1986. The enormously dramatic human impact of these and other industrial tragedies inspired the Permanent People's Tribunal (PPT) to begin the long process of drafting a human rights charter to address urgent human health issues and to protect future generations from the threat of exposure to such harmful levels of toxicants.

The PPT, established in 1979 by the International Foundation for the Rights and Liberation of Peoples, has its headquarters in Rome. It sees itself acting in the same tradition as did the International Military Tribunal at Nuremberg.

The Introduction to the *Charter on Industrial Hazards and Human Rights* says:

> The PPT is based in Rome, but its 75 judges come from all over the globe and include eminent persons whose reputations must be above reproach in art, culture, science, and politics, including a number of Nobel Prize winners. Individual hearings are initiated by aggrieved groups, and are normally heard by a bench of three to eleven sitting tribunal judges. Accused parties are invited to present their case at the hearings, and if they do not attend, the PPT appoints legal counsel to represent their case in a rigorous manner. The PPT applies principles of international law, and is bound by the Algiers Declaration on the Rights of Peoples as well as [by] its own Statute of operations.[58]

The charter was drafted and revised at four PPT assemblies: the first at Yale University in early 1991, the second in Bangkok in October 1991, the third in Bhopal a year later, and the final Tribunal in London in December 1994 (a date chosen to coincide with the tenth anniversary of the disaster at Bhopal). After this last meeting, the charter was again circulated to participants and experts all over the world before the final version was approved in early 1996.

Though the charter has not yet been formally ratified by the United Nations, this should not be seen as detracting in any way from its validity. The *Nuremberg Code*, after all, one of the earliest, most widely respected and most widely implemented international human rights documents in history, has never been formally ratified by the United Nations.[59] The *Charter on Industrial Hazards and Human Rights* will nonetheless at some point be "placed before the United Nations and other international bodies for official consideration." Still, even prior to its official recognition by international bodies, its charter, as its introduction affirms, clearly bases itself

> on the principle that official action is not enough: it calls upon individuals, community groups, trade unions, and public interests organizations to assert its rights as part of a common duty to take action against industrial hazards.[60]

This is exactly the same set of principles upon which the

Nuremberg Code was based at its inception. After it had been drafted as a result of the Doctors' Trials at Nuremberg, several decades passed before its principles began to be formally included in the legal statutes of nations. The long process of recognizing the inherent and independent validity of the *Nuremberg Code*, and then eventually implementing it in national law, is expected to be replicated in coming years in the case of the *Charter on Industrial Hazards and Human Rights*.

The charter[61] establishes itself on the same principles that underlie previous human rights documents such as the *Universal Declaration of Human Rights*, the *International Covenant on Civil and Political Rights*, the *Convention on the Elimination of All Forms of Discrimination Against Women*, the *United Nations Convention on the Rights of the Child*, and the *Declaration of Principles on Human Rights and the Environment*.[62]

The charter also arises out of a deep concern about the impact on human health of industrial hazards, both the large scale industrial accidents such as those that happened at Bhopal and Chernobyl, and "the widespread diffusion of hazardous products and processes resulting in industrial practices which cause human, social, and environmental destruction."[63] The charter is thus concerned with the human health effects of both high level acute exposures to toxicants and low level long-term exposures.

The term "industrial hazard" is not used narrowly in this document. The term should be understood to denote any synthetic chemical compounds or mixtures of compounds that may be biologically harmful to humans and other mammals. These industrial hazards would thus include, on the one hand, those chemical agents that have been deliberately manufactured for sale and use, such as solvents, insecticides and other pesticides, cleaning agents, artificial fragrances, artificial flavors, colorants, food preservatives and additives, and so on. On the other hand, the term "hazard" also includes those accidental and unwanted industrial byproducts which are released into the environment as unwanted consequences of manufacturing processes and which can then contaminate the air, water, food and soil. The charter is designed to define the rights of citizens vis-à-vis those industries and business interests that manufacture, produce, sell, transport, store, and use such hazards.

The charter is concerned with recognizing and identifying the rights of all the world's citizens. In addition, it is particularly concerned with recognizing the special vulnerabilities of women, whether of childbearing age or not. It says:

On account of the particular discrimination faced by women, both as waged and unwaged workers, attention should be given to the specific application of the rights stated below where women may be affected.[64]

The charter is concerned as well with the special vulnerabilities of children:

On account of their vulnerability ... special protection should be accorded to children exposed to industrial hazards.[65]

In addition to children and women, the document also notes the special protections that should be accorded to low income groups, to racial and ethnic minorities, and particularly to indigenous peoples.[66]

After noting (in Article 1) these especially vulnerable groups, and after underscoring the necessity for special measures to protect these groups, the charter devotes the remainder of its 38 articles to a variety of issues, a few of which, for our purposes, deserve special mention.

One of the most fundamental of the rights enunciated by this document is the right to live in an "environment free from [chemical] hazards,"[67] particularly when those chemical hazards have been imposed on individuals and societies by the behavior of industrial polluters.[68]

All persons have the right to a living environment free from [chemical] hazards. In particular, this right applies where hazards arise from:
(a) the manufacture, sale, transport, distribution, use and disposal of hazardous materials;
(b) any military or weapons application, regardless of national security.[69]

This right to an environment free from dangerous industrial and consumer toxicants applies to the environment in a person's home, in their place of work, in neighborhoods, in larger communities, and in the nation. Ultimately, of course, this must be recognized as a right that applies equally as well to the entire global environment, since environmental contaminants often do not stay in the geographical locale where they originated or were originally applied. They can readily migrate to very distant places via air currents, ground water, the food chain, and via the commercial transportation of goods around the world.

In order to protect their right to a living environment free from chemical hazards, citizens will need to have full access to all available information about those hazards. Thus, the charter establishes a clear right to adequate information about environmental contaminants and their specific risks.

> All persons have the right to regular and effective monitoring of their health and the living environment for possible immediate and long-term effects caused by hazardous or potentially hazardous economic enterprise.
> All persons have the right to be consulted on the frequency, character and objectives of environmental monitoring. The right to organise non-professional monitoring strategies, such as lay epidemiology, shall be protected. The rights of women, whose experience in providing health care may reveal otherwise unidentified consequences of hazards, are particularly affirmed.[70]

More specifically, citizens have a right to full information about any plan or intention to "establish, expand or modify"

> a hazardous industry in such location or in such a manner as may put at risk public health or the living environment....
> All persons have the right to be informed in their own language and in a manner which they are able to comprehend... of types and quantities of hazardous substances used and stored at the facility and emitted from the facility and contained in any final products. In particular, the right to information includes the right to regular toxic release inventories where appropriate. All persons living in the neighbourhood of hazardous facilities have the right to inspection of factory premises and to physical verification of hazardous substances and processes.[71]

This right to private monitoring of toxics and to full information about them is critical, of course, because without such a right citizens would be forced to rely only on the official (sometimes sanitized) statements given to them by an industry's public relations officers. It is well recognized that those industry-based sources—because of potentially large financial conflicts of interest—sometimes do not provide adequate information, and sometimes are not reliably accurate even in the little information they do provide.

Article 12 enunciates a "right to community education," i.e., a right to have community members, both children and adults, educated about potentially hazardous chemical pollutants. This education should be based on "the best available information and standards, drawn from both national and international sources."[72]

In light of this right to be educated, the charter urges states to "take effective steps to provide for" three different aspects of community education:

Labeling. The provision for "clear and systematic labeling of hazardous substances" is intended to provide community members with the information they need in order to make wise and careful choices about how much exposure to environmental toxicants they are willing to tolerate for themselves and their families. Without such clear and complete labeling citizens are effectively deprived of the ability and freedom to make those choices about their own lives.

Education. This provision for "appropriate education of the community, including children, on hazardous products and processes" is intended to provide the entire community with the kind of general knowledge about hazardous substances that they can then use to apply to specific situations. It is also intended to alert community members to the presence of chemical hazards of which they may not otherwise be aware.

Training. The provision for "training of police, medical professionals and other service providers on hazardous products and processes" is intended to give these community service agencies the information and practical operating principles they will need to protect themselves and those they serve from the adverse effects of exposure to toxicants.

Without such communitywide education about the hazards of toxicants, community members are effectively disenfranchised and not empowered to make decisions for themselves and their families about matters that could have long-term, irreversible, disabling, and sometimes life-threatening consequences. These provisions concerning citizen information, education and training affirm the right of individuals and families to have a significant level of self-determination over matters that directly affect their own health and well-being.

The charter further affirms the right of citizens and communities to be protected by scientifically based environmental management legislation, and effective enforcement of that legislation.[73] More importantly, the charter affirms the right of citizens and communities to have environmental laws that are "in compliance with the precautionary principle." The precautionary principle will be explained more fully in section five below. For our purposes here we need only outline its main theme: this principle urges that, when the scientific data about a chemical's toxicity are still incomplete, greater consideration should be given to concern about the health of citizens than should be given to concern about possible economic costs to businesses. That is,

> [W]here there are threats of serious or irreversible damage, lack of full scientific certainty shall not be used as a reason to postpone cost-effective measures to prevent [health] hazards and environmental degradation.[74]

This precautionary principle will turn out to be a very important one. Much current regulatory legislation about toxics in the U.S., for instance, clearly ignores and even flouts this principle. Because of this egregious failure to protect the citizenry's health we frequently see new scientific studies emerging which show marked adverse health effects from chemical products that have already been on the market for decades. One of the early and more blatant examples of our failure to apply the precautionary principle was illustrated by the work of Rachel Carson in exposing the toxicity and persistence of the organochlorine pesticides (such as chlordane, DDT and dieldrin).[75] Her work led eventually to legislation banning the use of most (though not all) of that class of pesticides in the U.S. (Unfortunately these products can, however, still be legally manufactured in the U.S. and then freely marketed anywhere else in the world.) The reason that policy mistakes of this sort can happen is because of our failure to adequately implement the precautionary principle into law.

The charter affirms the right of peoples everywhere to be protected by legislation that reflects this principle.

Article 17 affirms the right of workers to a working environment free from chemical hazards. This right extends to the pesticide applicator, to the aerospace laborer working with industrial solvents, and to office secretaries sharing their carpeted workspaces with computers, laser copiers, fax machines, and coworkers who may be wearing solvent-based artificial fragrances. Since workers spend such a large portion of their lives in their workspaces (second only to the amount of time they spend in their homes, more specifically, asleep in their bedrooms), it is crucial that work space be safe from toxicants. Many "tight" buildings today, in an effort to be energy efficient, have an insufficient exchange of outdoor air with indoor air—and indoor air is, almost without exception, grossly inferior to outdoor air.[76] (In addition, indoor air is not exposed to direct sunlight or to nature's heat, moisture, and winds which can sometimes work to break down and dissipate toxicants in the outdoor environment.) The corollary of this right to a safe workplace, of course, is that employers also have a corresponding duty to provide a healthy environment for their workers, free from mixtures of chemical toxicants that can cause adverse health effects. Furthermore, anyone who works in an environment from which it is virtually impossible to eliminate a certain amount of chemical hazard

> shall have the right to have provided, fitted free of charge and maintained in fully effective order, protective safety devices including personal protective equipment necessary to eliminate any such hazard as far as is possible. Employers may not refuse to provide the most effective equipment available on the grounds of cost or inconvenience.[77]

These occupational health and safety implications for employers are important, whether the occupation is one traditionally recognized as hazardous, such as pesticide application workers and chemical industry workers, or one not traditionally recognized as hazardous, such as office work or school teaching. In both instances, employers have an ethical obligation to provide a safe environment for their workers. (In addition, of course, it is to the employer's economic advantage for their workers to be safe and healthy, and for their capable functioning not to be impaired in any way by the presence of even low levels of neurotoxic contaminants in their workspace.)

Article 18 of the charter affirms the correlative right of workers to be given "reasonable notice of any proposed changes to their working environments which may pose a threat to worker health and safety." This would seem to be a relatively obvious right, one that should not be difficult to legislate, and one that should not require large resources to enforce. And yet there still seems to be significant resistance to implementing policies that would institute this right.

In 1997 and again in 1998, for example, a pesticide notification bill was introduced into the Washington State legislature,[78] and sponsors of the bill encountered enormous resistance, particularly from those associated with the agricultural pesticide industry, to even getting the bill out of committee to be heard on the floor of the House. Titled, "the Children's Pesticide Right to Know" bill, it would have required simply that workers and others in schools, in daycare centers, in state buildings and in apartment buildings be given 48 hours prior notice of any intent to apply pesticides inside their school or building. The bill would simply require that inhabitants of those buildings be told when the pesticide would be applied, which pesticide product would be used, and what the method of application would be. A memorandum in support of the bill describes its simple provisions:

> This bill requires posted notice 48 hours prior to pesticide applications in schools, daycare centers, workplaces, and apartment buildings. Signs must be placed at building entrances, notifying that a pesticide application will take place, and including information of the type and amount of pesticide as well as how to obtain additional information. The sign must also include a cautionary statement for individuals that may be especially susceptible to the adverse effects of pesticides.

This legislation would thus have allowed inhabitants of these buildings to be aware of their probable exposure to the pesticides that can adversely affect their health, in some cases quite dramatically. This legislation should hardly have been controversial. As Ashford and Miller explain, "At a minimum, regulators should require that application of chemicals, such as pesticides, be accompanied by adequate notice so that people can avoid the exposure."[79] And yet this bill, minimal as its provisions were, was defeated two years in a row by agricultural and pesticide interest groups before it even left committee. If nothing else, this defeat should properly be seen as a testimony to the power of agrichemical interests in a state that has substantial agricultural activity.

According to the *Charter on Industrial Hazards and Human Rights*, workers (and others in those buildings) do have a clear right to this kind of information, and employers and building managers do have a corresponding ethical duty to provide it. Workers also have a right to information about planned renovations in their place of work, about cleaning agents and solvents commonly used in their workspace, about the quality of their indoor air quality, and about any other issues which may have a direct bearing on their health and well-being.

Workers furthermore, according to the charter, have a right to participate actively and effectively in decisionmaking regarding matters that may directly or indirectly impact their health and safety in the workplace.[80]

Finally, Article 34 addresses the question about who should bear the burden of proof in cases where there is evidence that a person has been physically injured by exposure to toxicants.

As matters stand presently, when a person has been injured by exposure to toxicants (as at Bhopal), the burden of proof for showing that the injuries were indeed caused by that toxicant (or mixture of toxicants) is borne entirely by the injured party or parties. The legal presumption has been that it is the injured party's responsibility to prove, by collecting and presenting documented evidence, that the employer or business was at fault. The charter affirms instead that the burden of proof should *not* be on the injured party. Rather, the business should be required to prove that it was not negligent.

> Where there is prima facie evidence that death or injury was caused by an industrial hazard, the hazardous economic enterprise has the burden of proving that it was not negligent.
>
> No person adversely affected by hazardous activity shall be subjected to excessive documentation requirements or strict standards of proof in establishing that the hazardous activity caused their illness or symptoms. The link between hazards and illness shall be presumed if the affected persons establish
>
> (a) they suffer from symptoms commonly associated with any harmful substance, or any component thereof, which contaminated the environment; and
> (b) either
> (i) they were present within the geographical area of contamination during the period of contamination; or
> (ii) they belong to a group of persons commonly identified as secondary victims, including the siblings, partners, children or close associates of the original victims of the hazard.[81]

What this article means is that the person who has been made severely sick or disabled, who may no longer be able to earn a livelihood, and whose life may be irreparably disrupted and damaged by exposure to the toxicants in question, does not have the additional burden of taking their case up against the economic power and political influence of a large multinational corporate enterprise. As the 100,000 who were injured in the Bhopal explosion (as well as the families of the 2,000 who were killed) have learned, even a large class action suit, when put up against the self-protective economic and legal resources of a large transnational corporation, has almost no chance of being resolved in a timely manner, and even less chance of being resolved in favor of the injured parties. The affirmation of this right of injured parties—that industry should bear the full burden of proof—is a clear statement that present policy governing such toxicant injuries is ethically backward.

The charter concludes with articles clarifying the corresponding duties of individuals and organizations to uphold these rights, and the corresponding duties of states to implement these rights into national law. In the case of the *Nuremberg Code*, of course, it took two or three decades before national states began to implement its principles into statutory law. The same may turn out to be the case with the charter. Unfortunately, in its case, those who try to initiate such legislation will probably face enormous obstacles that did not stand in the way of the *Nuremberg Code*. They will especially have to face the opposition of highly organized transnational corporate interests which have enormous financial and legal resources at their disposal. Just as tobacco companies have fought every effort to pass legislation that would protect and promote the public health rather than their financial interests, so the chemical corporations can be expected to continue tenaciously opposing any attempts to implement into law the rights articulated in this *Charter on Industrial Hazards and Human Rights.*[82]

It thus becomes evident that one of the basic rights underlying all the principles in these documents is *the right to not be poisoned without your knowledge and without your consent.* This right is apparently so fundamental as not to even need expressing as directly and baldly as I have here expressed it. The right is simply assumed throughout these documents, and most readers can probably easily acknowledge its validity. Unfortunately, however, it is violated every day, sometimes in more dramatic and sometimes in less dramatic ways. Usually someone profits in some manner, directly or indirectly, from the processes that result in people being poisoned without their knowledge and without their consent. The profit is often economic, often very large, and it is not usually the people who are being poisoned who are reaping the profits.

We turn our attention now to two final documents, both of which articulate the internationally accepted ethical and human rights standards which govern all biological and medical research involving the use of human beings as research subjects.

THE *NUREMBERG CODE* AND THE WHO/CIOMS *INTERNATIONAL ETHICAL GUIDELINES FOR BIOMEDICAL RESEARCH INVOLVING HUMAN SUBJECTS*

We presently have very little adequate understanding of the

human health effects of long-term exposure to low doses of ambient toxicants and toxicant mixtures. Our ignorance about these 80,000 or so chemicals is, as we have seen, abysmal. "Even the most basic toxicity testing results cannot be found in the public record for nearly 75% of the top-volume chemicals in commercial use."[83] Clearly, more research is needed.

Fortunately, or perhaps unfortunately, much of this human research is already well under way. Large human populations, numbering in the tens or hundreds of millions, are already being exposed to, and hence are being tested for the health effects of, thousands of industrial and consumer toxicants and their mixtures. As Fagin and Lavelle explain, "We are all, in effect, involuntary participants in a vast, uncontrolled [toxics] experiment."[84]

It is well known that the only way we will ever come to any full understanding of toxicant induced health effects is by monitoring the effects of toxicants on large, actually exposed human populations, a process that is actually occurring in the world right now. Large human populations, at all ages and levels of human development (including intrauterine), are being daily exposed to an uncommonly wide variety of environmental toxicants and toxicant mixtures and they are, furthermore, being exposed for extended periods of time, i.e., for years and decades. If these populations are monitored for potential resulting health effects from those exposures—even if the monitoring is only of the passive informal sort that happens in hospital emergency rooms, in cancer wards, and in the offices of practicing physicians—then the entire process must be viewed as a series of ongoing experiments on the human health effects of long-term, low dose exposures to environmental toxicants. "The chronic exposure situation our nation has placed itself in is truly a vast experiment in the unknown."[85] Rachel Carson had already suggested this in 1962 in *Silent Spring*,[86] and today it is even more evident.

There are, in effect, multiple ongoing human subjects experiments under way, all of them testing for the health effects of exposure to toxicants. Some of these experiments involve industrial products and byproducts, some involve household consumer products, some involve pesticides, and so on. John Wargo, Associate Professor in the School of Forestry and Environmental Studies and the Department of Political Science at Yale University, states it very clearly: "pesticide licensing under conditions of such uncertainty [about their potential adverse health effects] has been an act of uncontrolled human and ecological experimentation."[87] This, unhappily, is not an exaggeration.

Though some in the past have not viewed these practices as human subjects experiments, in fact they are. The experiments are clearly posing (even if not deliberately or with much planning) a specific set of research questions about the long-term health effects of exposure to low doses of ambient toxicants and their mixtures. Most of the subjects are in effect blinded, since they are not fully aware of the chemicals to which they are being exposed. And the experimenters are partially blinded as well, since they do not know which specific subjects are being exposed to which chemicals.

Few of the experiments have any true control group (of unexposed subjects), since many of these chemicals are so ubiquitous that no one could possibly escape exposure to them. In fact, no human populations exist, even in the regions of the earth most remote from urban civilization, that have not been exposed to some level of modern environmental toxicants. Thus it would be difficult if not impossible to find a control group, and without one the experiments are not nearly as well designed as one would wish.

Nevertheless, these experiments are, in a sense, someday like a very large scale safety trial, analogous to the phase I safety trials for new pharmaceutical products. Yet in another sense, the experiments are analogous to phase IV postmarketing trials of pharmaceutical products, with the significant difference being only that there has not been, for most of these toxicants, any properly done preliminary phase I safety trials. Or to be more precise, the significant difference between all these toxicant trials and standard phase IV trials for pharmaceutical products is that *none* of the first three phases have been done. Nor has much of the required preliminary laboratory and animal research been done on most of these toxicants, all of which tests would have been necessary in order to consider these present trials ethically proper.

These large scale human subjects safety experiments, therefore, while poorly designed, and while missing much of the necessary preliminary test data, are in effect being conducted both by the transnational chemical manufacturing corporations and by the government agencies responsible for regulating them. Both the corporations and the government agencies probably hope that the outcomes of these experiments will be negative and that no adverse human health effects will be proven to result from exposure to these toxicants. They both probably hope to discover that none of these several thousand chemicals and chemical compounds will show any evidence of causing adverse human health effects, acute or chronic, at the doses to which people are daily exposed. Unfortunately, as we have seen in Chapter One, it does not appear that the results will be as benign as they are hoping.

Nonetheless, one key set of considerations has been noticeably missing from the thinking (or lack of thinking) that has led to these de facto trials: considerations about the ethical treatment of their human subjects. After all, well before a trial is even begun, its design must meet certain basic minimum ethical standards. In the case of experiments such as these which involve human beings as research subjects, there are, by international agreement, strict minimum ethical standards.

These ethical standards were first made explicit in the *Nuremberg Code*, a document drawn up as a result of the atrocities uncovered after World War II at the Doctors' Trials (1946–49) at Nuremberg. These trials found Nazi medical researchers guilty of conducting a wide variety of biological experiments on human beings with neither their full knowledge nor their free consent. Today, in precisely the same way, these ongoing toxics experiments are being conducted on human populations (us) that have not been given full information about the nature and extent of the experiments, have not been informed about their potential harms and benefits, and have not been asked for their consent to participate in the experiments.

When the Nazis felt need to justify their actions, either to themselves or to others, they often did so in utilitarian (i.e., in risk assessment) terms. For example, one of the Nazi doctors, Dr. Gerhard Rose, head of the Koch Institute of Tropical Medicine in Berlin during the war, expressed exactly these utilitarian rationalizations. He said that although he

> initially opposed performing lethal experiments on camp inmates, he came to believe that it made no sense not to involve 100 or 200 people in research, even lethal research, in pursuit of a vaccine for typhus when the Reich was losing 1000 men a day to this disease on the Eastern front. What, he asked, were the deaths of 100 men compared to the possible benefit of developing a prophylactic vaccine capable of saving tens of thousands?[88]

As we have seen, philosophers term this approach to moral decisionmaking—that is, the attempt to make moral judgments based on an estimated quantification of the anticipated costs and benefits of human acts—the utilitarian or consequentialist[89] approach. This approach has always particularly appealed to those who wish to find some way to quantify human well-being and suffering as a way of simplifying, or perhaps clarifying, moral decisionmaking. Risk assessment, as we noted earlier, is one popular modern incarnation of this utilitarian approach.

Because the Nuremberg Tribunals found this particular application of a utilitarian justification of human suffering so odious, at least in the way it was being applied to medical experiments in the camps, the ethical principles of the *Nuremberg Code* were formulated to require researchers to protect the health and well-being of each individual human subject in their experiments, regardless of any utilitarian rationalizations that may have been used to justify the experiments.

The principles outlined in the code are ethical requirements detailing the minimal proper conduct of researchers. There is very little room in these principles for the kind of "guesstimating" about the future, the attempts to predict possible future outcomes, and the weighing of varying competing interests that so characterizes environmental risk assessment strategies.

The philosophy behind the Doctors' Trials at Nuremberg was that all individual human beings have worth in themselves, and are not merely to be used as a means for the benefit of others, even if that benefit is very great. It is the German philosopher Immanuel Kant (1724–1804) who is most noted for enunciating this principle late in the 18th century: "So act as to treat humanity, whether in thine own person or in that of any other, in every case as an end withal, never as a means only."[90] The *Nuremberg Code* insists that every human person be treated with full respect for their humanity and for their right to self determination.

The core of the code is its insistence on applying the principle of informed consent. "The voluntary consent of the human subject is absolutely essential."

This means that the person involved should have legal capacity to give consent; should be so situated as to be able to exercise free power of choice, without the intervention of any element of force, fraud, deceit, duress, overreaching, or other ulterior form of constraint or coercion, and should have sufficient knowledge and comprehension of the elements of the subject matter involved as to enable him to make an understanding and enlightened decision. This latter element requires that before the acceptance of an affirmative decision by the experimental subject there should be made known to him the nature, duration, and purpose of the experiment; the method and means by which it is to be conducted; all inconveniences and hazards reasonably to be expected; and the effects upon his health or person which may possibly come from his participation in the experiment.[91]

The document thus clearly requires that each individual subject involved in the experiment have full legal capacity to give consent. It will be clear to everyone that infants and minor children do not have such legal capacity, and that some other classes of people do not either. Today's large scale corporate-government toxics experiments which are already so fully under way in the world clearly violate this central norm of informed consent in the *Nuremberg Code*.

The code also clearly requires that each person "be so situated as to be able to exercise free power of choice." This means that there must be no coercion or "undue inducement"[92] involved in getting subjects to participate in any experiments, including the present toxics experiments.

At present, however, it is virtually impossible for anyone to avoid being a participant in these experiments, just as it was impossible for the prisoners in the Nazi camps to avoid being participants in those experiments. No one today is able to freely choose whether to participate in the experiments or not. They do not have the freedom to say, "No, I would rather not participate and I would rather not have my children participate either in these chemical experiments." In this way, today's experiments also violate the central foundational norm of the *Nuremberg Code*, the principle of free consent from each fully informed individual subject.

The code further requires that each person be given "sufficient knowledge and comprehension of the elements of the subject matter involved as to enable him [or her] to make an understanding and enlightened decision." Unfortunately, no one in today's ongoing toxics experiments is given sufficient information about the potential risks of exposure to these toxicants; nor are they given information about the nature of the chemical contaminants to which they will be exposed. In some cases, notably in the case of pesticide compounds and artificial fragrance compounds, manufacturers deliberately and strenuously fight to oppose laws that would require them to disclose even the names of the chemicals in their products. Nor do they wish to disclose the nature, characteristics, and possible adverse health effects of these chemicals. Furthermore, people and communities are not given information about the quantities of *any* of these ambient chemicals to which they may be exposed (except for the very few on the U.S. Toxics Release Inventory, as we saw above), nor are they given information about the known adverse health effects those chemicals may be expected to cause. Subjects in these experiments are therefore suffering from a significant dearth of information about the contaminants to which they are being daily exposed. In this way, therefore, the chemical corporations, the manufacturers and distributors of these toxicants, and the government regulatory agencies that have been failing to adequately protect communities from chemical injury, are already violating the central principle of the *Nuremberg Code*: the principle of informed consent.

This requirement to inform people about the experiment in which they may be participating also requires that there be made known to them "the nature, duration, and purpose of the experiment; the method and means by which it is to be conducted; [and] all inconveniences and hazards reasonably to be expected." Citizen-participants in today's ongoing toxics experiments have been given no information about how long the experiments will last (indefinitely?); they have not been told the purpose of the experiments (corporate profit? Social betterment?); they have not been made aware of the method and means by which the experiments are to be conducted (expose large numbers of people to a wide variety of toxicants via a wide range of pathways, then monitor for adverse health effects, using a highly passive monitoring system?); and they have clearly not been fully informed about the "inconveniences and hazards reasonably to be expected," (some of which have been noted above in Chapter One). None of this information has been effectively made known to any of the world's peoples who are daily participating as human subjects in these experiments.

The code also requires that each person be fully informed about the potential "effects upon his health or person which may possibly come from his participation in the experiment." I suspect that many people, had they been provided with a full awareness of the potential effects on them and their children (cancer, asthma, MCS, immune system and endocrine system dysregulation, for example), might wisely have chosen, if they had had the freedom to make such a decision, to not participate in these toxics experiments.

And finally, the code requires that each subject should "be at liberty to bring the experiment to an end" whenever they wish. That is, each subject must be able to freely withdraw from the experiment at any time, for any reason at all (or even for no reason). Unfortunately, today it is virtually impossible to avoid exposure to a very wide variety of ambient environmental toxicants, and it is thus no longer possible to "withdraw from the experiment." So in this way, the current toxics experiments violate yet another of the key provisions of the *Nuremberg Code*.

In fact, today's large scale toxics experiments, which are in essence using almost every person on the planet as a subject—women, infants, the elderly, the sick and the well—are effectively violating every ethical norm outlined in the *Nuremberg Code*. Subjects have not been informed about the nature of the experiments, have not been told any of the possible risks to their health or person, have not been asked for their consent to participate, have not been given the freedom to choose whether to participate or not, and have not been allowed to withdraw from the experiment at any time. In these ways, participants in the current ongoing toxics experiments are similar to the concentration camp prisoners who were forced to participate in the Nazi medical experiments. So all the subjects in today's toxics experiments are in a situation very like that which the *Nuremberg Code* was designed to prevent.

The WHO/CIOMS document, *International Ethical Guidelines for Biomedical Research Involving Human Subjects*, promulgated in 1993, is in effect a fuller and much more detailed iteration of the principles expressed in the *Nuremberg Code*. It too insists on full compliance with the principle of informed consent.

In addition, it more fully develops the concept of "vulnerable populations," i.e., populations that need special protections due to their special vulnerabilities. Infants and children, for example, need special protections due to their unique biological vulnerabilities and due to their inability to protect themselves. Pregnant women may need special protections as well. Certain populations in some developing nations, people with certain mental or behavioral disorders, and any other persons whose ability to comprehend information, or whose ability to give free consent, has been potentially compromised in any way may also need protections against being exploited by researchers.

Today's toxics experiments, with their inclusion of virtually every human being on the planet as a research subject, have shown no regard for vulnerable populations. All the world's vulnerable populations and groups have been fully enrolled as subjects in the experiments, without any attempt at all to inform them about the potential hazards, and without any pretense of requesting their free and uncoerced consent. The experiments thus clearly violate virtually every provision of the WHO/CIOMS *International Ethical Guidelines for Biomedical Research Involving Human Subjects.*

Telford Taylor, lead prosecutor in the Doctor's Trials at Nuremberg, Robert Drinan, and others have recently argued eloquently and persuasively that "a permanent international tribunal is needed to judge and punish those who commit war crimes and crimes against humanity."[93] Two reasons supporting this suggestion are obvious.

> 1. Statements, even authoritative statements, of ... ethics are not self-enforcing and require active promulgation, dissemination, and enforcement.
> 2. The world has no effective mechanism for promulgating and enforcing basic medical ethics and human rights principles.[94]

The Permanent People's Tribunal discussed above in this chapter (section 3., 3) may well be a beginning step toward such a permanent international tribunal.

Annas and Grodin have suggested that there should be an analogous permanent international tribunal to hear cases related to research ethics. They have argued that

> the world needs an international tribunal with authority to judge and punish those physicians who violate international norms of medical conduct, as well as an independent body to conduct ongoing surveillance and to develop a rapid response capacity. Without these, the world is as [it was] before Nuremberg.... In addition, the courts of individual countries, including the United States, have consistently proven incapable either of punishing those engaged in unlawful or unethical human experimentation, or of compensating the victims of such experimentation. Primarily, this is because such experimentation is often [considered to be] justified on the basis of national security or military necessity.[95]

In the case of the present testing of the health effects of ambient toxicants on large human populations, the justification, should one ever be offered, would probably not be based on national security or military necessity—it would almost certainly be couched in terms of the economic value said to accrue to certain parts of the market.

Annas and Grodin's proposed permanent tribunal would ideally be supported and sanctioned by the United Nations, would be politically neutral, and would be composed of a large panel of respected and distinguished judges from around the world. The Permanent

People's Tribunal as proposed seems to fit these criteria rather well, with the exception of being officially supported and sanctioned by the UN. The UN should perhaps consider whether this tribunal should be the one designated as the official organ for prosecuting human rights violations related both to biomedical research ethics and to environmental toxicants.

The five human rights documents we have examined in this section all provide a foundation for the acceptance of certain fundamental rights that might be termed "life integrity rights," i.e., the rights necessary for a person to be able to live in an environment and under conditions that do not destroy their ability to keep their lives, health and well-being intact. As Barry Levy, president of the American Public Health Association, has said: "Everyone, regardless of race, nationality, religion, gender, age or political belief, is entitled to 'life integrity rights'"[96] of just the sort that have been outlined in the five documents we have examined.

We turn now to a more specific consideration of the ethical principles that both underlie and ground the principles enunciated in these human rights documents, and to some principles that can clearly be derived from these documents.

HUMAN RIGHTS AND THE VIRTUE OF JUSTICE

The simplest and clearest definition of justice comes down to us from a tradition much older even than Plato. He quotes the idea (in his *Republic*) as coming down to him from "the ancients," and indeed it is found even as early as Homer. According to this notion, justice means that each person must be given what is properly due to them. Injustice, on the other hand, "implies that what belongs to a man is withheld or taken away from him—and, once more, not by misfortune, failure of crops, fire or earthquake, but by man."[97]

If human rights documents are to mean anything, they must be universally accepted as clear statements that the rights laid out in them are properly due to human beings, and that not insuring those rights to people does true injustice.

4. The Golden Rule, Silver Rule, and Sufferings of the Other

The Golden Rule—to do unto others as you would have others do unto you—is accompanied in most of the world's religions by its corollary, the Silver Rule—do not do unto others what you would not wish others to do unto you.[98] The golden and silver rules have been long recognized, from earliest antiquity to the present, as two of the most fundamental principles for guiding human conduct if people wish to live well. It might well be argued that all other ethical norms actually ultimately derive from these two.

What these two ethical norms ask us to do, in effect, is to view others and to treat others as deserving of the precise same level of personal respect and concern that we recognize ourselves to deserve. They ask us to view the Other as another self.

Radical as it may seem, public policy should perhaps also be based, at least to some degree, on these two principles. This would mean that in forming legislation and public policy, legislators and policymakers should put themselves in place of the Other, and even attempt to anticipate the Other's concerns. Policymakers and regulatory agencies should arrange matters as best they can to see that no one, not even the decisionmakers in transnational corporations, should do to others what they would not wish others to do to them. An old joke says that the golden rule means that whoever has the gold makes the rules. This perverted version may be the one that has too often held sway in some matters, but it should not hold sway in matters related to the environment and public health.

If these two principles, the golden and silver rules combined, guided legislation and policymaking, the planet and its peoples might see significant improvement in their prospects for the future.

5. The Precautionary Principle

Most by far of the chemical compounds and industrial byproducts in widespread use today, and virtually all of the compounds being proposed for use, do not yet have anything approaching adequate scientific data to substantiate any claims of safety. Nor are there any adequate data on the possible toxic effects of the chemical mixtures to which people are daily exposed, and it will almost certainly be at least several decades or more before such data become available. As we saw above, testing for the health effects of mixtures of just the 1,000 most toxic chemicals, in mixtures of three, would require 166 million experiments to be performed, and that would provide data only on the health effects of those particular mixtures on one species of animal, at one dosage level, and at one stage in their lives. Much more research would clearly need to be done in order to answer the questions to which we most need answers: about dose-response relationships, health effects of exposures at different stages in life, long-term health effects, subsequent health effects on offspring, and so on.

Thus, a question to be faced by policymakers and government regulators in the meantime is whether chemicals, both new ones and those in present use, should be licensed for use and dispersal in the environment when we lack adequate scientific data regarding their impact on human health. Which stance should society take on chemical agents about which there is not yet a sufficient body of multiple, large scale, replicable studies? Should we allow such chemicals to be used and dispersed into the environment, even though we do not yet have adequate evidence concerning their effects on human health? Or should such chemical products not be licensed until there are adequate studies (undertaken and funded by the developer or manufacturer of the product) proving that the product is not a threat to the public health? In short, in the absence of adequate toxicity data, should we license or not?

Those in the manufacturing camp and those in the public health camp frequently come down on opposite sides of this question. The position taken by most chemical manufacturing corporations, chemical marketers, and some commercial users is that when we do not have strong evidence showing that a chemical or compound is clearly toxic to human beings, to wildlife, or to the environment, manufacturers should be allowed to market it until it is proven to be. Unless there is convincing evidence that a given compound is toxic, they feel, it should be regarded as safe and should be made available to all who wish to use it. The corporations thus seem to feel that chemicals, like people, should be considered innocent until proven guilty.

According to author Christopher Hood, there are two opposing schools of thought in this issue: anticipationism, and resilience.[99] The resilience—or bouncing back—school of thought holds that the earth is (and organisms are) highly resilient and able to bounce back from any assaults made on them. It claims to be based on the belief that, "While limited to only one past and one present, every society is faced with a multiplicity of potential futures."[100] We can anticipate but cannot predict the future, it says, since the multiple interactions of such an enormous multiplicity of variables cannot be foreseen before they actually come to pass. Because we cannot predict the future, we would be better off making the best judgments we can, but should be prepared to "bounce back" should any untoward consequences develop.

This resilience school of thought, which is more likely to be favored by the chemical corporations, is countered by what Hood calls anticipationism, and what we have been calling

> The *Versorgensprincip*, or precautionary principle, originally enunciated by the West German government in 1976, has gradually become a focus for creative thinking on these subjects throughout the EEC [European Economic Community] and more widely. The precautionary principle is proactive in that it advocates the implementation of controls of pollution without waiting for scientific evidence of damage caused by the pollutant(s), and without necessarily requiring consideration of the relative costs and benefits of regulation to industry or the public.[101]

This precautionary principle (usually supported by those working in public health) stands firmly opposed to the bouncing-back school of thought and holds instead to the anticipationist school of thought. Anticipationism urges us to make every effort to anticipate and avoid problems, particularly those that give evidence of being serious or irreversible. Albert Einstein has been quoted as saying that "a clever person solves a problem; a wise person avoids it."[102] And Albert Schweitzer worried that, "Man has lost the capacity to foresee and to forestall. He will end by destroying the earth."[103] Advocates of the precautionary principle hope that this is not true, and that some wise policymakers do still have the ability to foresee and to forestall.

The precautionary principle (in line with the anticipationist school of thought) therefore affirms that when there is inadequate scientific data to clearly determine a chemical's safety or toxicity, the operative presumption should be in favor of protecting the public health rather than in favor of protecting the manufacturers' interest in dispersing the product into the marketplace and the environment. Precaution urges that, in the face of scientific uncertainty, we should worry more about protecting the physical health of citizens than about insuring the economic benefit that might accrue from marketing the product. The precautionary principle thus takes the position of "being protective when uncertain."[104]

The principle was adopted internationally at the global United Nations Conference on Environment and Development (UNCED) in

Rio de Janeiro, Brazil, in 1992. Principle 15 of the *Declaration of Rio* states that "where there are threats of serious or irreversible environmental damage, lack of full scientific certainty shall not be used as a reason for postponing cost-effective measures to prevent degradation." This formulation was then incorporated (and somewhat expanded) into the 1996 *Charter on Industrial Hazards and Human Rights'* as we have seen above.

The precautionary principle has, unfortunately, not been incorporated into policy. The tobacco industry, for instance, commonly cites the "lack of adequate scientific evidence" as a reason to justify the continued minimalist regulation of tobacco sale and use.

In fact, "More research is needed" is the persistent refrain of both the tobacco companies and the chemical corporations. Does tobacco cause lung cancer? "We do not know for sure; more research is needed." Does it cause cardiovascular disease? "More research is needed." Do pesticides cause neurologic, endocrinologic, or immunologic dysfunction? "More research is needed."

This common refrain should raise in our mind the key policy question: what regulatory and policy stance should nations and communities take when toxicity questions are still scientifically undetermined, and when more research is still needed? The precautionary principle, as we have seen, urges that we exercise caution in the face of scientific uncertainty. "Better safe than sorry," we might say, especially when the adverse toxicological effects may well be serious, irreversible, untreatable even with palliatory measures, permanently harmful or disabling, and sometimes fatal, to large numbers of people.

The Center for Ethics and Toxics (CETOS), a private research and advocacy organization, expresses the precautionary principle thus:

> Where the introduction of a new toxicant or expanded use of one already in commerce threatens risk of irreversible or serious damage to health or the environment, the existence of scientific uncertainty about safety shall be used to *limit* such introduction or use.[105]

The precautionary principle has also been defined as "a preference for avoiding unnecessary health risks instead of unnecessary economic expenditures when information about potential risks is incomplete."[106]

While commerce in chemicals and chemical compounds can sometimes provide economic benefit for both manufacturers and consumers—a consideration which should not be lightly dismissed—

the health of the people in a community is a more fundamental concern and should clearly take precedence over near-term economic
interests when the toxicological data on new chemicals is incomplete. As the old saying has it: "protection delayed is protection
denied."

In conclusion, the precautionary principle is one that ought to
be taken as a clear guide in toxics policymaking, in legislation, and
in regulatory enforcement.

6. Nonconsensual Exposure[107]

The CETOS *Toxics Bill of Rights* affirms, as one of the most
fundamental rights of individuals and communities, that, "Human
beings deserve the maximal protection under the law from non-consensual exposure to toxic substances."[108] While this may seem like
an obvious right that people should and do have, as matters stand
now, both in industrialized and developing nations, most people
would find it virtually impossible to avoid nonconsensual exposure
to quite a large variety of toxicants. While they may be able to avoid
a certain amount of exposure in their foods by buying (if they can
afford it) only foods that are grown without pesticides and have no
chemical additives, they will find it virtually impossible to avoid
breathing air that is polluted with pesticide residues and drift, the
byproducts of industrial processes, and vehicle exhaust. Some people may be able (if they can afford it) to avoid the chemical contaminants in their drinking, cooking, and bathing water by installing
water filters in their homes or by purchasing bottled spring water.
However, they will probably not be able to avoid the residues and
drift from pesticides sprayed in their neighbors' yards, along their
neighborhood streets, along all county and state roadways, in city,
county, and state parks, on golf courses and in cemeteries, on farms,
inside their shopping malls and grocery stores, around and inside
their public buildings, around and inside their children's schools,
and also sprayed aerially over enormous acreages of private timber
and private agriculture. For those people sensitive to pesticides, and
for the growing number of people who want to protect themselves
and their families from becoming excessively sensitized to toxicants,
it is virtually impossible to avoid exposure to widespread drift
residues of herbicides and insecticides, as well as to a wide variety
of industrial pollutants and other ambient environmental toxicants.

This right to be safe from nonconsensual exposure to toxics, then, affirms that individuals and communities have a fundamental right to avoid being exposed, if they so wish, to toxicants that they have reason to believe may do them physical harm. This principle supports the tenet that forced exposure to environmental toxicants is morally wrong. Synthetic chemical poisons of whatever quantity should not be forced on anyone—male or female, adult or child, pre-natal or postnatal, young or old, sick or well. Toxics should not be forced on anyone against their will.

7. *Tragedy of the Commons*

Though Garrett Hardin's classical formulation of "the tragedy of the commons"[109] originated in the context of world hunger issues, it can also be used as a fruitful analogy for conceptualizing environmental issues.

In Hardin's thinking, the commons is any public area which everyone in the community may use equally (for example, to graze their herds), yet any profits made by an individual as a consequence of using the commons can rightfully accrue solely to him as an individual. According to Hardin, this "commons" system works quite well as long as the commons is abundant and plentiful, and is not damaged or depleted by use.

Problems arise, however, when the commons is in short supply or is easily damaged or depleted by overuse. In situations of such scarcity, when an individual strives to profit individually by using the common area for their own benefit, it may have the ultimate effect of damaging, depleting or perhaps destroying the commons. Once the commons has been ruined, no one is able to profit from its use at all. One person is thus able to ruin the commons for every-one. Unless each individual cares for the commons equally, eventu-ally a time will come when the commons will have been destroyed. According to Hardin, this is a relatively frequent outcome, particu-larly in the modern world, once a commons is put to unregulated use for individual (or corporate) profit.

His solution—a somewhat controversial one—is to simply par-cel up the commons into individual units of private property.[110] Though this solution may be workable for Hardin's purposes (the economics of food production), it would hardly be feasible as a solu-tion for environmental issues.

Our air and water are clearly a part of the environmental "com-

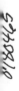

mons," and "air is the element most diffuse, most shared, most invisible, least controllable, [and] least understood."[111] Air is also, in some ways, the most contaminated. Steingraber says in *Living Downstream*:

> Air is by far the largest receptacle for industrial emissions. Of all of the toxic chemicals released by industry into the nation's environment each year, more than half [are] released into air. These emissions include about seventy different known or suspected human carcinogens.... And while air pollution in the United States has markedly improved over the past quarter century, more than a hundred urban areas still fail to meet national [minimum] air quality standards. In other words, nearly one hundred million Americans breathe air that is officially illegal.[112]

In addition to the airborne toxicants that originate from sources within the boundaries of a given nation, the air at any given point on earth also contains toxicants that have been released into the atmosphere by people and industries far removed from that point in space and time. Because pesticides and other toxicants can drift on air currents for hundreds, sometimes thousands, of miles[113] from their point of origin, some of the chemical contaminants we carry in our tissues "are pesticides sprayed by farmers we have never met, whose language we may not speak, in countries whose agricultural practices may be completely unfamiliar to us."[114]

Furthermore, air and water are both clearly not in infinite supply; nor are they infinitely regenerable. One unfortunate but common misperception about the earth and the environment—a misperception fostered by the chemical manufacturing interests and by the "resilience" school of thought discussed above—is that they *are* almost infinitely regenerable and resilient.[115] As Marc Lappé explains,

> the flawed belief in the earth's resilience (as in our own) has blocked inventive and essential solutions.... To count on the earth to heal itself is as foolhardy as counting on the body to process all toxic molecules into innocuous ones.[116]

Once we have recognized the air and water as a commons—as resources available for everyone's use, and from which some individuals (and corporations) can and do profit—we see that we are dealing with Hardin's classic tragedy of the commons. The question then becomes: what can be done about it?

The present system in the U.S., in which each corporate entity is allotted a certain quantity of pollution credits for their use, is somewhat like parceling out the air to private parties. When any given industry or corporation is then also allowed to sell a portion of its pollution credits to other corporations when it does not intend to use all of them, then the system seems even more as if it were parceling out air into privately owned quantities. (A further criticism of this system is that it simply encourages an arrangement in which the maximum allowable pollution will actually be dispersed, since any reduction of pollution by one corporation simply allows another corporation to pollute more.)

Clearly, however, this parceling is a kind of illusion. The air and water cannot actually be parceled into separate individual units for private purchase and ownership. Clean air and clean water are not in infinite supply. And some industries exploit them as dumping grounds for their chemical wastes. If they do this to the point of damaging the air and water to the extent that others cannot even safely breathe and drink them—in other words, if we are clearly suffering from Hardin's classic "tragedy of the commons"[117]—by what means can we protect the air and water from even more serious and irreparable damage caused by those who would exploit it for their own economic benefit?

This "commons" way of conceptualizing environmental issues may prove fruitful in our effort to understand the social justice and human rights concerns surrounding the manufacture, transport and use of toxics.

8. Absence of Evidence Is Not Evidence of Absence

The need for more research on the potential health consequences of synthetic toxicants is, as we have seen, obvious. However, one of the ways that chemical corporations try to imply that their products are safe for use is to claim that "there is no evidence that product X causes any adverse health effects." Or, "there is no evidence that our product is carcinogenic." Or, "there is absolutely no evidence of neurotoxicity associated with use of our product." These claims can sometimes sound persuasive to the citizens who will be making the decisions about whether to purchase or use product X in their daily lives.

But the claim that there is no evidence of toxicity is not the same as the claim that there is evidence of nontoxicity. It is important to realize that these claims about a lack of evidence of toxicity can continue to be made only as long as there are so few studies examining the toxic effects of chemicals and their mixtures. The less knowledge we actually have, and the fewer studies that are actually done, the more easily chemical interests can continue to make the claim that "there is no evidence of toxicity."

As a matter of fact, of the 80,000 (or more) chemicals now in common commercial use in the U.S., according to Steingraber,

> only about 1.5–3 percent (1,200 to 1,500 chemicals) have been tested for carcinogenicity. The vast majority of commercially used chemicals were brought to market before 1979, when the federal Toxics Substances Control Act (TSCA) mandated the review of new chemicals. Thus, many carcinogenic environmental contaminants likely remain unidentified, unmonitored, and unregulated. Too often, this lack of basic information is paraphrased as "there is lack of evidence of harm," which in turn is [mistakenly] translated as "the chemical is harmless."[118]

A similar problem has arisen in relation to Gulf War Illness—the cluster of symptoms suffered by some 10,000 veterans who served in the Gulf War. The U.S. Departments of Defense and Veterans Affairs have issued reports claiming that they found "no evidence" that exposure to chemicals was responsible for the veterans' diseases. However, the House of Representatives Committee on Government Reform and Oversight adopted (unanimously) a report that strongly criticized the two departments for "the weakness of their efforts to establish the cause or causes of Gulf War Illness."[119] The departments' behavior, says the report, has been "plagued by arrogant incuriosity and a pervasive myopia that sees a lack of evidence as proof."[120] Tautologous as it may sound, a lack of evidence is not evidence.

A similar complaint might well be made about the toxicity studies that come from those scientists who are in the employ of the chemical manufacturing corporations. These studies sometimes seem to be characterized less by a desire to find the truth than by a desire to not find any evidence of toxicity.

In sum, what this principle urges us to clearly remember is that the absence of evidence for something is not evidence of the absence of that something.

9. Moderation in All Things

Finally, Aristotle's principle of "moderation in all things" (perhaps even moderation in applying the principle of moderation) may also be operative in matters of environmental health policy. "Nothing to excess" might be a better way of expressing it, and yet it seems that in the years since World War II we have failed to apply this principle to our manufacture and use of toxics. We have instead seen an immoderately excessive reliance on chemical technologies for dealing with an enormously wide variety of problems. The industrialized world came to embrace the advertising slogan, "Better living through chemistry," and has even seemed to be operating on the questionable assumption that "if some is good, then more is better." However, as Aristotle reminded us 2,300 years ago, more is not always better. More is sometimes worse, and sometimes more is deadly.

One intriguing theory from the field of evolutionary biology may provide us with a useful metaphor for understanding the modern world's overreliance on chemicals. The theory to which I'm referring[121] is an old attempt to suggest one possible evolutionary mechanism by which some species may have deadapted and become extinct.

This theory claims that sometimes a unique specialization which allows a given species to survive and reproduce can become, over countless generations, overdeveloped to such an extreme that it no longer has any positive survival value at all, and may in fact have negative survival value. One example of this process may be the simple gross bodily mass of the ruling reptiles. These dinosaurs' enormous body size was a unique adaptation that originally probably had great survival value for them. According to this theory, however, their body size continued to grow until it increased far beyond its point of species usefulness. It was almost as if the species had caught on to the value of this size specialization, and so continued to develop it until the great size was so exaggerated that it was no longer a benefit, but instead became a detriment, ultimately leading to the disappearance of the species. This is one instance where more was not necessarily better; in fact, more was lethal.

Another example of a genetic specialization developing past its point of usefulness may be the upward curving tusks of the ancient woolly mammoths. These large curved tusks were useful for fighting and for digging (according to the author of this theory), and thus were an adaptation that had great survival value for the mammoths. But over hundreds or thousands of generations, the tusks continued to curve further and further upward until they had curved so far upward that they were no longer useful for anything. They had overevolved, and thus may have helped account for the ultimate disappearance of the woolly mammoths.

Whether this theory has any validity (or whether it still has any adherents) is not my point. It can still prove useful as a metaphor for the human species and its present overuse of synthetic chemical agents.

Our use of some insecticides, for example, and of some antibiotics, antifungals, and rodenticides seems to have proven quite useful in our ability to cure or prevent the spread of certain diseases, and hence in our species' ability to survive and reproduce. Our moderate use of these compounds was a valuable adaptation that had significant survival value for us. But as the human species discovered the value of synthetic chemicals, we apparently theorized (perhaps unconsciously) that if some is good, more is better. And, in the process of a huge overproduction and overuse of these and other synthetic chemical compounds, we may well be taking what was originally an effective survival specialization and magnifying it to its destructive extreme. What once worked for the benefit of the species may turn out to be working toward its ultimate detriment.

One pesticide researcher, Mark Winston, says it clearly.

> The extent and impact of our current dependence on pesticides for both agricultural and nonagricultural purposes is staggering. In 1993, [an estimated] 1.1 billion pounds of active pesticide ingredients [i.e., not counting the so-called "inert" ingredients] were used in the United States, and 4.5 billion pounds world-wide. The U.S. figure translates to about 4 pounds of pesticides for every man, woman, and child in America. Considering that toxic dosages of most pesticides to humans are about one hundred thousandth to one millionth of a pound, that's a considerable amount of poison.[122]

With this quantity of exposure, we should not be surprised that we are seeing the kinds of emerging health effects outlined in Chapter One above. After all, "spraying a billion pounds of anything across the United States [every year] is bound to have side effects, let alone spraying that much of a potent chemical."[123]

Thus, the 20th century's experience with the gross overuse of synthetic chemicals of all sorts may be just one more example of the enormous destructive power of excess. Our failure to appreciate Aristotle's principle of moderation may turn out to be more than a moral failure; it may turn out to be a public health failure, and perhaps in the long run an economic failure. It could even ultimately work toward the detriment of the human species as a whole.

10. Summary

Here in Chapter Two, our analysis of guiding principles began with an outline of what risk assessment is and what its (rather severe) shortcomings are. Risk assessment, as the only method that guides policymaking about the manufacture, use and dispersal of environmental toxicants, is in desperate need of a very heavy counterbalance if the interests of communities and their health are to be sufficiently protected. The human rights approach to policy making provides that needed counterbalance.

In Chapter Three now, we address the following question: if the ethical principles we have examined above were to be taken seriously by legislators, elected officials and regulatory agencies, what would be some of the policy recommendations that a thoughtful and moral society would want to implement in order to protect the health, happiness, and well-being of its citizens?

Notes

1. D. Satcher, "CDC's First 50 Years: Lessons Learned and Relearned," *American Journal of Public Health*, 86, #12 (December 1996) 1705–08. p. 1706.
2. *Haemophilus influenzae* type B, a bacterial infection.
3. D. Satcher.
4. *Ibid.*
5. *Ibid.* Emphasis added.
6. "Poll: Definition of public health unclear to most Americans," *The Nation's Health* (February 1997) 24.
7. *Ibid.*
8. Noted in a speech by Gil Omenn, Dean of the School of Public Health and Community Medicine, University of Washington, delivered at the meeting of Grantmakers in Health, Fort Lauderdale, Florida, February 27, 1997. Cited in P. Montague, "Immune system toxins," *Rachel's Environment and Health Weekly*, #536 (March 6, 1997).
9. Ignaz Semmelweis (1818–65), the Hungarian physician who practiced at a Viennese lying-in hospital in the mid 19th century.
10. J. Mann, "Health and Human Rights: If Not Now, When?" *Health and Human Rights*, 2, Number 3 (1997) 113–20. p. 117.
11. Quoted in "Panel urges medicine to stess prevention, public health," *The Nation's Health*, XXVII, No. 1 (January 1997) 3.
12. *Healthy People 2010*, Office of Disease Prevention and Health Promotion, U.S. Department of Health and Human Services, Sept. 15, 1998, p. 54.
13. I am excluding, for now, the virtue-vice and character approaches to philosophical ethics.

14. J.S. Mill, *Utilitarianism* (London: 1863).

15. The term "harm" can sometimes be used as an approximate synonym for "cost."

16. The phrase "risk-benefit" is not a parallel linguistic construction, whereas the term "cost-benefit" is a parallel construction, according to Robert J. Levine, *Ethics and Regulation of Clinical Research*, second ed. (New Haven, CT: Yale University Press, 1986, 1988) 452+xx. This distinction, while not of crucial importance, is also not a trivial distinction. The term "risk," after all, means merely a *potential* cost, whereas the term "cost" means an actual real cost. The term "benefit," on the other hand, does not denote a potential benefit, but an actual benefit. Thus, when researchers use the phrase "risk-benefit" (rather than "cost-benefit") they are in effect weighing the merely *potential* costs (viz., risks) against the real *actual* benefits. This practice gives substantially more intellectual weight to the benefit side of the analysis (since the benefits are actual), and less intellectual weight to the cost side of the analysis (since "risks," after all, are only *potential* costs). The term "hazard," as used here, is approximately equivalent to the term "risk." Hazard is sometimes expressed as a probability of some specific harm or cost to some specific group of persons over some period of time.

17. The practice is only a few decades old, and outlined in National Research Council, *Risk Assessment in the Federal Government: Managing the Process* (Washington, D.C.: National Academy Press, 1983). The most recent set of guidelines for environmental risk assessment is G.S. Omenn, *Framework for Environmental Health Risk Management*, Presidential/Congressional Commission on Risk Assessment and Risk Management, January 1997. It can be found on the worldwide web at http://www.riskworld. com. I say "stepchild" only because Mill's work was primarily focused on philosophical considerations about the nature of right and wrong, and about the foundations of ethical decisionmaking. Today's risk assessment methods, in addition to their (relatively minor) concern with ethical issues, are more likely to be concerned with economic and power issues, and with weighing the concerns of corporate interests against the concerns of public health advocates. Today's risk assessment thinking, at least as evidenced in the relevant government documents, is also much less philosophically sophisticated than either Bentham's or Mill's work.

18. G.S. Omenn, *op. cit., p. 1.*

19. *Ibid.,* p. 15.

20. *Ibid.,* p. 18.

21. *Ibid.,* p. 10.

22. *Ibid.,* p. 9–10.

23. "The environmental justice movement of the 1980s and 1990s initially focused on claims that race and poverty are involved in the siting of undesirable facilities. Today, the charge has broadened to include all issues of environmental degradation." J.M. Guralnik and S.G. Leveille, "Comment: Environmental Racism and Public Health," *American Journal of Public Health*, 87, Number 5 (May 1997) 730–31.

24. In Chapter Two, section 3, below.

25. Quoted in P. Montague, "1997 Snapshots—Part 2," *Rachel's Environment and Health Weekly*, #579 (January 1, 1998).

26. G.J. Annas and M.A. Grodin, eds., *The Nazi Doctors and the Nuremberg Code: Human Rights in Human Experimentation* (New York, NY: Oxford University Press, 1992) 371+xxii. p. 267–68.

27. See Chapter Two, section 3, 3), below, for one Nazi doctor's words precisely to this effect.

28. An ethical analysis of exposure assessment might ask, for example, whether there are any significant socioeconomic or ethnic differences in the exposed and nonexposed populations (which groups, for example, are more likely to use city parks), and whether socioeconomic discrimination is something to be considered by decisionmakers. Such an analysis might also ask whether infants and young children, whose rates of respiration and metabolism are different to adults, and whose organ systems are immature and still in the process of development, might more likely be exposed to such herbicides, and whether possible discrimination against children should be considered by decisionmakers.

29. I hope to have made it clear that such public health considerations have not commonly been part of the risk assessment process in the past, and that the new *Framework* does not even suggest that these considerations be weighed into the equation in the future. I include it here in this illustration only as a possible "best case" scenario, not as a scenario that is likely to actually occur.

30. A correspondent tells me that Ottawa and its suburbs have passed legislation proscribing application of pesticides in city parks on city properties. She tells me that a suburb of Montreal has done the same.

31. M.H. O'Brien, "The Need to Assess Alternatives to the Production and Release of Dioxin." A speech presented at the San Francisco Bay Regional Water Quality Control Board workshop, Oakland, CA. (May 7, 1997).

32. G.S. Omenn, *op. cit.*, p. 32.

33. Quoted in B. Levy, "Public Health Requires Both Science and Advocacy," *The Nation's Health* (Feb. 1997) 2.

34. G.J. Annas and M.A. Grodin, eds., *op. cit.*, p. 53, 58.

35. "For example, exposing a pregnant rat to dioxin on day 15 of pregnancy causes effects that do not occur if the rat is exposed on day 14 or 16. This makes laboratory research on endocrine-disruptors a great deal more complex (and therefore more costly) than typical toxic chemical research." P. Montague, "The Weybridge Report," *Rachel's Environment and Health Weekly*, #547 (May 22, 1997).

36. P. Montague, "The Weybridge Report."

37. P. Montague, "The Weybridge Report."

38. For a very readable and detailed account of one example of this particular conflict, see C. Van Strum, *A Bitter Fog: Herbicides and Human Rights* (San Francisco: Sierra Club Books, 1983) 288+x.

39. A. de Tocqueville, *Democracy in America*, trans. Heffner, Richard D. (New York, NY: Penguin Books, 1835, 1840, 1984) 317. p. 105.

40. J. Mann, *op. cit.*, p. 113.

41. Preamble.

42. *Universal Declaration of Human Rights.* United Nations: 1948. 6. Preamble.

43. Preamble.

44. See, for example, J.B. Berkson, *A Canary's Tale: The Final Battle, Politics, Poisons, and Pollution vs. the Environment and the Public Health* (Hagerstown, MD: Self-published, 1996) 452+xviii. See also R. Jerome and M. Nelson, "Toxic Avenger," *People*, February 9, 1998: 113–15.

45. The assumed standard against which the health effects of toxics are measured is the 155 pound adult Caucasian male. Children, women, fetuses, the elderly, and even perhaps other ethnic groups, may well have quite different responses to a given dose of toxicant exposure. However, none of these possibilities are normally examined in standard toxicology testing.

46. See J. Harr, *A Civil Action* (New York: Random House, 1995) 500, for a clear and highly readable account of personal harm from chemical pollutants in the municipal water supply of one small town.

47. See Chapter One, section 15 above for one example. See also R. Jerome and M. Nelson, *op. cit.* See also J.B. Berkson, *op. cit.*

48. M. Lappé, *A Toxics Bill of Rights*, Center for Ethics and Toxics, 1996, Article 2.0.

49. *Draft Declaration on Human Rights and the Environment.* United Nations, 1994. Preamble.

50. *Ibid.,* Article 5.

51. *Ibid.,* Article 7.

52. *Ibid.,* Article 22.

53. *Ibid.,* Article 8.

54. *Ibid.,* Article 14.

55. *Ibid.,* Article 25.

56. *Ibid.,* Article 15.

57. J. Wargo, *Our Children's Toxic Legacy: How Science and Law Fail to Protect Us from Pesticides* (New Haven: Yale University Press, 1996) 380+xvi. p. 3. As a footnote to this disaster, "Emergency medical efforts were frustrated by the fact that no one knew what the chemical was." S. Steingraber, *Living Downstream: An Ecologist Looks at Cancer and the Environment* (Reading, MA: Addison-Wesley, 1997) 357+xvi. p. 101. Laws implementing the principle of full disclosure of information about toxics may well have been helpful in this incident.

58. Introduction to *Charter on Industrial Hazards and Human Rights.* Permanent People's Tribunal, 1996. p. 1–2.

59. G.J. Annas and M.A. Grodin, "Medicine and Human Rights: Reflections on the Fiftieth Anniversary of the Doctors' Trial," *Health and Human Rights*, 2, No. 1 (1996) 7–21. p. 9.

60. Introduction to *Charter on Industrial Hazards and Human Rights.* p. 2.

61. Replicated in Appendix V of this book.

62. *Charter on Industrial Hazards and Human Rights.* Preamble.

63. *Ibid.*

64. *Ibid.*, Article 1.

65. *Ibid.*

66. *Ibid.*, Article 15. It states: "Indigenous peoples have the right to protect their habitat, economy, society and culture from industrial hazards and environmentally destructive practices by economic enterprises."

67. Of course no environment is free from hazards, because life is not free from hazards. However, the context of this document is specifically the hazards that have resulted from the production of synthetic chemical agents, whether chemical agents are those deliberately produced as in the case of pesticides, or are unwanted byproducts of industrial processes, such as dioxins.

68. J. Wargo, *op. cit.*, p. 298.

69. *Charter on Industrial Hazards and Human Rights*. Article 8.

70. *Ibid.*, Article 11.

71. *Ibid.*, Article 9.

72. *Ibid.*, Article 12.

73. *Ibid.*, Article 14.

74. *Ibid.*

75. I believe that lindane is the only organochlorine insecticide still available for use in the U.S., though there have been arguments for banning it as well.

76. See, for example, N. Ashford and C.S. Miller, *Chemical Exposures: Low Levels, High Stakes*, first ed. (New York: Van Nostrand Reinhold, 1991) 214. p. 11–16 and 64–70.

77. *Charter on Industrial Hazards and Human Rights*. Article 17.

78. House Bill 1775, State of Washington, 55th Legislature, 1997 Regular Session. By Representatives Cole, Conway, Cody, Fisher, Wood, Cooper, Hatfield, Romero, Blalock, Keiser, Mason, Wolfe, Boldt, Doumit, O'Brien, Tokuda, Murray and Lantz. Read first time 02/07/97. Referred to Committee on Agriculture and Ecology. An act relating to notification of pesticide application.

79. N. Ashford and C.S. Miller, *Chemical Exposures: Low Levels, High Stakes*, second ed. (New York: Van Nostrand Reinhold (John Wiley & Sons, 1998) 440+xxiii. p. 159.

80. *Charter on Industrial Hazards and Human Rights*. Article 19.

81. *Ibid.*, Article 34.

82. For one illustration of how much money and effort chemical corporations are willing to put into opposing these rights, see J. Harr, *op. cit.*

83. D. Roe, et al. *Toxic Ignorance*. Environmental Defense Fund, 1997. Executive Summary. Consider also: "No toxicity data or minimal data are available for 66 percent of pesticides and their supposedly inert ingredients, 84 percent of cosmetic ingredients, 64 percent of drugs, 81 percent of food additives, and 88 to 90 percent of chemicals in commerce. Thus, scientific data concerning health effects of the vast majority of chemicals are woefully lacking." N. Ashford and C.S. Miller, *Chemical Exposures: Low Levels, High Stakes*, 2nd ed., p. 61–2.

84. D. Fagin and M. Lavelle, *Toxic Deception: How the Chemical Industry Manipulates Science, Bends the Law, and Endangers Your Health* (Secaucus, NJ: Carol Publishing Group, 1997) 294+xxvi. p. 3.

85. C. Duehring, "Overexposure from legal pesticiding: a generation at risk," *Medical and Legal Briefs*, 3, No. 6 (May/June 1998) 1–4. p. 3.

86. "This policy, Carson argued, had turned us into a nation of industry guinea pigs." J. Wargo, *op. cit.*, p. 82.

87. "Review of John Wargo, *Our Children's Toxic Legacy*," *American Journal of Public Health*, 87, Number 3 (March 1997) 473. The review explains that this experimentation "has placed children at risk because they are more vulnerable and more often exposed to certain pesticides than are adults."

88. G.J. Annas and M.A. Grodin, eds., *The Nazi Doctors and the Nuremberg Code*. p. 267–68.

89. Sometimes also termed the "teleological" approach.

90. I. Kant, *Fundamental Principles of the Metaphysic of Morals*. Vol. 42 of Trans. Thomas Kingsmill Abbott (Chicago: *The Great Books of the Western World*, Encyclopædia Britannica, Inc., 1785, 1952). p 272.

91. See Appendix II.

92. While the term "undue inducement" does not explicitly appear in the *Nuremberg Code*, the later WHO/CIOMS *Guidelines*, do include it in Guideline Number 4.

93. G.J. Annas and M.A. Grodin, "Medicine and Human Rights: Reflections on the Fiftieth Anniversary of the Doctors' Trial." p. 15.

94. *Ibid.*, p. 17–18.

95. *Ibid.*, p. 15.

96. B. Levy, "Conditions in which people can be healthy," *The Nation's Health*, 27, Number 4 (April 1997) 2.

97. J. Pieper, *The Four Cardinal Virtues: Prudence, Justice, Fortitude, Temperance* (Notre Dame, IN: University of Notre Dame Press, 1966) 234+xiii. p. 44.

98. This "silver rule" can be found in the teachings of virtually all of the world's great spiritual traditions. A few examples: "What you don't want done to yourself, don't do to others." (Confucian, 6th century BC.) "Hurt not others with that which pains thyself." (Buddhism, 5th century BC.) "Do not do unto others all that which is not well for oneself." (Zoroastrianism, 5th century BC.) "Do naught to others which if done to thee would cause thee pain." (Hinduism, Mahabharata, 3d century BC.) "What is hateful to yourself, don't do to your fellow man." (Rabbi Hillel, Judaism, first century BC.) Etc. from Editor, *The Bulletin of the King County Medical Society*, 73, #12 (December 1994) cover.

99. C. Hood and JDK C, eds., *Accident and Design: Contemporary Debaters in Risk Management* (London: UCL Press Limited, 1996) 253+xiv. p. 10–13.

100. Quoted *ibid.*, p. 14.

101. Quoted from Tait & Levidow *ibid.*, p. 10.

102. Quoted in T. Swearingen, "Activist Mom Wins Goldman Prize," *Rachel's Environment and Health Weekly*, #542 (April 17, 1997).

103. Quoted in J.B. Berkson, *op. cit.*, p. 171.

104. From p. 50 of the June 1996 preliminary draft of G.S. Omenn. *Framework for Environmental Health Risk Management.*

105. M. Lappé, *op. cit.*, article 2.4. My emphasis.

106. G.S. Omenn, *op. cit.*, p. 60.

107. This recommendation is taken from article 2.5 of M Lappé, *op. cit.*

108. *Ibid.*, article 2.0.

109. G. Hardin, "Carrying Capacity as an Ethical Concept." *Lifeboat Ethics: The Moral Dilemmas of World Hunger.* Eds. G.R. Lucas, Jr., and T.W. Ogletree (New York: Harper & Row, 1976) 120–31.

110. This is a gross oversimplification of Hardin's position.

111. S. Steingraber, *op. cit.*, p. 178.

112. *Ibid.*, p. 179.

113. "[R]esearchers also found pesticides that were thousands of miles away from where they had been sprayed. Trees in the Arctic, for example, were found to carry traces of insecticides used in tropical areas." *Ibid.*, p. 176.

114. *Ibid.*, p. 179.

115. M. Lappé, *Chemical Deception: The Toxic Threat to Health and the Environment* (San Francisco: Sierra Club Books, 1991) 360+xvi. p. 237–55.

116. *Ibid.*, p. 254.

117. We might think of soil and other environmental media as a commons as well.

118. S. Steingraber, *op. cit.*, p. 99–100.

119. M. Wadman, "Critics claim U.S. inquiry was 'irreparably flawed,'" *Nature*, 390, # 6. November 6 (1997) 4.

120. Quoted *ibid.*

121. I first came across this theory in ATW Simeons, *Man's Presumptuous Brain: An Evolutionary Interpretation of Psychosomatic Disease* (New York, NY: Dutton, 1960, 1961) 290.

122. M.L. Winston, *Nature Wars: People vs. Pests* (Cambridge, MA: Harvard University Press, 1997) 210+x. p. 11.

123. *Ibid.*, p. 12.

THREE

Modest Proposals

Where there is no vision, the people perish.
—Proverbs 29:18

It will be important to develop a central vision concerning what steps need to be taken to address the public health complications associated with the now burgeoning human exposure to toxics around the world.

In 1993, the Union of Concerned Scientists, headquartered in Cambridge, Massachusetts, issued a "World Scientists' Warning to Humanity," a document which had been signed by 1,670 scientists from 71 different countries around the world. Signatories included 104 Nobel laureates, which is a majority of the living recipients of the Prize in the sciences. The document warns that:

> Human beings and the natural world are on a collision course. Human activities inflict harsh and often irreversible damage on the environment and on critical resources. If not checked, many of our current practices put at serious risk the future that we wish for human society and the plant and animal kingdoms, and may so alter the living

154

world that it will be unable to sustain life in the manner that we know. Fundamental changes are urgent if we are to avoid the collision our present course will bring about.[1]

This document urges "fundamental changes" if the earth and its peoples are to avoid the damage predicted by these scientists. The signatories may well be correct about the need for fundamental changes in global policy regarding toxics, but my own recommendations here in Chapter Three are much more modest and, I hope, are more likely to be considered acceptable. Despite their moderateness and reasonableness, however, we will see in Chapter Four that these changes can be expected to face significant opposition from some very powerful and very interested parties.

We must keep in mind that, as Dr. Irving Selikoff says, "These are no longer scientific problems [alone]. They are social problems, they are political problems, and they are problems in which the scientist can only make a contribution, which, however necessary, is not sufficient."[2] I would add only that these are ethical problems as well, problems that demand an ethical analysis as well as a political and scientific analysis, problems that give rise to questions such as: What is ultimately best for us? What is the right course of action for us to take? What would the morally good society do in the face of these questions and issues? What choices would the morally just legislator make? These are the kinds of questions to which we now turn.

We begin with the almost universal recommendation, "More research is needed."

1. Research

Virtually everyone agrees that more research is needed. More research will need to be funded in a wide range of areas of concern. Some of these studies will be expensive, of course, but, according to a U.S. interagency draft report on chemical sensitivity disorders, "researchers and funding centers must accept these expenses as part of the price of sound public health science."[3]

Furthermore, as scientist René Dubos explains,

> The time has come to give to the study of the responses that the living organism makes to its environment the same dignity and support which is being given at present to the study of the component parts

of the organism.... Exclusive emphasis on the reductionist approach will otherwise lead biology and medicine into blind alleys.[4]

Until physicians and biologists understand how bodies react to the materials they encounter in their environments we will not fully understand the total impact of toxicant induced illnesses. We will, therefore, need to undertake research into environmental epidemiology, toxicology, delayed effects of toxicants on various body systems, clinical treatments for toxicant induced illnesses, the true total impact of toxics on human economies, and research into less toxic alternatives (especially to pesticides and to certain industrial chemicals and chemical byproducts). An enormous amount of research needs to be done, more than could be detailed in this short space. However, two or three areas deserve special mention.

BIOMEDICAL RESEARCH ON MCS

One of the 12 major recommendations urged by the 1992 WHO consultation on *Allergic Hypersensitivities Induced by Chemicals* was:

> New problems allegedly linked to hypersensitivity should receive rigorous scientific investigation to confirm the existence and nature of syndromes such as multiple chemical sensitivities.... Research should also facilitate the early detection of new and unknown allergens and chemicals in the environment and diet.[5]

Fortunately, the conceptual design for much of this research has already been well outlined. For example, research "to confirm the existence and nature of syndromes such as multiple chemical sensitivities," one of the more controversial disorders, has been outlined by Dr. Claudia Miller in much of her work.[6] Her design would employ one of the most rigorous and powerful experimental protocols it is possible to use in biomedical research involving human subjects—double-blind, placebo controlled, human challenge studies.[7]

These studies, as Miller outlines them, would need to be performed in a hospital-based Environmental Medical Unit (EMU). Unfortunately only one EMU presently exists in the U.S., the one that is housed in William Rea's Environmental Health Center in Dallas, Texas.[8] But there are efforts under way to finance and construct other EMUs for research purposes.[9]

An EMU is an in-hospital individual dwelling unit specially designed, constructed, furnished, and operated so as to minimize exposure of the inhabitant to airborne (as well as to waterborne and foodborne) toxicants. Ventilation systems are designed to provide the maximum fresh, filtered outside air so that the inhabitant is exposed to only minimal particulate and fume contamination. CS Miller has described an EMU thus:

> By definition, an EMU is in a hospital where patients can remain 24 [hours] a day in a clean environment for up to several weeks. Like an intensive care unit or a coronary care unit, the EMU would be a specialized, dedicated hospital facility. The EMU must be in a hospital to accommodate very sick patients; [conventional toxicology] exposure chambers do not offer comparable levels of care. Because chemical challenges may precipitate bronchoconstriction, mental confusion, severe headaches, depression, and other disabling symptoms, these patients should not be tested in an exposure chamber on an outpatient basis.
>
> Conventional exposure chambers do not reduce background chemical exposures for extended periods (up to several weeks) so the effects of a particular challenge in a patient can be assessed accurately. This is the central limitation of [conventional] exposure chambers and the reason they should not be used to rule in or rule out chemical sensitivity. If subjects are not kept in a clean environment for several days before and during challenges, false positive responses may occur because of interfering exposures and false negative responses may occur because of masking. In contrast to [a conventional] exposure chamber, an EMU would minimize interfering exposures before and during challenges, thus maximizing the reliability and reproducibility of test responses.[10]

The design of these human challenge studies would be quite straightforward, and would look something like the following. A subject who is suspected of being sensitive to certain environmental incitants would be housed in an EMU and provided with chemically less-contaminated food and water for some period of time, perhaps four to seven days, before challenge studies were initiated. This preliminary period provides the subject with an opportunity to be less exposed to ambient toxicants, in order to "unmask" and to have their chronic symptoms diminish or clear, so that effects of the administered incitants will be more robust and noticeable.

After this period of time has elapsed, subjects will then be challenged with various incitants, in a double-blind, placebo controlled manner, and monitored for symptomatic responses to those challenges.

This experimental methodology would provide clear empirical

evidence that researchers could use "to determine in the most direct and definitive manner possible whether chemical sensitivities exist."[11] The EMU could thus be used as a research tool for questions relating health effects to etiology in general, and it could also be used as a diagnostic tool for individual patients to determine which incitants are most likely to cause them to have which physical reactions.

The methodology is based on a set of research postulates laid out by Claudia Miller—we will refer to them as Miller's postulates—that are analogous to Robert Koch's four postulates for determining which (and whether) infectious agents were responsible for diseases such as tuberculosis, anthrax, cholera and so on.

Very briefly, Koch's four postulates for determining whether a given microbe is etiologic for a given disease are, in rough form, the following:

1. That unique microbe must be found present in all cases of the disease.

2. That unique microbe must be able to be taken from the host and isolated in a pure culture.

3. Inoculations of that cultured microbe into animal hosts must then produce in those hosts the identical disease.

4. That unique microbe must then be able to be taken from the new hosts and again isolated in pure culture.

In other words, if you find the same microbe in all cases of a disease, if you are able to culture that microbe and inject it into another host so that that host too gets the same disease, and if you are then able to culture that microbe out of all the newly diseased hosts, then at that point you can safely say that that microbe is etiologic for that particular disease. That bug causes that disease.

Claudia Miller's four analogous research postulates would be used similarly to determine etiologicity with respect to environmental chemical incitants and patient symptoms. Miller's postulates would, if met in a strictly controlled EMU environment, "confirm (and it not met, refute) that a person's symptoms were caused by a particular substance."[12] Her four postulates are:

1. When a subject simultaneously avoids all chemical, food and drug incitants, remission of symptoms occurs (unmasking).

2. A specific constellation of symptoms occurs with reintroduction of a particular incitant.

3. Symptoms resolve when the incitant is again avoided.

4. With reexposure to the same incitant, the same constellation of symptoms reoccurs, provided that the challenge is conducted within an appropriate window of time. Clinical observations suggest that an ideal window is 4 to 7 days after the last exposure to the test incitant.[13]

It will be crucial in these experiments to rigorously control for the phenomenon of masking, since if this is not adequately taken into account, then data from the testing could be entirely unreliable; i.e., if researchers do not control for the effects of masking, there would be a much greater likelihood that the tests would yield false negatives.

The phenomenon of masking can best be explained thus: when subjects are exposed to a variety of incitants in their environment, they may be experiencing simultaneous physical reactions to several of those incitants, all in varying degrees. It will be, in that situation, much more difficult to isolate the physical effects of any one particular incitant because of the ongoing "background noise" of reactions to the other incitants. If a person normally drinks ten to fifteen cups of coffee in any given day, for example, and one wishes to test for the effects on that person of just one cup of coffee at 1:00 P.M., the effects of that one particular cup of coffee may be "masked" by the nearby effects of all the other previous cups. That is, any physical effects that may be caused by the 1:00 P.M. cup may not be robustly evident because those effects could have been covered up (masked) by the lingering background effects of all the previous cups. That person may then mistakenly report that an individual cup of coffee at 1:00 P.M. has no, or almost no, effect on them. This may actually, however, be a case of a false negative. If the subject were to refrain from drinking coffee for perhaps four to seven days prior to the challenge test, so that the masking effects of coffee stimulation and withdrawal could subside, then the physical effects of the one cup may become much more clinically evident.

Miller describes the phenomenon of masking in this way:

> Masking and unmasking are colorful lay terms for which there is no scientific equivalent. Nevertheless, investigators' abilities to understand masking and unmasking and manipulate these variables knowledgeably may determine the success of studies in this area. When chemically sensitive patients follow a diet free of their problem foods and live in a relatively chemical-free home in the hills of central Texas

where there are no major agricultural or industrial operations or air contaminants, they say they are in an unmasked state. Under these circumstances they claim that if a diesel truck drove by they could identify specific symptoms due to the diesel exhaust, for example, irritability, headache, or nausea.

On the other hand, the patients report that when they travel to a large city like Houston or New York City, stay in a hotel room, and eat in restaurants, they become masked. In the presence of many concurrent exposures (exhaust, fragrances, volatiles offgassing from building interiors, various foods) in New York City many report feeling chronically ill, as if they had the flu. If a diesel truck drove by under these circumstances, most report they would not be able to attribute any particular symptoms to the exhaust because of background noise from overlapping symptoms occurring as a consequence of overlapping or successive exposures.[14]

At least in theory, says Miller, "such background noise or masking hides the effects of individual exposures—responses are blurred."[15] For this reason, it will be important for investigators to control for the effects of masking, and the only truly effective way to do this is by use of the EMU.

The challenge testing in these trials must be done in a blinded fashion as well. This means that both incitants and placebos must be administered at doses well below the olfactory threshold so that subjects are not able to detect by smell whether they are being challenged or not. (The more rigorous form of these challenge tests will be double-blinded so that the person who administers the challenge substance and observes the consequent effects on the subject also does not know whether the challenge substance is a toxicant or placebo.)

In addition, all clinical precautions must be taken to help subjects recover as quickly as possible from any symptoms that may result from these direct challenge exposures. Any techniques (such as the administration of trisalts, for example,[16] or buffered vitamin C) that can help a subject recover more quickly from the effects of their exposures should be made available to them.

Apart from these scientific and clinical considerations, there are ethical considerations. All these research protocols would require that each prospective subject be fully informed about any potential risks to their health and well-being that could possibly result from their participation in the research, as well as about the possible benefits to them and to the human community. Every precaution must be taken to insure that subjects are able to freely give or deny consent for participation in these protocols, in accord with the provisions of both the *Nuremberg Code* and the 1993 WHO/CIOMS *International Ethical Guidelines for Biomedical Research Involving Human Subjects*. Moreover, in the case of human challenge studies (where human beings will be directly exposed to a pathogenic agent), special care must be taken to insure that subjects are aware of the adverse effects they may suffer as a result of the direct challenges (with toxicants). For many chemically sensitive subjects, they will already be acutely aware of what some of their particular physical reactions are to toxicant exposures; many of them suffer those effects almost daily during the course of their regular lives. It is thus likely that it will not be difficult for such EMU studies, despite the fact that they are direct challenge studies, to meet all the necessary requirements for ethically proper protocols.

If protocols such as these are undertaken, the test results should make abundantly clear the associations between exposure to toxicants and the subsequent clinical symptoms. Indeed, a body of such tests, if they were to yield positive results, would be strong evidence for actual causality—that those chemical incitants used in the challenge do in fact cause those symptoms experienced by the patient.

While the philosopher David Hume (1711–1776), in *An Enquiry Concerning Human Understanding*,[17] may be quite correct in his epistemological claim that we do not ever directly experience unmediated causality, still we may at least deduce (with varying degrees of confidence) the existence of some instances of causality. Sir Austin Bradford Hill, in a classic study entitled *the Environment and Disease: Association or Causation*,[18] offered nine criteria which, if met, would be sufficient to deduce cause and effect.[19] These criteria are: (1) strength of the association between the exposure and the illness; i.e., how closely are exposure and illness associated with each other? (2) Consistency; i.e., "Have different people in different places and times observed the association?"[20] (3) Specificity of the association. (4) Temporality; "Does the exposure precede the illness?"[21] (5) Biological gradient; "An association that follows a biological gradient or dose-response curve strongly suggests causality."[22] (6) Plausibility; "Hill comments that it is helpful if the causation we suspect is biologically plausible, but that what is plausible depends upon the biological knowledge of the time: 'in short, the association we observe may be new to science or medicine and we must not dismiss it too light-heartedly as just too odd.'"[23] (7) Coherence; "The cause-and-effect relationship under scrutiny should not conflict with other generally known facts about the disease." (Miller adds: "Since so little research has been done on MCS, so far this has not been a problem.")[24] (8) Experiment; the EMU experiments outlined above can be expected to provide the kind of data to which Hill is referring here. (9) Analogy; sometimes cause and effect can be inferred by analogy. For example, "The sensitivities reported by MCS patients are reminiscent of the heightened sensitivity to tobacco smoke reported by those who have recently quit smoking. Likewise, there are close parallels between MCS and addiction [to intoxicants]..."[25] (10) Miller then adds a tenth criterion which, if met, would also help establish causality: unique symptomatology. She explains:

> The more obscure or unique a symptom is, particularly if it is reported by several independent exposure groups (for example, industrial workers, white collar professionals, Gulf veterans), the greater the likelihood of causation. For MCS, it would be difficult to imagine that the curious symptom of odor intolerance, which has been reported by demographically diverse groups following various exposure events, could be "invented" by all of them. Equally unexpected and counterintuitive are MCS patients' practices of avoiding fragrances, foods, alcoholic beverages, etc., that they formerly relished. Why would anyone who really liked pizza, chocolate or beer give them up unless they made them ill? Why would a mechanic who loved his job and used to think that WD-40 would make a wonderful perfume, suddenly report that odors at work made him ill, if in fact they did not? Why would doctors, lawyers, teachers and others say they quit their professions because of severe mental confusion around fragrances and engine exhaust, if this weren't the case? Scientifically, it would be absurd to dismiss such eccentric behaviors in otherwise sane individuals without searching *exhaustively* for a plausible biological basis.[26]

Hill makes it clear that no one of these nine (or ten) criteria are completely sufficient in order to infer causation, and none is a *sine qua non*. Rather, in aggregate, the criteria help us in determining probable causality.

With the help of Hill's criteria, Miller's postulates, and the EMU described above, investigators should be able to determine what some of the causal agents are which both sensitize people to chemicals, and which then trigger symptoms in those who have already become sensitized.

ECONOMIC IMPACT STUDIES

In addition to this kind of clinical and biomedical research, economic and social impact studies should be done for toxicant induced illnesses. For example, Ashford and Miller recommend that the U.S. federal government "undertake controlled studies of the economic and social effects of indoor air quality on the workplace."[27] The 1992 WHO consultation also strongly urges that, "The true personal and financial costs of human disease due to environmental chemical allergens should be analyzed."[28] After all, "the health care costs [alone] associated with these conditions are undeniably enormous."[29] Health care costs in the U.S. alone have risen gigantically in recent decades, "from 5.3 percent of the GDP in 1960 to 13.9 percent in 1993, with a dollar value exceeding $1 trillion, nearly $4,000 per person. An important question is, how much does toxicant-induced loss of tolerance contribute to this sum?"[30] The larger question is, how much do all the combined toxicant induced illnesses outlined in Chapter One (including MCS) contribute to this sum?

We clearly do need studies that will analyze the economic impact, both direct and indirect, of these diseases on local and national communities and economies. It should, after all, become increasingly clear to society that it "has an interest in preventing and limiting the problem of chemical sensitivity"[31] and other toxicant induced illnesses. For instance, one study has concluded that asthma alone costs the economy in one U.S. city (Seattle) approximately $40 million annually just in lost work alone.[32] Other cities may find the economic impact of such environmentally induced respiratory disorders equally severe. However, a true economic impact study would look at much more than just lost work statistics, important as that factor is. A fuller study would examine the total impact of toxicant induced disorders on an economy, including the ongoing medical costs to families, lost time in school, lost work both for the person who has the disorder and for their caregivers and lost productivity in other spheres. The ripple effects of that lost productivity on other aspects of the economy would also need to be taken into account.

One economic analyst who looked at the total impact of toxicant induced disorders associated with poor indoor air quality has found that the impact is not small. James Woods, a consultant on indoor air pollution, has estimated that "$60 billion in income and productivity is lost annually [in the U.S.] because of employees' falling sick from MCS and other problems linked to sick-building syndrome."[33]

Studies such as this one, if done with sufficient scope and exactness, may help policymakers in their legislative efforts to minimize the likely impact of toxicants on people's health and consequently on the economy.

EPIDEMIOLOGY, TOXICOLOGY, AND TREATMENT STUDIES

In addition, more epidemiological studies to determine the prevalence and increasing incidence of toxicant induced illnesses are also needed. One such study entitled "Ecology of Increasing Disease: Population Growth and Environmental Degradation," appeared in the October 1998 issue of the journal *Bioscience*. This study, based on data from sources such as the World Health Organization and the U.S. Centers for Disease Control and Prevention, concluded that an estimated 40 percent of deaths each year can be attributed to various environmental factors, particularly organic and chemical pollutants. If these findings are corroborated by future research, it would also be data worth including in studies that attempt to analyze the total economic impact of toxicant induced illnesses.[34]

Studies which could provide a fuller toxicological understanding of these chemical substances—both for single chemicals and for the mixtures of chemicals to which people are regularly exposed in their day-to-day lives—are also needed. Any such studies which use human beings as research subjects must, of course, be designed in such a way as to meet all ethical requirements for the protection of those subjects.[35] Evidence has emerged suggesting that some pesticide manufacturing companies have already begun to test some of their products using methods of direct challenge in human subjects, and the ethical propriety of these experiments has been questioned.[36] Any such experiments done with human beings as subjects will run the risk of being ethically very complex.

Research into new treatment modalities to help those who are already suffering from toxicant induced conditions is also desperately needed, especially since current treatment options are so limited and have such checkered success.

Such studies are clearly needed sooner rather than later because, as one report on chemical sensitivity concludes, "the sooner ... research is funded to better understand, treat, and perhaps even prevent the illness, the lower [will be] the cost to the economy, health, and life in the long run."[37]

Finally, the results of such research need to be widely disseminated so that they can be made available to a wider audience than just the medical specialists directly associated with chemical injury. Family physicians and other primary health care providers, for example, should be able to readily access the results of research related to chemical injury. Some of the best work in the effort to widely disseminate such original research was undertaken by Cindy Duehring and her Environmental Access Research Network (EARN), the central publication of which is the bimonthly journal *Medical and Legal Briefs*.[38] Ms. Duehring's work in the publication of current medical research and legal decisions related to toxicant induced illnesses was given high recognition some years ago when she received Sweden's highly regarded Right Livelihood Award (widely considered to be the alternative Nobel Prize) in December 1997.[39]

Our first recommendation, therefore, is that research into toxicant induced illnesses should become a high priority. We turn our attention next to a recommendation involving how clinicians should approach toxicant induced illnesses.

2. Initial Clinical Presumptions

Initial clinical presumptions should favor those diagnostic interpretations of patient symptoms that claim organic etiologies rather than those that claim psychological etiologies.

This means simply that when a patient presents in a physician's office with certain physical complaints, the physician's initial presumption should be that the cause of these complaints is in the realm of the physical rather than in the realm of the psychological. The primary reason for this presumption lies in the high risk of physiologic damage to the patient if clinicians were to presume a psychological diagnosis while an underlying organic condition was ignored and therefore continued to go unrecognized, undiagnosed, and untreated.

This is actually one of the fundamental and generally-accepted principles of standard clinical diagnosis,[40] that any possible organic etiologies for the patient's condition should first be conclusively ruled out before settling on a psychological diagnosis. Unfortunately, however, this "has simply not been done for illnesses associated with low-level chemical exposure."[41]

According to this principle, the full range of laboratory assays, examination by relevant specialists, and reviews of appropriate current research literature should be fully explored before concluding that a condition is psychogenic. One example of how this principle operates is nicely described in a little book by Berton Roueché, a collection of true stories of diagnostic medical detective work.[42] The story in question occurred in 1979 and involved Mrs. McBride, a 43-year-old woman, widowed and with three teenage daughters, who presented to an internist (on referral from her gynecologist) with the following symptoms: besides the low hemoglobin (for which the gynecologist had referred her to the internist), she also suffered from

> [p]ains in her stomach, and a burning sensation lower down ... [in] the left upper quadrant of the abdomen. She said she also seemed to be tired most of the time. She couldn't do her regular exercises. Her muscles ached, and she had occasional dizzy spells. And everything seemed to irritate her, especially her children.[43]

In addition, on physical examination, the woman's spleen was slightly palpable. This was not considered entirely normal, but also was not considered clearly diagnostic of any specific conditions. In the internist's view,

> There was nothing remarkable about any of Mrs. McBride's complaints. They could all very well have been functional [psychological] in origin. But somehow she [the internist] didn't think they were. Mrs. McBride just didn't impress her as a neurotic type. An instinct told her that those pains and aches, the dizzy spells and the fatigue, the irritability and the myalgia had some organic root.[44]

A variety of lab tests were eventually ordered which did reveal an organic disorder but did not reveal anything about its possible cause. Only after an enormous amount of dedicated detective work on the part of the internist, including numerous lab tests and a personal visit by her and another physician to Mrs. McBride's home (which included her art studio), was a diagnosis of lead poisoning finally confirmed.

According to the internist, Mrs. McBride's symptoms could easily have been diagnosed as psychogenic, particularly given her challenging situation as a widow with three teenage daughters. In addition, the internist could perhaps have concluded that as an artist Mrs. McBride may have been possessed of a somewhat "sensitive" or "artistic" personality, and thus may perhaps have been more susceptible to psychosomatic complaints. But the internist did not make these psychological presumptions. Instead, her (the internist's) initial clinical presumption favored an organic etiology, and this indeed did turn out to be an accurate presumption, though it took dedicated and caring detective work on her part to prove it. Beginning with the presumption of an organic etiology is an important precaution for diagnosticians to keep in mind.

Again, the reason for this precaution is that, if an underlying organic condition is ignored or missed as a result of a too hasty diagnosis of psychogenicity, organic damage may continue to occur—and may continue to be ignored.[45] Such an overhasty psychological diagnosis would then have caused unnecessary, and perhaps irremediable, physical harm to the patient.

This precaution is thus an expression of one of the most fundamental original principles of medical ethics—"First do no harm" (*primum non nocere*). This principle means that the first thing the clinician should be concerned about is to at least not make things worse. Physicians who initially presume, and too soon conclude, psychogenicity may easily miss underlying organic disorders, and thereby—as a result of their too hasty psychological diagnosis—cause further untreated organic damage.

Therefore, in the absence of being able to absolutely verify a clear psychological etiology for a given condition, the basic *primum non nocere* principle of medical ethics requires that the initial clinical presumption should always favor interpretations that claim an organic etiology. This principle will particularly apply in cases of newly emerging diseases and newly emerging disease etiologies. Some clinicians may be tempted, of course, when they see a patient with a set of symptoms they have not seen before, to start with an initial presumption that the condition is probably psychogenic, particularly if some of the symptoms seem to be analogous to psychogenic symptoms they have seen before. Our "organicity" principle, however, argues that such a presumption is wrongheaded and potentially dangerous. As Claudia Miller points out,

> There are about 37,000 psychiatrists and 241,000 psychologists in the United States. Any theory of disease so bold as to suggest that depression, anxiety, panic attacks or fatigue might be caused by chemical exposures should expect a less than enthusiastic reception. Yet, most would agree in principle that organic bases for illnesses should be ruled out before psychological explanations are invoked.[46]

This organicity principle should especially be applied in the case of any diseases which have become highly politicized. Many of the emerging toxicant induced disorders have become, for various reasons, highly politicized, much like HIV/AIDS became so highly politicized in the early years of that pandemic. This politicization has largely been a consequence of opposition by chemical manufacturing corporations, and the public relations firms which serve them. MCS, GWS, CFS, FMS and other toxicant induced conditions have all become highly politicized. And in many cases clinicians have been rather too quick to diagnose people suffering from them as having disorders with a psychological, rather than a physiologic, etiology.

It should not come as any great surprise to see, along with the emergence of so many new chemical technologies, the simultaneous emergence of new medical symptomologies. Along with the burgeoning proliferation of new synthetic chemical toxicants in our food, water, air, and soil, and with the consequent enormous increase in human exposures to such a wide variety of ubiquitous chemical agents, as well as exposures to an even greater variety of environmental mixtures of those chemical agents, clinicians rather should probably be surprised if they did not see new pathologies. They should certainly not be surprised to see some old diseases (such as asthma) beginning to show up with newly emerging etiologies (such as Reactive Airway Disease Syndrome).

For these reasons, a recent set of guidelines for health professionals was issued jointly by EPA, the U.S. Consumer Product Safety Commission, the American Lung Association, and the American Medical Association. It clearly states that "the current consensus is that in cases of claimed or suspected MCS, complaints should not be dismissed as psychogenic, and a thorough workup is essential."[47]

Yet another factor contributing to this failure of physicians to recognize organic etiologies for toxicant induced illnesses such as MCS is that "most physicians do not usually obtain [adequate] occupational or environmental histories on their patients, and patients themselves may not be fully aware of possible precipitating events or exposures."[48] In the absence of such data about effects of physical exposures to toxicants, it may simply be easier for clinicians to conclude that a psychological etiology is perfectly acceptable for their diagnostic purposes.

After all, as Susan Sontag has pointed out so well in her classic *Illness as Metaphor*,[49] the less that is understood about a disease the more likely it is that the disease will be characterized as having a psychological etiology. In this study Sontag examines the common perceptions of tuberculosis in the 19th century as a disease of the overly passionate and of those with sensitive and artistic temperaments. These psychological explanations could only be plausible, of course, prior to 1882 when Robert Koch published the first paper in which he described his discovery of *Mycobacterium tuberculosis* and established its role in the cause of TB.[50] As soon as the microbial causes of TB became well understood, the psychological characterizations of the disease began to fall away almost immediately. Sontag then analyses the common misperceptions of cancer—and "the cancer personality"—in the 20th century in the same way that she analyzed the perceptions of TB in the 19th. She concludes that, "Theories that diseases are caused by mental states ... are always an index of how much is not understood about the physical terrain of a disease."[51] The more we understand about diseases, the less we resort to psychological interpretations to make sense of them.

"Moreover," she adds, "there is a peculiar modern predilection for psychological interpretations of disease, as of everything else."[52] One of the problems with such explanations of diseases is that psychological explanations sometimes tend to "undermine the 'reality' of a disease."[53] And perhaps worse than that,

> Psychological theories of illness are a powerful means of placing the blame on the ill. Patients who are instructed that they have, unwittingly, caused their disease are also being made to feel that they have deserved it.[54]

"Punitive notions of disease have a long history,"[55] unfortunately, and perhaps satisfy a certain need in all of us, physicians and nonphysicians alike, to help us feel that we understand something which we in fact do not understand. Such (blame the victim) theories perhaps also serve a perverse comforting function for certain people—somehow assuring them that they, at least, since they do not deserve it, will not contract the disease in question—regardless of the harm these theories may do to others.

In any case, regardless of the unfortunate comfort that such psychological interpretations of disease may offer, clinicians have an obligation to make all efforts to discover or rule out every possible organic cause of disease before they turn to psychological explanations.

In sum, this "organicity" principle simply requires that clinicians always initially presume an organic etiology for the symptoms of their patients, and only later—only after exhaustive labwork, consultations with specialists, and reviews of recent relevant research literature have ruled out all possible physical causes—only then should clinicians entertain the diagnosis of a psychological rather than physical etiology for their patients' symptoms.

3. Informed Consent

Practices implementing the principle of informed consent and the right to know should become general policy and should be reflected in normal business and consumer practices.

Since 1988, to offer one small example, the U.S. federal government has required warning labels on all wines that contain more than 10 parts per million of total sulfites because it is known that a certain small percentage of people in the U.S. are allergic to sulfites. People who are allergic to them can experience headaches, hives, asthma, cramps, flushing, and other such symptoms on exposure to levels as low as 20 ppm. The U.S. FDA reports that approximately 0.4 percent of the U.S. population, or about one million people, are highly allergic to sulfites.

The purpose of the warning labels is to inform wine drinkers of the presence of sulfites so that they can themselves decide whether to take the risk of being exposed to a substance that may cause them to develop physical symptoms.

Labels informing consumers about the presence of sulfites in wines are not, of course, the only warning labels required by law. Cigarette manufacturers are required to include a warning on each package of cigarettes—and in each advertisement for cigarettes— informing purchasers of potential adverse health effects from using their product. Dentists in California are required by state law to inform all their patients about potential adverse health effects that may result from the use of mercury in silver amalgam dental fillings. This warning, which must be posted in all dental offices, reads:

> This dental office uses amalgam filling materials which contain and expose you to mercury, a chemical known to the state of California to cause birth defects and other reproductive harm. Please consult your dentist for more information.[56]

This requirement is based on California's Proposition 65, passed in 1986, which "mandates the public be informed about products that pose a health risk."[57]

Another state, Massachusetts, has recently passed a law which, according to the *Nation's Health*, [requires] tobacco manufacturers to identify the additives in each brand of cigarettes or smokeless tobacco sold in the commonwealth and to reveal how much nicotine those products yield.... Manufacturers must disclose not only the amount of nicotine before burning, but other variables that affect nicotine delivery, such as the pH of the smoke and the percentage of ventilation in the filter.[58]

Tobacco companies, predictably, strongly opposed these right-to-know laws, but a federal court (in the Massachusetts case) subsequently upheld the state's right to regulate tobacco products.[59]

Of course, not everyone who drinks wines with sulfites experiences adverse symptoms, and not everyone who smokes cigarettes develops cancer or cardiovascular disease, but a certain percentage of people do. The purpose of warning labels and notices is to inform citizens about potential health risks so that the power of choice, and the ability to take responsibility for their own health-related decisions, lies with them rather than with the state or with a product's manufacturer or distributor.

Laws requiring such labeling are thus based on the idea of freedom of choice. The philosophical foundations for the idea of freedom of choice are the twin ethical principles of autonomy and respect for persons. These two principles together require that all people "who are capable of deliberation about their personal choices should be treated with respect for their capacity for self-determination."[60] These principles require that citizens be allowed the power, the information, and the freedom to make their own decisions about matters which directly concern their own and their family's health and safety.

These twin principles—autonomy and respect for persons—are two of the fundamental operating principles upon which modern democratic states are based, and these deserve, therefore, to be reflected in the public policies of those states. For the most part they have been. In matters related to toxics exposures, however, they have not, at least not always. They should be.

As the CETOS *Toxics Bill of Rights* expresses this principle, "Labeling, disclosure and explanation of testing, ingredients or components with potential toxicity in any commercial commodity shall be conveyed voluntarily and fully without regard to proprietary privileges."[61] This means that information about potentially harmful ingredients in a product must be fully disclosed by the manufacturer, regardless of whether that information might be considered proprietary, or protectable as a trade secret.

In the world of medical ethics, these twin principles have been reflected in the principle of informed consent. The principle of informed consent is operative in biomedical research, in clinical medicine, and in our purchase and use of pharmaceutical products; it clearly states that it is unethical to expose a human being to any procedure, substance, or risk without that person's informed consent. This means that the person in question must be fully informed about the nature and extent of the potential risks and potential benefits. They must be given the opportunity to reflect on that information, and finally must be given the opportunity to freely give or deny consent to accept that risk.

Statutory requirements that citizens be given all relevant information about potential health risks of the products to which they may be exposed, as recommended here, would simply be public policy's reflection of the principles of informed consent, autonomy, and respect for persons.

These same principles would also require that citizens be informed about potential threats to their and their family's health and well-being in the form of pesticides, industrial solvents, industrial byproducts and toxics releases, building materials, consumer products (such as bedding, padded furniture, clothing, household products, artificial fragrances, cleaning materials, and so on), as well as toxicant residues in food and water. Citizens should be allowed to make their own informed decisions about these matters directly related to their own (and their family's) health and well-being, and they should be given *all* relevant information so they can make wise choices. Government agencies should not have the power to make these decisions for them.

Writing in the context of her work with herbicide issues, Carol Van Strum argues that,

> Instead of politically vulnerable government agencies making such decisions in secret, based on secret information, the public itself could decide whether to accept the risk of cancer, birth defects, genetic damage, miscarriages, neurological and other disorders in return for redder apples, dandelion-free lawns, cheaper lemons, or a higher allowable timber harvest.
>
> To those who bear the risk, exposure to poisons is a matter of life and death. Decisions about poisons which disrupt the basic mechanisms of life and the integrity of future generations raise profound moral questions. Society cannot afford to entrust such decisions to corporate or political entities that exempt themselves from the restraints of morality and ethics.[62]

Implementing the principle of informed consent in public policy would mean that individual citizens, in fact and not just in principle, would have both the information and the power necessary to make their own risk-benefit judgments about the products and services available for their use.

Unfortunately, some legislators in one state (Oregon), acting in consort with the wishes of corporations who do business there, attempted in 1998 to pass a law specifically *opposing* the principle of informed consent. The Oregon House of Representatives bill 3281 reads in part:

> No city, town, county, regional authority or other political subdivision of this state shall adopt or enforce any ordinance, rule or regulation requiring collection or reporting of information relating to the use, storage, possession, transportation or composition of hazardous substances if a primary intent of such ordinance, rule or regulation is the distribution of the information to the public.[63]

Any corporations involved in the manufacture, distribution, use, storage, or disposal of toxics would likely be pleased if legislation like this were to be enacted. But such laws would clearly not serve the health interests of the community at all. Nor would they serve the principles on which modern democratic states have been founded. Wise judgments can be effectively made only when an electorate has been adequately and properly informed about the matters on which they are asked to vote. This means that citizens have a clear right to have access to full and accurate information about matters that could directly affect their and their family's physical health and well-being.

This principle of informed consent, based as it is on the fundamental principles of autonomy and respect for persons, seems so fundamental to the workings of a modern democratic state that some in the U.S. have suggested that it be made part of the law of the land, and be added as an amendment to the U.S. *Constitution*. Van Strum says:

> An informed-consent amendment could provide that no law nor [sic] court shall limit or impair the people's right to obtain on a timely basis full disclosure of information about matters which may affect them; nor[,] except to protect from a clearly greater harm[,] shall any person be unnecessarily deprived, in time of war or peace, of the right to ... informed consent before being exposed to a potentially harmful substance or energy form.[64]

Van Strum, one of the proponents of such an amendment, believes that, "The campaign for this reasonable constitutional right could provide a positive focus for the many citizen groups now exhausting themselves in separate battles for the same thing."[65] She is fully aware, of course, that "[i]ndustry and government would understandably find informed consent distasteful. They would proclaim it," she continues,

> impractical and expensive, and inimical to public welfare—claims which have little more credibility than unfounded claims of pesticide safety. In opposing informed consent, industry and government would have to [in effect] admit that toxic exposure does occur and that people have no right either to know about it or to stop it. They would have to convince the public that ignorance and helplessness are preferable to knowledge and control.[66]

She also believes that a campaign to draw up and ratify an informed consent constitutional amendment, even if the process ultimately did not succeed in accomplishing ratification, would still serve as an important educational process in itself, and may even have some effect on people's market expectations and purchasing behaviors.

We will look briefly at one specific example to illustrate how an informed consent amendment (or law) could operate in public policy. A current controversy, described at some length by Stauber and Rampton in their book *Toxic Sludge Is Good for You*, will serve as our example. This controversy concerns the present use of sewage sludge for agricultural fertilizer.

The solid waste that remains after sewage treatment is called raw sewage or sludge. It usually contains, in addition to human biological waste matter, significant concentrations of toxic industrial wastes, including PCBs, chlorinated pesticides (such as DDT and lindane), other chlorinated compounds (such as dioxins), heavy metals (such as arsenic, cadmium, lead, and mercury), biological contaminants (such as bacteria, viruses, protozoa, parasitic worms, and fungi[67]), and sometimes asbestos, petroleum products, and various industrial solvents.[68] The problem of disposing of this sewage sludge became suddenly more critical only a few years ago when, in 1988, the U.S. Congress passed the Ocean Dumping Reform Act, which mandated "a complete end to ocean dumping by June 1991, and [imposed] fines of up to $500,000 per day if New York failed to comply."[69] One proposed solution that municipalities then came up with was to spread the treated sewage sludge on fields as agricultural fertilizer for food crops.

Over the objections of public health advocates, and despite the intense opposition of some citizen groups in the targeted agricultural areas, there soon developed large scale programs to dispose of this sludge by using it as fertilizer. Municipal sewage sludge from Milwaukee, Wisconsin, for example, had already been packaged and sold as fertilizer for several decades. This sludge, marketed as "Milorganite," contained high levels of cadmium (a heavy metal) so package labels carried the warning: "Do not use on vegetable gardens, other edible crops or fruit trees. Eating food grown on soil containing Milorganite may cause damage to health."[70] Stauber and Rampton note, however, that

> Under current federal rules ... most sludge products carry no such warning. Consumers are largely unaware that tens of thousands of acres, from Midwest dairy land to Florida citrus groves and California fruit orchards, are routinely "fertilized" with byproducts of industrial and human sewage.[71]

The lead levels alone in such sludge can apparently be cause for concern. According to Dr. Stanford Tackett, "a chemist and expert on lead contamination,"[72]

> The use of sewage sludge as a fertilizer poses a more significant lead threat to the land than did the use of leaded gasoline.... All sewage sludges contain elevated concentrations of lead due to the nature of the treatment process.... Lead is a highly toxic and cumulative poison. Lead poisoning can cause severe mental retardation or death.[73]

This information suggests that the agricultural use of sewage sludge may present some rather notable risks to the public health. Such health problems did recently begin to emerge, in fact, in the small town of Lynden, Washington. Stauber and Rampton wrote that even before dairy farmers Linda and Raymond Zander noticed difficulties with their own health, they noticed problems with the health of their cattle. Within a year of the sludge being spread on fields adjacent to their farm, "'we noticed ... lameness and other malfunctions [in our cattle],' said Linda Zander."

> Tests found heavy metals in soils at the sludge disposal site and in water from two neighborhood wells that serve several families. Since then, Raymond Zander has been diagnosed with nickel poisoning,

and several family members have shown signs of neurological damage which they believe is linked to heavy metal poisoning including zinc, copper, lead and manganese. Sixteen neighboring families have experienced health problems ranging from flu symptoms to cancer. Linda Zander formed an organization called "Help for Sewage Victims," and began to hear similar stories of sickness and death from farmers near sludge sites in Virginia, Pennsylvania, North Carolina, Georgia and other parts of the country.[74]

If industrial waste and human biological waste were treated in different processes, then the toxicity problems may be more manageable. But as it is, with the current single process, extremely high levels of industrial waste remain in much sewage sludge residue. Karl Schurr, professor of toxicology at the University of Minnesota, says that "some of the same chemicals found in sewage sludge were also employed by Cesare Borgia and his sister Lucrezia Borgia in Italy during the 1400s to very slowly poison their opponents."[75]

There is evidence, therefore, that the practice of spreading sewage sludge on agricultural food crops may pose some level of risk to the public health. If further evidence continues to corroborate this, then the principle of informed consent, if it were implemented into law, should doubtless require that foods grown in fields fertilized with such sludge should be so labeled. Such informed consent laws should also require that labels list some of the potential health risks that may result from eating foods grown in fields fertilized with municipal sewage and industrial sludge.

"Biosolids" is the euphemistic term that public relations experts for the sewage treatment industry would rather see us use in place of the term "sludge,"[76] even though that term is not entirely accurate. The term is not accurate because a significant portion of that sludge is actually industrial rather than biological waste.

The food processing industry has already shown evidence of strongly opposing any implementation of the principle of informed consent in relation to the practice of fertilizing food crops with municipal sewage sludge. According to Rick Jarman, a representative of the powerful National Food Processors Association, "consumers don't need to know whether their food has been grown in sludge."[77] If the principle of informed consent were to be implemented in public law, then regardless of Rick Jarman's opinion, consumers would have the legal right to know whether the food they buy for their families had been fertilized with municipal sewage sludge.

Naturally, the complex controversies surrounding this practice have been much oversimplified in this brief summary: those with an interest in a fuller description of the problem can turn to Stauber's and Rampton's book as well as to other available sources.[78] I offer this simplified account only as an illustration of how one possible application of the principle of informed consent, if it were enacted into law, might directly benefit the public health.

In any case, the principle of informed consent does seem important enough that it should be expressed in some form of enforceable public law. As one activist says, "[W]hether we are making decisions about a cancer treatment, breast-feeding our children, or taking a plane ride, we are entitled to the information available. It is both our right and our responsibility to be educated and to make informed decisions."[79]

Moreover, if our political ideals hold that democratic governments are—or at least ought to be—based on the consent and judgments of the governed, then we would want those citizen judgments to be as well informed as possible, and to be based on true knowledge of the actual risks and potential benefits of any given policy. Thomas Jefferson expressed it well.

> I know of no safe depository of the ultimate powers of society but the people themselves, and if we think them not enlightened enough to exercise their control with a wholesome discretion, the remedy is not to take it from them, but to inform their discretion.[80]

If Jefferson was correct in this assessment that the discretion of the people should be well informed, then by whatever means seems best, the principle of informed consent should indeed find full and proper expression in the laws, policies, and perhaps even constitutions of modern democratic states.

Surprisingly, even some large corporations are beginning to see the validity of this principle. In the wake of the commercial development of some genetically altered food crops (corn, soy beans and potatoes, for example), activists have been demanding that when these food products arrive in the stores they should be fully labeled *as* genetically altered so that customers will be able to make up their own minds about purchasing them. One of the largest biotechnology firms in the world, Novartis, the Swiss corporation formed by the merger of Sandoz and Ciba-Geigy in 1996, explained its support for the clear labeling of such foods. According to one report,

Company officials acknowledge that there is no need for labeling from a scientific and safety standpoint [sic], but say that if the industry believes in the consumers' right to choose, it "cannot reasonably argue against labels facilitating this choice."[81]

This recognition in at least one corporation is certainly a positive step. One hopes that it might set a precedent—for Monsanto, for instance, and its heavy investment in the development of genetically engineered food crops.

Monsanto Corporation has developed some genetically engineered food crops that are able to withstand the effects of being sprayed with substantial quantities of Monsanto's profitable glyphosate herbicide, "Roundup." These genetically altered crops can be sprayed with much heavier doses of Roundup than the natural crops without experiencing any noticeable ill effects. Whether human health will suffer any long-term adverse effects from eating such genetically engineered, "Roundup ready" food crops, or from ingesting higher doses of herbicide residues, has not yet been adequately studied.

Until these questions have been answered (and perhaps even afterwards), consumers may well feel that they should be informed about which of their foods have been genetically altered or sprayed with heavier doses of herbicides or both. In the absence of informed consent laws, customers currently have no way of knowing which foods have been altered and sprayed and which have not, and hence have no way of making their own decisions about which kinds of foods they will eat and feed to their families. The decisions have instead already been made for them, by corporate executives and by the inaction of legislators and government regulatory agencies.

A Special Case: Pesticide Labeling

Implementing the principle of informed consent in matters related to the marketing and use of pesticides in particular, should be given the highest regulatory priority, not only because of their toxicity but because of their volume. And their volume is enormous, as illustrated by D.C. Vacco in the *Secret Hazards of Pesticides*.

Pesticides are widely used throughout the United States in non-agricultural settings—in[side] homes, outside homes, in offices, schools, and recreational areas. Over 70 million pounds of pesticides are applied on lawns alone every year. The use of lawn care pesticides is increasing at about 5 to 8 percent annually. In fact, four times as many pesticides are used on home lawns as are used to grow food crops. Commercial lawn care is now a $1.5 billion industry. In addition, according to a 1985 study, pesticides used on golf courses accounted for nearly 12 million pounds nationwide.[82]

As matters stand now, pesticide manufacturers are not required to disclose even the names of most of the chemicals in their pesticide compounds. They are instead allowed to designate only one or two of the ingredients as "active," and all the rest as "inert," whether these other ingredients are biologically inert or not. By law they are required to provide on the label the names of only the so-called "active" ingredients.[83] These often comprise only one to four percent of the total compound. Nor are manufacturers required to provide information about the known adverse health effects of exposure to any of those active ingredients. All the remaining chemicals—often 96 percent or more—which are perhaps designated "inert,"[84] "include some of the most dangerous substances known."[85] A small sample of some of the chemicals used as so-called inerts in various pesticide products include carbon tetrachloride, chlorobenzene, chloroform, ethylbenzene, ethylene dichloride, methyl bromide, phenol, 1,1,2-trichloroethane and toluene.[86] According to a 1996 report from the New York State Department of Law, the known adverse health effects of some of these inerts include such effects as central nervous system disorders, kidney and liver damage, carcinogenicity, brain damage, convulsions, vomiting, respiratory depression, anemia, headache, hyperactivity, chromosomal aberrations, numbness, paralysis, blood cell disorders, gonadal atrophy, fetal resorption, fetotoxicity, difficulty breathing, unconsciousness, coma, and death.[87]

Manufacturers are not required by any agency to disclose even the names of those ingredients they have chosen to designate as inert. They are allowed to protect them as "proprietary secrets," and the public is not allowed to know the identity, characteristics, purposes, or potential health hazards of any of these ingredients, despite the fact they "are neither chemically, biologically, or toxicologically inert."[88] Some of the chemicals used as inerts in pesticide products are also used in other products and industrial processes, and in some of those uses they can be regulated (to some extent) by other laws. However, "[e]ven though some laws limit human exposure to these chemicals by restricting their release into air, water or the workplace, there is no way of knowing when the same chemicals are [unrestrictedly] released as inert ingredients in pesticides."[89]

Pesticide manufacturers have fought strenuously in the courts and in legislatures to avoid being required to disclose even the names of these inert ingredients, or the potential adverse health effects of exposure to these chemicals. They seem to believe that people do not need to know about these things, even if they want to know, and even if they strongly petition legislatures and the courts to be given access to the information. Monsanto Corporation's Ortho Weed-B-Gone Lawn Weed Killer, for instance, "is labeled with its active ingredient, as the government requires: sodium 2,4-dichlorophenozyacetate. What is not mentioned on the label is that this popular weed-killer, known as 2,4-D, is also suspected of being carcinogenic and otherwise toxic to the neurological and reproductive systems."[90]

Monsanto believes that people do not need to know these facts about the active ingredient in the weed-killers they put on their lawns each spring and summer, even though Monsanto knows that children, pregnant mothers, and pets will subsequently be playing and rolling on those lawns. The principle of informed consent says that Monsanto is simply wrong about this. People do deserve to be informed of the full complement of chemical ingredients—both active and "inert"—in the pesticides they purchase and use. And they deserve to be told as well about the known and suspected adverse health effects that can result from being exposed to those ingredients.

Fortunately, a U.S. District Court decision by Judge James Robertson determined that the EPA may no longer "routinely conceal the identity of certain pesticide ingredients."[91] This court ruling would mean, if it survives the appeals process, that the EPA will henceforth be obliged to require the disclosure of the identity of the inert ingredients in the six pesticide products named in the suit: Roundup, Aatrex 80w, Weedone-LV4, Velpar, Garlon 3A, and Tordon 101.

The suit was pressed by both the Northwest Coalition for Alternatives to Pesticides (NCAP) and the National Coalition Against the Misuse of Pesticides (NCAMP). The manufacturers of these pesticides argued that the secrecy of the chemical composition of the products should be protected as proprietary information. Plaintiffs argued, however, that any competitors could easily learn the exact composition of these products by readily available "back engineering" techniques, and that, therefore, there was no significant commercial value—except in hiding the identity of these chemicals from the public—in keeping the so-called "inert" ingredients secret. On the other hand, they said, there may well be, significant public health benefits in allowing consumers to be aware of the ingredients (and of their potential health effects) in the products they are using and to which they and their families are being exposed.

Some consumers, in fact, if they were made aware of the full list of these ingredients and their health effects, may perhaps choose not to expose themselves, their families, their neighbors, and their pets to the products which include them, only a very few of which have been adequately tested for safety.[92]

This ruling in favor of NCAP and NCAMP was a ray of hope for those who believe in the principles of informed consent and of citizens' right to know. The ruling is, of course, being aggressively appealed by the pesticide manufacturers. Monsanto (manufacturer of Roundup) and other pesticide manufacturers have an enormous economic interest in not disclosing all the ingredients in their pesticide products. They know that some consumers could become so concerned when they see the names and health affects of the solvents and toxicants in these products that they would refuse to purchase and use them. Mothers may even decide, eventually, not to bring their children to parks or playgrounds where these products have been used. They may insist that the schools their children attend stop using these products anywhere inside or around the school buildings where their children spend their days, or on the fields where their children romp and play. People may insist that their employers no longer spray these products anywhere in or around the buildings in which they work. They may petition their country clubs to stop using these products in such high quantities on the golf courses. They may pass laws requiring that road crews seriously cut back on the practice of spraying these products along state, county, and municipal roadways. Manufacturers realize all this, and they fully understand the negative economic repercussions. So it is little wonder they have so strenuously opposed any attempts to implement informed consent legislation.

But courts and lawmakers should not be fooled by the opposition of the chemical industry. They should recognize that their primary responsibility is to the citizenry and to their right to have full information about the chemical products to which they may be exposed. The contest truly is between the narrow self-interests of the chemical manufacturing corporations and the right of citizens to have full information about the products with which they and their families may come into contact.

The 1996 U.S. Food Quality Protection Act (FQPA) may turn

out to be one small step in the right direction. A major provision of this law, which will be administered by EPA, requires that agency

> to develop consumer information, to be displayed in grocery stores, on the risks and benefits of pesticides used in or on food, as well as recommendations to consumers for reducing dietary exposure to pesticides while maintaining a healthy diet.[93]

It will be interesting to see how much influence the pesticide industry and agricultural interests will have when it comes to the actual wording of these notices.

This law also requires that EPA "reassess roughly 9000 existing tolerances (maximum legally permissible [pesticide] residue levels in food.)"[94] While this is an admirable goal, and certainly one to be supported by all the human rights principles outlined in Chapter Two, we have to wonder how many decades it will take before even preliminary minimal health testing is completed and new regulatory policies can begin to be negotiated. The EPA, after all, simply does not presently have the resources for a task of this size, and even if it did, it would likely encounter such a barrage of resistance from the pesticide interest groups that the task would be made extremely daunting indeed.

The FQPA further requires that these pesticide tolerances and other food-related health risks be assessed independently for potentially more sensitive populations, such as infants and children.[95] This is another laudable requirement, yet one which will unfortunately add decades more to the length of time of testing, and hence before implementation of the relevant health safety regulations.

In fact, "the FQPA calls for a comprehensive overhaul of pesticide policies,"[96] and this, should it actually come to pass, would be a very good thing. However, as we will see in more detail in Chapter Four, the transnational corporations which manufacture pesticide products would stand to lose a great deal if there were to be much strengthening of pesticide policy in the U.S. We can expect, therefore, that they will make every effort to weaken attempts to implement this law in ways that are not likely to diminish their production and the public's use of the pesticide products that are so lucrative for them.

We can only hope that lawmakers and EPA administrators will have the wisdom, foresight, and courage to implement pesticide policies that are *primarily* designed to protect the population's health, and not primarily designed—as they are now—to protect the economic interests of the corporations.

In addition to the FQPA, another small step has been taken toward implementing the principle of informed consent. A few years ago, the U.S. Occupational Safety and Health Administration (OSHA) began seeking public comment about how best to provide workers and employers worldwide with information about, and identification of, chemical hazards with which they may come into contact, in order to best protect their health.[97] This effort is in accord with agreements made at the 1992 UN Conference on Environment and Development (UNCED), and is a movement in the right direction. This project, however, is focusing primarily on high dose hazards encountered in the workplace, and does not address the issue of informing people about the dangers of long-term, low dose exposures to environmental toxicants to which they are exposed in their daily life. But OSHA's effort does at least represent one small step forward in the slow implementation of the principle of informed consent.

Carol M. Browner, EPA Administrator, summed it up well: "Arming the public with basic information about toxic chemicals in their communities is among the most effective, common-sense steps to protect the health of families and children from the threats posed by pollution."[98]

4. Burden of Proof

The burden of proof for determining product safety should lie entirely with the developers of those products, and adequate demonstration of that safety should be made well before the product is ever brought to market.

The CETOS *Toxics Bill of Rights* expresses this principle clearly when it says that "no substance shall be introduced into commerce without a full evaluation of its short- and long-term effects, including those on neurological and immunological development."[99]

The American Public Health Association (APHA) has urged the same thing. It recommends that "every chemical [should be] considered potentially dangerous until the extent of toxicity is sufficiently known."[100] This recommendation is clearly in contrast to the current unreflective regulatory practice which assumes instead that chemicals should be considered harmless until they are proven to be toxic. The APHA recommendation would have the effect of properly placing the burden of proof for demonstrating safety on the developer of the chemical product. The APHA believes that "this [new] alternative approach reflects an attitude of risk avoidance, instead of the attitudes of risk regulation or risk acceptance implicit in the TLV [threshold limit values] concept."[101]

At present, the burden of proof for determining the safety or toxicity of any given new industrial chemicals or chemical compounds, new consumer products, or new byproducts of an industrial process (new pesticides excepted) often lies with the relevant regulatory agency, which in the U.S. is often the EPA. The current operating assumption is that new chemical products[102] or byproducts are presumed to be biologically safe until they have been proven toxic by rigorously designed scientific trials undertaken by, and funded by, the relevant regulatory agency. No philosophical or scientific justification has ever been proposed for making this peculiar legal presumption of safety, probably because no justification would likely be very persuasive. Instead, the principle of *caveat emptor* (buyer beware) has tended to prevail in today's chemical business undertakings.

The *caveat emptor* principle, however, was found to be ethically inappropriate when it was applied to foodstuffs, food additives, and medications, so the U.S. Food and Drug Administration (FDA) was formed as a kind of consumer protection agency to protect all those who eat commercial foods and those who use commercial pharmaceutical products. The *caveat emptor* principle was considered inappropriate when applied to foods and medications because it was felt to be so easy for manufacturers or hucksters to dupe a public that was sometimes not as fully educated about foods and medications as it might have been, and hence was more liable to be taken advantage of. Now, in order to protect ordinary citizens from the unethical claims of manufacturers and marketers who might feel their own financial gain to be a higher priority than the safety of the consuming public, the FDA requires that manufacturers and distributors of foods, food additives, and medicines prove that their products are safe for human consumption.[103] Only then will a license for manufacture and distribution be issued.

Our recommendation here is that in the same way, those who stand to gain financially from the introduction of a new chemical product should be required to prove that their product is biologically safe before it can be licensed for a given specified use. This should apply to manufacturers of all new chemical products (including detergents, cleaning agents, artificial fragrances and fragranced products, fabric softeners and paints) as well as to manufacturers of products that offgas volatile organic compounds into the air (for example, new carpeting, mattresses, new padded furniture, new clothing, new building and remodeling materials, inks used in books, magazines and newspapers, products made of polyvinylchloride—also called vinyl, or PVC—including some children's toys, mattress covers and water pipes).

As things stand now, manufacturers have almost no incentive to test their products for safety prior to marketing and distributing them. In fact, manufacturers have an incentive *not* to test their products for adverse health effects. The reason is this (as we will see below): that if they did test their products and found them to be risky to human health, they could then be found liable in court for either negligence or intent to harm.

There is simply too little case law at present to support claims that would hold manufacturers liable for harm caused by the presence of toxic agents in their products, even if that harm could have been prevented by the manufacturer's testing the product for toxicity, and then labeling it with warnings about the potential hazards.

And yet, in one recent case the 12th Judicial District Court in Louisiana did find E I DuPont de Nemours and Company at fault for failing to test their newly developed (and newly marketed) carpet, DuPont Certified Stainmaster Carpet, for potential health hazards. The plaintiff in the case, Mr. Andre Caubarreaux, had been in good health before the carpet was installed in his home but soon after the installation he experienced sinus and respiratory problems which eventually developed into fulminant chronic asthma and bronchitis. According to an article in *Medical and Legal Briefs*.

> On two separate occasions after the installation, Caubarreaux traveled away from his home. During those trips his condition improved, but worsened again upon returning home. His health continued to deteriorate until he suffered respiratory failure which required hospitalization. In the hospital, away from the carpet, his health improved again.[104]

The DuPont Company had not undertaken even rudimentary tests for the safety of their new carpet product. This despite the fact that there have been thousands of health complaints against carpet manufacturers over the years, despite the well-publicized accounts of the many employees at EPA headquarters who suffered adverse health effects after the installation of new carpeting in their offices,[105] despite the fact that EPA subsequently removed that carpeting because of its toxicity, and despite the fact that DuPont had itself received over 100 telephone complaints about this particular product, the Certified Stainmaster Carpet, and another 150 written complaints about it. Despite these fairly obvious reasons to test their new product for potential health hazards to insure the safety of the people who bought it and installed it in their homes and offices, DuPont still chose not to test it.

Subsequent testing of the carpet using the standard, well-accepted methods of gas chromatography and mass spectrometry (GC/MS) detected the clear presence of a variety of chemicals known to play a significant role in respiratory problems. These same tests also identified "42 other chemicals offgassing from Caubarreaux's DuPont Certified Stainmaster Carpet." The article went on to say that,

> A summary of the testing report states Caubarreaux's carpet "probably offgassed organics at a rate of up to 100 times or higher than what would have been expected of a 'normal' carpet. Such offgassing could be expected to produce significant exposure effects.[106]

The court therefore concluded:

> Considering the testimony of the treating physicians regarding the carpet's cause of injury to the plaintiff and the unrebutted testimony of the scientists which tested the carpet and found it to be dangerous, the weight of the evidence easily preponderates to a finding that the DuPont Certified Stainmaster Carpet was unreasonably dangerous in construction and composition.... Furthermore, because DuPont witnesses agreed that there were no design parameters used to insure that only safe chemicals were used in the production of the final product, ... the evidence also preponderates to a finding that the carpet is unreasonably dangerous.[107]

The court thus found that, "A manufacturer cannot bury its head in the sand and later claim that it did not and could not have known of the danger which it is causing...."[108] The plaintiff was awarded $2.25 million for general damages, $1.9 million for economic losses, $22,000 for medical expenses, and $50,000 for loss of consortium, for a total of just over $4.2 million.

DuPont is sure to appeal the decision, so the ultimate fate of this case is still uncertain. Should it be upheld, however, cases such as this could ultimately have the effect of supporting a requirement that the burden of proof for showing convincing evidence of product safety should lie with the product's developer or manufacturer.

As matters stand now, with the burden of proof lying on the regulatory agency to prove that a product is unacceptably toxic to human health, it is clearly in the manufacturer's interest to have that testing delayed for as long a time as possible. After all, as Van Strum writes,

> a chemical [or other product] may continue to be manufactured, sold, and used until the regulatory process is completed, which usually takes years. Industry protects its profits by prolonging that process as long as possible, challenging agency actions at every turn.... During the years that a chemical may be in the process of reevaluation—perhaps for grave health reasons—its manufacturer continues not only to sell it, but to promote it with [the] safety claims already called into question by the regulatory agency.[109]

It is in the manufacturer's interest to delay testing like this only because, unlike the situation with food additives and pharmaceuticals, the burden of proof presently lies with the regulatory agencies. If the burden of developing and presenting evidence to support the claims of safety lay with the manufacturer, then it would be in the interests of the manufacturer to see that testing was accomplished in the shortest possible time.

In assessing the safety of a new chemical product which is being considered for licensure, full consideration should be given to the following seven factors:

1. Its potential adverse human health effects.
2. Persistence of that product in the environment.
3. Potential for dispersal of the product or byproduct throughout the environment, and how local climate and weather conditions (e.g., winds, temperature and precipitation) could affect that dispersal.
4. Its effects on nonhuman organisms (including agricultural crops, other plants, wildlife, pets and soil organisms).
5. The variety of pathways by which human beings would be exposed to the product (via ambient air, the water supply, residues on vegetation, foodstuffs, and in food animals).
6. The level of toxicity liable to affect human health.
7. The product's persistence in human tissues and the potential for bioaccumulation in tissues.

In addition to the obvious manifestations of short-term acute toxicity, potential long-term health effects (such as those outlined in Chapter One) should, of course, also be considered.

When sufficient satisfactory evidence has been properly presented by the manufacturer to the relevant regulatory agency showing that a product is adequately safe for manufacture and use, then it would be available for licensure and for dispersal into the marketplace. Label warnings would be required to reflect any potential adverse health consequences of use, just as labelings and inserts in pharmaceutical products today inform consumers of their potential adverse effects.

The precise same arguments for placing the burden of proof on developers and manufacturers to determine the safety of new pharmaceutical products that individuals use for medical purposes, apply to manufacturers of new chemical products; but they apply even more forcefully because the use and dispersal of new chemicals in the environment are so much more difficult to control. A pharmaceutical product, after all, is controlled, both *de jure* and *de facto*, by physicians who prescribe (or do not prescribe) it, and by the pharmacists who distribute it. Physicians also regularly monitor for potential adverse health effects of the pharmaceuticals they prescribe. In this way, any adverse effects of a new product can be caught before too many people have been harmed. In addition, the product's dispersal into the environment is relatively well controlled by these practices.

Moreover, once a medication has been ingested by a human being, metabolic processes break down a certain proportion of the drug so that its subsequent impact on the ambient environment, and hence on other people who have not chosen to use it, is somewhat lessened. So the environmental fate of most pharmaceutical products is fairly well controlled, and the exposure to that medicine of others is minimized. Individuals are thus able to determine to some degree the extent to which they are exposed to any given pharmaceutical product.

(And yet even this is not entirely the case. As early as 1977, a study entitled "Drugs and drug metabolites as environmental contaminants"[110] found residues of pharmaceutical products in sewage sludge at the Big Blue River sewage treatment facility in Kansas City, and "sewage sludge provides a major pathway by which drugs enter the environment."[111] More recent studies have found that, "Pharmaceutical drugs given to people and to domestic animals—including antibiotics, hormones, strong pain killers, tranquilizers, and chemotherapy chemicals given to cancer patients—are being measured in surface water, in groundwater, and in drinking water at the tap."[112] This all becomes understandable when we realize what an article in *Rachel's Environment and Health Weekly* makes clear:

> When a human or an animal is given a drug, anywhere from 50% to 90% of it is excreted unchanged. The remainder is excreted in the form of metabolites—chemicals produced as byproducts of the body's interaction with the drug.[113]

Thus, even though we may believe that we have a choice about whether to ingest pharmaceutical products, the case seems to be not quite as clear as we may have thought.

The case is entirely different, however, and much more dramatic, when it comes to applied pesticide products, airborne byproducts of industrial processes, other toxic releases, and even the offgassing of chemical compounds in bedding, furniture, and clothing. Individual citizens cannot at all easily determine to what degree they will be exposed to those compounds. Thus, there is all the more reason for government agencies to take strong precautions to insure that chemicals released into the atmosphere and water, where people will be exposed to them whether they wish to be or not, are safe for everyone who may be exposed to them. This protection of the health interests of citizens should be recognized as an ethical duty incumbent on governments, and particularly on governments of those democratic states which have strong traditions of protecting the rights of individuals. And again, to emphasize, the burden of providing convincing evidence of a new product's safety should rest primarily with the developers and manufacturers who stand to gain financially from its production and use.

Thus, when a new product (or byproduct) is proposed for licensing, the first concern should be to provide strong, convincing evidence that it is safe for those who will be using it, as well as for those who may be inadvertently, and without their consent, exposed to it during and after use. These people, especially the people who are *not* using the product but who will be exposed to it inadvertently and nonconsensually—perhaps due to drift, volatilization, seepage, runoff into streams and rivers (which supply homes and cities with their water), or other means of dispersal—have the right to be protected from the adverse effects of a product they have not chosen to use or be exposed to, and have perhaps even consciously chosen not to use.

At present, this scenario of unprotected and nonconsensual exposure to toxicants is played out almost daily with pesticides (particularly in spring and summer months), usually because of the high quantity of pesticide drift. Pesticide residues, especially those applied aerially, but even those applied closer to the ground, can (as we have seen above) drift hundreds and sometimes thousands of miles on winds and air currents, exposing large numbers of unsuspecting people along the way. This nonconsensual exposure to biocidal toxicants is one of the more blatant examples of human rights violations. All the basic principles of human rights outlined in Chapter Two clearly require that no one in a free democratic state should be required to breathe or ingest poisons against their will. As Rachel Carson has said so well:

> If the [U.S.] Bill of Rights contains no guarantee that a citizen shall be secure against lethal poisons distributed whether by private individuals or by public officials, it is surely only because our forefathers, despite their considerable wisdom and foresight, could conceive of no such problem.[114]

Surely, had the founding fathers foreseen such a possibility, she implies, a constitutional provision for protecting ordinary citizens against nonconsensual exposure to ambient poisons—spread by neighbors, by local businesses, by agricultural or timber interests, or even by their own government—would have been at least considered for inclusion in the Bill of Rights.

Members of the American Public Health Association have proposed a policy resolution urging the adoption of a constitutional amendment that recognizes "citizens' rights to clean water, clean air, [and] freedom from toxin-induced illness."[115] This resolution "urges the states and Congress to pass a constitutional amendment which will assure all Americans the right to clean air, clean water and the protection of the other natural resources of the nation."[116] The fact that a similar initiative is under way in over 40 states,[117] indicates that the APHA is not the only body that believes this resolution to have merit.[118]

To sum up, a large step in the direction of providing protection for citizens from the chemical toxicants to which they may be unwittingly and unwillingly exposed would be to reverse the present burden of proof requirement, and place it on chemical developers and manufacturers who stand to profit financially from introduction of new chemical products and byproducts.

5. Disaggregated Safety Standards

Product safety standards, indoor air quality (IAQ) standards, and chemical exposure standards should be determined separately for infants and children, for females (especially pregnant females), for the elderly, and for other groups with unique vulnerabilities.[119]

The following point made by the APHA is perhaps not well enough known:

> [O]ccupational exposure limits (OELs) were established 15 to 40 years ago; [and] historically, these values have been set near the maximum acutely tolerable level, with little regard for the risks of long-term serious or irreversible damage for men, women, and children such as cancer or reproductive health effects, effects on growth and development, and toxic illnesses....[120]

It is probably also not well enough known that these exposure standards were not determined by disinterested medical and public health professionals, but were instead determined largely by representatives of chemical manufacturing corporations. In fact, according to the APHA, the minutes of the committee that set these threshold limit values (TLVs) clearly indicate that

> starting in 1970, employees of various multinational chemical companies have played central roles as committee members in developing TLVs for over 120 chemicals; and that this company role was not balanced by those representing workers' interests, such as union representatives.[121]

Because of these considerations, the APHA has urged that regulatory agencies responsible for setting workplace health standards "[re]evaluate the effects on more sensitive populations not previously considered in standard development."[122] This APHA recommendation may apply primarily to chemical exposure standards in the workplace, but it should apply equally, if not even more stringently, to schools, day care settings, hospitals, and other places where infants and children may spend any significant amount of time. After all, as the Centers for Disease Control and Prevention has warned, "children have an increased susceptibility to [pesticides], and low level pesticide poisoning may mimic sudden infant death syndrome."[123]

This recommendation should apply equally to nursing homes and other extended care facilities where older citizens, or the medically compromised, may spend extended periods of time.

What is being proposed here is simply that the standard 70 kilogram (155 lb.) Caucasian adult male should not be considered the only standard for determining toxicity and health effects of environmental toxicants. Certain more vulnerable groups may require more stringent standards in order to protect their health.

Safety standards for the whole variety of different human groups, therefore, should not be aggregated into one single standard, and that standard should not be based solely on the adult Caucasian male. Safety standards should be disaggregated to allow for the unique physical vulnerabilities of infants and children, females, the elderly, and so on.

6. Safe Schools

Schools especially should be made as free as possible from all chemical pollutants that could adversely affect students' health, learning abilities, abilities to think clearly and concentrate, and physical comfort levels.

Reasons for this recommendation may best be approached purely from a human rights perspective, citing the 1990 international *Convention on the Rights of the Child*, now ratified by 187 out of 193 countries. Article 24 of the convention declares that governments "recognize the right of the child to the enjoyment of the highest attainable standard of health."[124] Schools, as the environment in which children spend the greatest amount of time aside from their homes, should be as healthful as possible.

Paragraph three of Article 24 of the convention states that governments "shall take all effective and appropriate measures with a view to abolishing traditional practices prejudicial to the health of children."[125] Thus, if there are traditional procedures and practices in schools that put the child's "highest attainable standard of health" at risk, then those procedures and practices should be modified or eliminated.

And yet, in addition to looking at the question of schools from a purely human rights perspective, we might just as fruitfully look at it from a teleological or utilitarian perspective. It is of critical importance to acknowledge that students in schools should be able to concentrate, learn, think clearly, and be comfortable, and that schools should therefore be completely free of any chemical pollutants that have been shown to, or may possibly, put children at risk of having those abilities compromised. The costs to children and to societies of not insuring our schools' health and safety is potentially enormous.

The World Health Organization's Expert Committee on Comprehensive School Health Education and Promotion issued a set of recommendations that they said would, if followed, help schools become the "health-promoting schools"[126] they ought to be. Two of WHO's key recommendations are: "Schools should be healthy places in which to work...."; and "Schools must provide safe water and sanitary facilities and protection from diseases...."[127] These two recommendations, though perhaps originally intended primarily to address protection from infectious diseases caused by microbial agents, should now also be taken to include protection from chemical contaminants in the indoor air, in the water supply, in the food, in the soil, and in or on the products with which children come into contact during the course of their school day.

Implementing these recommendations would probably mean, among other things, the avoidance of certain harsher kinds of cleaning agents, avoiding artificially scented products and school supplies of any sort, unsafe synthetic carpeting materials (especially when new), artificially scented room deodorizers, toxic whiteboard markers, certain kinds of art supplies, certain kinds of biology laboratory preservatives and so on.

The State of New York in 1994 issued a report entitled *Recommendations to Improve the Environmental Health and Safety of Schools*. One of its recommendations was, "Schools shall develop guidelines to reduce exposure to chemical fragrances which can cause possible adverse reactions in some individuals."[128] These guidelines should be written to include not only the obvious artificial fragrances in perfumes, colognes, lotions and hairsprays, but also the artificial fragrances included in cleaning products, in laundry detergents, in whiteboard markers, in hand soaps, and in bathroom deodorizers.

If chemically toxic materials cannot adequately be removed from all learning spaces, and if it is not possible to find low-toxicity replacements for these materials (for example in certain science or art areas), then students should be provided with physical barrier protections (such as gloves, goggles, masks and respirators), during those periods in their school day when they are more likely to be exposed to these toxicants, in order to minimize potentially damaging exposures.

Implementation of these recommendations would also mean a significant reduction in schools' use of synthetic pesticides, both indoors and outdoors, and a greater reliance on integrated pest management practices. Most schools today routinely spray pesticides both indoors (sometimes even on school days when children are present), and outdoors. Herbicides are frequently used on school grounds, on athletic fields, on flower and shrub beds, and on sports tracks.[129] Many school districts spray these areas in the spring when school is still in session, and again in the late summer shortly before school resumes.

Children can be personally exposed to these herbicides by several biological routes. The most common route of exposure would be by inhalation of pesticide drift residues on the day of, and in the days immediately following, an application. Other routes would include dermal absorption, perhaps while playing on sprayed grounds and athletic fields, oral ingestion from putting contaminated fingers or objects in the mouth, and tracking pesticides from the grounds into the classroom after each play period, where these chemicals are then absorbed into the carpet fibers (if the classroom is carpeted) and can volatilize into the indoor air. These pesticides and residues are likely to persist much longer indoors than they do outdoors where they are exposed to sunlight, wind and rain, and where they are much more likely to disperse and become less concentrated. Indoors they are more likely to accumulate and concentrate over time, particularly if school floors are carpeted, and if it is common practice (as it is in virtually all schools) for children to wear their shoes indoors as well as outdoors.[130]

The more we become aware of how much modern schools expose our children to toxicants[131] the more we realize how little legal protection children have against exposure to toxics in their schools. One laboratory animal research professor complains that, "We protect our lab rats better than we do our children. In order to expose lab animals to what our children are being exposed to on a daily basis, I need to receive permission," he said.

One school in Australia, designed especially for children who already suffer from toxicant induced chemical sensitivity, has undertaken measures, including establishing a fragrance-free policy for all students, faculty and staff,[132] to insure that students and staff are able to avoid prolonged exposure to toxics. Some residential universities in the U.S. have also begun to design and build special dormitories for their students who suffer from various allergies and chemical sensitivities.[133] Other schools are considering doing so as well.[134] Ashford and Miller recommend that the U.S. Department of Education should "assist states in establishing special classrooms for chemically sensitive children."[135]

Many of the toxicants which so dramatically affect people with chemical sensitivities can also be toxic, though perhaps less noticeably so, to persons who have not yet developed such sensitivities. As more people come to understand this risk to themselves and their children, more parents and school boards will realize the importance of taking precautions to insure that their children do not develop toxicant induced pathologies. At that point we will begin designing schools with an eye to reducing toxicant loads in students and staff in order to protect them from neurologic, immunologic, respiratory, endocrinologic, reproductive, and carcinogenic harm.

My own school, North Seattle Community College, has realized that some of its students (as well as some of its faculty, administrators, and staff) do suffer varying degrees of adverse health effects from ambient toxicants found in the air in campus buildings (even though our campus has a history of being much more concerned than most about toxicants and health). In response to this need to protect the campus community from exposure to toxics, the school has taken a significant step in dealing with this problem by implementing an Indoor Air Quality (IAQ) policy. This policy (reproduced in Appendix I of this book) specifically requires that building managers always use the least toxic cleaning agents available for any given cleaning need. It also requires that any possible release of toxicants, or use of pesticides, or indeed any procedure that may involve risk to the IAQ of campus buildings must be preceded by a 48 hour notice to the entire campus community. In addition, everyone who works on the campus and who attends classes there is urged to observe the fragrance-free campus policy while on campus. Campus administrators, furthermore, are required to provide substantial IAQ education to the entire campus community on a regular and ongoing basis.

The Evergreen State College in Olympia, Washington, has an almost identical policy,[136] and a few other colleges and universities around the country—such as the School of Social Work at the University of Minnesota—have also implemented policies restricting the use of artificial fragrances in their buildings in an attempt to improve the quality of their indoor air.

If schools are intended to be places where students engage in the work of learning, and if certain toxicants have a pronounced and measurable compromising effect on the ability of certain persons to learn, then exposure to those toxicants should be minimized or completely avoided in schools. It's that simple.

7. Safe Workplaces

The same principle holds true as well for our offices and work spaces. Workplaces should also be made as free as possible from chemical pollutants that can adversely affect workers' physical comfort, as well as their abilities to focus adequately and to have enough energy and mental clarity to perform their work well and responsibly.[137]

Ambient levels of toxicants in the workplace have generally been regulated by reference to certain official occupational exposure limits (OELs). However, as we saw above, 75 percent of these OELs were established at least 15 and as many as 40 years ago, set largely by representatives from the chemical manufacturing industry, and were historically set "near the maximum acutely tolerable level without regard for the risks of long-term serious or irreversible damage for men, women and children"[138]

Recognizing the fundamental inadequacy of relying on standards established largely by private chemical company interests, and set mainly to protect only against immediate acute exposures rather than against long-term chronic exposures, the American Public Health Association, in November 1996, issued a policy statement entitled, "The precautionary principle and chemical exposure standards for the workplace." This policy statement concluded that "current U.S. workplace chemical-exposure limits often fail to adequately protect the health of workers."[139]

This policy also "encourages the development of a workplace chemical-exposure, including pesticide-exposure, prevention policy based on the ... precautionary principle."[140]

In making these recommendations, the APHA is explicitly referring to the precautionary principle discussed in Chapter Two. This principle, to restate it, affirms that when there is a current lack of adequate scientific evidence to prove that a chemical is safe at the levels to which human beings will be exposed, we should err, if it is erring, on the side of caution. That is, we must assume that the chemical is not safe, in order to protect the public health. The principle also explicitly states that when evidence exists that there is some risk of serious or irreversible harm, lack of scientific certitude must not be used as an excuse for postponing measures to prevent such harm. The potential damage inflicted on human beings (as well as on pets, wildlife, fish, and other species) by some toxicants can be both serious and irreversible, and thus this principle is clearly an appropriate one.

(The recommendations outlined in the APHA's policy statement on the workplace should probably also apply, and perhaps even more stringently, to chemical exposure limits in schools, where equally important work is being performed.)

Furthermore, simply from the viewpoint of common sense, if certain toxicants do have (as we have seen above) a compromising effect on the abilities of certain persons to think clearly, to make thoughtful decisions, and to accomplish a high quality of work, then those toxicants should simply not be permitted in our places of work and business. If our workers are creating products and performing services on which society depends, and if we want our workers to do that work well, then we should not expose them to toxicants that may have a compromising effect on their ability to do that work. This should not be a difficult concept for business executives and building managers to accept.

As more and more employers become aware of this, they will want to provide their workforce with a physical atmosphere and air quality that is conducive to good work and high productivity, and not with an atmosphere that compromises some of their workers' abilities to perform well.

8. Transparent Processes

Regulatory agencies charged with assessing and managing the environmental risks to communities and consumers should ensure that the risk assessment processes used for making environmental health decisions are fully transparent and entirely public. Written records should be kept of all discussions and should be, with their conclusions, made easily and readily available to all interested people in the community.

9. Full Disclosure

Full written public disclosure, by researchers, of all financial interests in the results of their research should be required by journals which publish that research. Furthermore, disclosure of the sources of their research funding, as well as the formal affiliations of all the organizations which have provided that funding, should also be required.

Environmental research today is often funded by corporations and industries which have a clear financial interest in the outcome of the research. The Tobacco Institute, for example, regularly sponsors research that is intended to support the tobacco industry's point of view on tobacco use, a practice which has been aptly termed "cigarette science." The result is that the questions, methods, and data in these experiments may well be sullied, or at least seriously slanted. The Tobacco Institute clearly has a potential conflict of interest in the outcome of the research which they choose to fund. Such potential conflicts of interest may affect at least the questions posed by researchers, and may also affect the study design and methods, if not the actual data. Any published research findings by scientists who were funded by the Tobacco Institute therefore should, in the interests of full disclosure, include clear acknowledgment of the sources of that funding so that readers can be made aware of them. This principle should hold for authors of all articles published in peer-reviewed scientific journals.

In the judicial systems of most national democratic states, judges are expected to be, to every extent possible, impartial and objective agents in the processing of a case. Since it is well recognized that a financial conflict of interest may compromise a judge's ability to deal with a case objectively, judges are normally proscribed from sitting on cases in which they may be financially interested parties.

In the same way, scientists are expected to be, to every extent possible, impartial and objective agents in the research endeavors in which they are engaged. It may be unrealistic for society to expect that researchers would never undertake research in which they have a financial interest, but we might at the very least presume that they should disclose the full extent of their financial interests in the research. If the chair of toxicology at a leading research university, for example, has been funded by Dow Chemical Corporation, it would be appropriate for that fact to be made clearly visible to the whole faculty, to students, and to readers of any research articles published by the professor who holds that chair.

How many scientists who conduct and publish scientific research actually have a financial interest in the outcomes of their studies? It appears that many do. A study of almost 800 scientific articles which were published in peer-reviewed journals in 1992 found that "one third of lead authors had a direct financial interest in the published research."[141] This is probably a somewhat higher percentage than many of us might have expected. According to an article in *Nature*,

> George Lundberg, the editor of *JAMA* [Journal of the American Medical Association], says that financial conflicts of interest among scientific authors are "widespread" but that readers are largely unaware of them "because so many editors are not following what we consider to be good editorial practices of requiring and publishing financial disclosures routinely."[142]

The study just mentioned, undertaken by Sheldon Krimsky, professor of urban and environmental policy at Tufts University in Medford, Massachusetts, outlined the definition of "financial interest."

> "Financial interest" was defined as: the author being listed as an inventor in a patent or patent application closely related to the published work (this occurred in 22 per cent of the articles studied); serving on a scientific advisory board of a company developing products related to the author's expertise (20 per cent); or serving as an officer or major shareholder of a company with commercial interests related to the research (7 per cent).
>
> Consultancies, personal financial holdings and honoraria were excluded, on the grounds that such links could not be adequately documented.[143]

This definition of "financial interest" does not include as much as I believe it should. For example, I believe that researchers whose work is directly funded by interested parties should disclose the sources of that funding. While such funding may not constitute "financial interest" according to the above limited definition, it does at least constitute a clear financial factor that may have an influence on, or at least may be perceived to have an influence on, the outcomes of that scientist's research.

A more recent study in the *New England Journal of Medicine* "shows pretty clearly that scientific and medical experts who take corporate money hold opinions that differ significantly from experts who don't take corporate money."[144] The study examined articles published in peer-reviewed medical journals between March 1995 and September 1996 on the subject of a then current controversy about the safety of calcium-channel antagonists. In only two of the articles did authors publicly "divulge their connections to corporations."[145] In this *NEJM* study articles were "reviewed and classified as being supportive, neutral, or critical with respect to the use of calcium-channel antagonists."[146] Not surprisingly, the study found a strong correlation between the position taken in the articles and the authors' financial relationships with the pharmaceutical industry.

> Authors who supported the use of calcium-channel antagonists were significantly more likely than neutral or critical authors to have financial relationships with manufacturers of calcium-channel antagonists (96 percent, vs. 60 percent and 37 percent, respectively; P<0.001). Supportive authors were also more likely than neutral or critical authors to have financial relationships with any pharmaceutical manufacturer, irrespective of the product (100 percent, vs. 67 percent and 43 percent, respectively; P<0.001).[147]

The study found, in other words, that there was "a strong association between authors' published positions on the safety of calcium-channel antagonists and their financial relationships with pharmaceutical manufacturers."[148] Dr. George Lundberg (editor of *JAMA*) says that he found the results of this study "disturbing."[149]

Whatever the reasons, there is a correlation between the conclusions of published articles and the financial relationships the authors have with industry. Readers deserve, therefore, to be made aware of these relationships, and on the same basis funding sources should be fully disclosed.

Not everyone agrees with this proposal to require such financial disclosures, of course. Kenneth Rothman, Professor of Public Health at Boston University, and current editor of the journal *Epidemiology*, is one who disagrees with it. He believes that if editors were averse to publishing work by scientists who had a financial interest in their research and declined to disclose it, this would have the effect of "diminish[ing] scientific interchange, in the long run reduc[ing] objectivity, and harm[ing] scientific method."[150]

I don't find this argument persuasive. I believe, in fact, that if journals began to require such financial disclosures of their authors, it may well *increase* the objectivity in research, and thereby increase faith in the scientific enterprise and actually enhance scientific interchange. And if faith in the scientific enterprise has languished in recent years (which seems to be the case), it would not hurt at least to buoy that faith somewhat, which I believe would be achieved by scientific journals disclosing the financial interests of their authors. This view is in line with that expressed in the conclusion of the *NEJM* study: "[F]ull disclosure of relationships between physicians and pharmaceutical manufacturers is necessary to affirm the integrity of the medical profession and maintain public confidence."[151] In any case, requiring some level of financial disclosure by the authors of scientific papers simply seems the right thing to do.

Fortunately, some leading scientific journals have begun, just in the past few years, to require such financial disclosures by their authors. *The New England Journal of Medicine*, for example, was the only one of the 14 journals included in Krimsky's study that required financial disclosure in 1992. Since then, *Science* has initiated a financial disclosure policy, the *Lancet* introduced such a policy in 1994, and the *Proceedings of the National Academy of Sciences* introduced one in 1996.[152] If other journals follow their lead, we might soon expect to see fair, equitable, and ethically appropriate financial disclosure by authors of papers in peer-reviewed scientific journals.

A related issue is the disclosure of the funding sources of all-expenses-paid seminars and vacations for federal judges. A *Washington Post* news story revealed a few years ago that:

> Federal judges are attending expenses-paid five-day seminars on property rights and the environment at resorts in Montana, sessions underwritten by conservative foundations that are also funding a wave of litigation on these issues in federal courts.
>
> Funding for the seminars, run by a group called the Foundation for Research on Economics and the Environment (FREE), also comes from foundations run by companies with a significant interest in property rights and environmental issues, Internal Revenue Service records show.[153]

These seminars were intended, according to advance letters sent to judges to advertise the seminars, to "explore the role of property rights, incentives, and voluntary cooperation in achieving environmental goals." The letters also indicated that "time is provided for cycling, fishing, golfing, hiking and horseback riding."[154]

Judges who attended these seminars later indicated that they were not aware of the nature of the private interests that provided the funding for them. I believe they should have been made aware of this, and that all funding sources for seminars such as these should be fully disclosed in the advertising materials. This principle, moreover, should apply to the seminars, workshops and training sessions for government risk managers, and for personnel in any government regulatory agencies.

10. Access to Public Spaces

As the incidence of chemical sensitivity disorders continues to grow, issues of equal access to public spaces such as shopping malls, office buildings, theaters, churches, schools and workplaces will become increasingly important. That is, as the number of people who are physically unable to tolerate exposure to pesticides and the toxicants in artificial fragrances continues to escalate, communities will need to rethink their concepts of public access.

If in the past the number of such chemically sensitive persons was small, societies could consider the issue of their restricted access to public spaces unimportant. With the growing incidence of chemical sensitivity disorders, however, the matter can no longer be considered unimportant. Epidemiological surveys indicate that the number of people who are made physically sick by exposure to the toxicants in pesticides and artificial fragrances is approaching one-quarter of the population. "Several large surveys [some of which surveyed several thousand people] suggest that between 15 percent and 34 percent or up to one-third of Americans consider themselves especially sensitive, allergic, or unusually sensitive to certain chemicals."[155] In one survey of over 4,000 households, 6.3 percent answered "yes" when asked, "Have you ever been told by a doctor that you had environmental illness or chemical sensitivity?"[156] In another survey of 200, four percent "reported that they had extreme chemical intolerances that had been diagnosed by a physician."[157] The most commonly seen estimate of the prevalence of MCS comes from an independent consultation of the National Research Council. In its study of MCS in America the NRC estimated that approximately 15 percent of the population was chemically sensitive.[158]

Regardless of which of these studies are the most accurate, none of their estimates are trivial. Even the smallest of the estimates, the one that indicates that 4 percent of the population has been formally diagnosed with MCS, is not trivial. If the population of the U.S. is approximately 265 million , then even that most conservative study would indicate that 10.6 million Americans have become hypersensitized to a multiplicity of chemicals. We might estimate that similar numbers would apply to other industrialized countries. (Whether the numbers of chemically sensitive people in nonindustrialized countries are higher or lower is not yet known. They may be lower because of the lesser presence of industry, or they may be higher because of less regulation of toxics and heavier use of pesticides—including some pesticides that have been banned in the U.S. and other industrial-ized nations. Epidemiological studies in non-industrialized countries still need to be done.)

In any case, we can probably assume that the number of peo-ple who actually are chemically sensitive is somewhat larger than the number who have been formally diagnosed, just as the number of people who actually have cancer is probably somewhat larger than the number who have been formally diagnosed with it.

If significant numbers of people do find their lives restricted by their sensitivities to the toxicants that they commonly encounter in public spaces, particularly pesticides and artificial fragrances, the question societies will eventually need to grapple with is whether it is to be considered acceptable for this number of people to be effectively excluded from significant participation in public life. Peo-ple who are made sick by exposure to these toxicants—people who may have an asthma attack in the presence of artificial fragrances, for example, or who may develop severe migraine headaches in the presence of even low levels of pesticide residues, or who may faint in the presence of such chemicals—simply cannot go into spaces where they are likely to encounter them. They do not go to the malls, to theaters, or to schools. Many have had to quit their professions because of an inability to tolerate exposure to certain chemicals. Many have had to stop going to church, synagogue, temple or mosque because they know there will be strong artificial fragrance residues in the air in those spaces.

It will eventually be important for societies to squarely face these questions about equal access to public spaces. Many public build-ings do provide wheelchair ramps, electric door openers, and wheel-chair-accessible toilet facilities for people with certain kinds of phys-ical disabilities because societies have decided that these disabilities should not exclude people from public spaces. Several colleges and universities around the country, as well as some K–12 schools, have begun to develop and implement fragrance-free policies for their campuses, and "the current trend is leaning toward hospitals devel-oping policies to accommodate the health needs of patients with MCS" too.[159] If people with chemical sensitivities constitute some nontrivial proportion of the population, then it should probably be incumbent on societies to begin to address these questions of equal access now.

The questions, of course, are not easy ones. When it came to making public spaces accessible to persons in wheelchairs, it was more a matter of modifying curbs, stairways, entrances to buildings, elevators, restrooms and so forth in order to make those spaces accessible. The costs involved were primarily financial, not personal. But now, making public spaces accessible to those who are made sick by toxicants may involve facing different social issues.

For example, questions about pesticide usage and notification will need to be faced and dealt with. Questions about some people's right to wear artificial fragrances to the theater, to work or to church versus other people's right to not be made sick by those fragrances will need to be squarely faced. Some of these questions are in certain ways analogous to the issues surrounding exposure to second-hand tobacco smoke: the conflict between some people's right to smoke tobacco in public places versus other people's right to not be made sick by that smoke is a perfect instance.

These questions are complex and difficult and will not be easily solved. But it is probably time for denial to end and for societies to face the truth and begin formulating policies that will be as fair as possible for all their members.

11. Additional Proposals

CHLORINE

In 1993 the American Public Health Association passed a resolution urging the gradual elimination of synthetic chlorinated chemical compounds, and advocating research that would lead to the development of safer alternatives.[160]

The International Joint Commission on the Great Lakes issued an almost identical resolution recommending the gradual elimination of chlorine-containing compounds. Such persistent and harmful chemicals, they said, should no longer be allowed to exist in the ecosystem "whether or not unassailable scientific proof of acute or chronic damage is universally accepted."[161] In taking such a stand, the commission made a clear declaration in strong support of the importance of the precautionary principle.

Whether such a policy is the one that is actually eventually chosen, national and international public health agencies should at least begin to seriously consider introducing regulatory policies that would drastically reduce worldwide production and use of chlorine and chlorinated chemical compounds.

In Utero Torts

Tort claims should be allowed against employers for chemical injuries sustained by a child *in utero* while the child's mother was working in a place or manner that caused her to be exposed to contaminants.

A recent ruling by the California Court of Appeal, Fifth Appellate District, held that an injury "sustained by a child while *in utero* from the mother's chemical exposure at work 'is actionable in tort to the same extent as any nonemployee's direct injury by the employer.'"[162] In this case,[163] the mother sued her employer for damages after her child was born with cerebral palsy. The mother had been chronically exposed, while pregnant, to "fumes from a propane gas-powered buffing machine used without adequate ventilation and monitoring."[164]

The *Charter on Industrial Hazards and Human Rights* which we examined in Chapter Two clearly supports this position in its Article 24.

> All persons injured or otherwise detrimentally affected by any hazardous economic activity have the right to swift, comprehensive and effective relief. This right applies to all persons affected by hazards or potential hazards, including persons not yet born at the time of injury or exposure, and those injured, bereaved or economically and socially disadvantaged, whether affected directly or indirectly.

In addition, article 2.1 of the CETOS *Toxics Bill of Rights* affirms that, "Incipient persons shall be protected from potentially harmful exposures during embryonic development and post-natal life."[165]

It thus seems that both legal and human rights considerations concur on this question, and would support the claims of injury to an embryonic child caused by its mother's exposure to toxicants while working in a toxic environment.

Imported Chemical Residues

Products arriving in the U.S. from other parts of the world should be monitored for residues of pesticides and other chemical compounds that have been outlawed for use in the U.S.

Products showing evidence of contaminants which have been prohibited from being used in the U.S. should either be banned from entry, or should be brightly labeled with prominent warnings.

SUMMARY

The modest proposals outlined in Chapter Three are only a few of the policy changes that need to eventually emerge to deal with the growing threat of toxicant induced illnesses. The proposals are intended to be moderate and common sense rather than radical and dramatic. While some may believe that much more radical policy changes will be necessary in order to adequately protect the health of the world's citizens, the modest proposals suggested here would be at least a good and necessary beginning.

Modest or not, however, these proposals can be expected to face, indeed have already had to face, obstacles and challenges so formidable as to sometimes seem almost impossible to overcome. Because these obstacles have been so formidable, our examination of them in Chapter Four is titled "Brick Walls."

Notes

1. From "World Scientists' Warning to Humanity," 1993. Quoted in J.B. Berkson, *A Canary's Tale: The Final Battle, Politics, Poisons, and Pollution vs. the Environment and the Public Health* (Hagerstown, MD: Self-Published, 1996) 452+xviii. p. 222.

2. L. Gayle, "Mother's Milk—as Safe as Apple Pie?" *One in Three: Women with Cancer Confront an Epidemic.* Ed. J. Brady (San Francisco and Pittsburgh: Cleis Press, 1991) 79–87. p. 84.

3. *Draft Report on Multiple Chemical Sensitivity*, Interagency Workgroup on Multiple Chemical Sensitivity (Agencies represented on the workgroup included the Department of Defense, Department of Energy, Department of Health and Human Services, Department of Veterans Affairs, and the U.S. Environmental Protection Agency), August 24, 1998. p. 41.

4. Quoted in N. Ashford and C.S. Miller, *Chemical Exposures: Low Levels, High Stakes*, 2nd ed. (New York: Van Nostrand Reinhold / John Wiley & Sons, 1998) 440+xxiii. p. 147.

5. J.G. Vos, M. Younes and E. Smith, eds., *Allergic Hypersensitivities Induced by Chemicals: Recommendations for Prevention* (London: CRC Press [on behalf of the World Health Organization Regional Office for Europe] 1996) 348. p. 13

6. For example, C.S. Miller, et al., "Empirical Approaches for the Investigation of Toxicant-induced Loss of Tolerance," *Environmental Health Perspectives*, 105, Supplement 2 (March 1997) 515–19. See also N. Ashford and C.S. Miller, *op. cit., passim.*

7. Edward Jenner's first direct challenge experiments testing the protective efficacy of cowpox inoculation for immunizing people against contracting smallpox were, I believe, the first scientifically designed biomedical

experiments involving human subjects in the history of modern scientific medicine. For an ethical examination of Jenner's experiments, see T.A. Kerns, *Jenner on Trial: An Ethical Examination of Vaccine Research in the Age of Smallpox and the Age of AIDS* (Lanham, MD: University Press of America, 1997) 104.

8. For a full discussion of the EMU, see W. Rea, MD, *Chemical Sensitivity*, 4 (Boca Raton, FL: Lewis Publishers, and CRC Press, 1992–97) 2924, vol. 4, p. 2187–2284. See also C.S. Miller, "Toxicant-induced Loss of Tolerance—An Emerging Theory of Disease?" *Environmental Health Perspectives*, 105, Supplement 2 (March 1997) 445–53. p. 450–51.

9. C.S. Miller, Personal communication. May 20, 1997.

10. C.S. Miller, "Toxicant-induced Loss of Tolerance—An Emerging Theory of Disease?" p. 451.

11. *Ibid.*

12. *Ibid.*, p. 450.

13. *Ibid.*

14. *Ibid.*, p. 448.

15. *Ibid.*

16. W. Rea, MD. Alka Seltzer products also help some people recover from the effects of an exposure.

17. D. Hume, *An Enquiry Concerning Human Understanding*, 1748.

18. A.B. Hill, "The Environment and Disease: Association or Causation?" *Proceedings of the Royal Society of Medicine*, 58 (1965) 295–300.

19. These criteria are also synopsized by Miller in C.S. Miller, "Chemical Sensitivity: symptom, syndrome or mechanism for disease?" *Toxicology*, 111 (1996) 69–86, p. 81–3.

20. C.S. Miller, "Chemical Sensitivity: symptom, syndrome or mechanism for disease?" p. 82.

21. *Ibid.*

22. *Ibid.*

23. *Ibid.*

24. *Ibid.*

25. *Ibid.*, p. 83.

26. *Ibid.*

27. N. Ashford and C.S. Miller, *op. cit.*, p. 164.

28. J.G. Vos, M. Younes and E. Smith, eds.

29. C.S. Miller, "Chemical Sensitivity: symptom, syndrome or mechanism for disease?" p. 83.

30. *Ibid.*

31. N. Ashford and C.S. Miller, *op. cit.*, p. 158.

32. L.K. Varner, "Alarm over asthma," *Seattle Times,* February 22, 1998, E1,5. p. E1.

33. D.M. Blank, "A Growing Sensitivity to What's in the Air," *New York Times,* February 22, 1998, BU 11.

34. D. Pimentel, "Ecology of Increasing Disease: Population Growth and Environmental Degradation," *Bioscience* (October 1998).

35. Cf. especially *Nuremberg Code* and *WHO/CIOMS International*

Ethical Guidelines for Biomedical Research Involving Human Subjects.
Both appear as appendices to this book.

36. J.H. Cushman, Jr., "Group wants pesticide companies to end testing on humans," *New York Times* (July 28, 1998). A9.

37. C. Duehring, "The global problem of MCS part one: overview of investigative reports' findings," *Medical and Legal Briefs*, 2, Number 5 (March/April 1997) 1–5. p. 5.

38. *Medical and Legal Briefs,* PO Box 1089, Minot, ND 58702-1089. Phone (701) 837-0161.

39. R. Jerome and M. Nelson, "Toxic Avenger," *People* (February 9, 1998) 113–15. Cindy Duehring died of MCS-related complications on June 29, 1999.

40. P.R. Gibson, "Environmental Illness/Multiple Chemical Sensitivities: Invisible Disabilities," *Women and Therapy,* 14, Number 3/4 (1993) 171–85. p. 177.

41. *Ibid.*

42. B. Rouché, *The Man Who Grew Two Breasts: And Other True Tales of Medical Detection* (New York: Truman Talley Books/Dutton, 1995) 197.

43. *Ibid.,* p. 38.

44. *Ibid.*

45. Other considerations may be important as well: "Pursuing the psychiatric route first may subject the patient to the complexities of establishing a therapeutic relationship and/or the prescribing of psychoactive drugs, and both may generate doubts concerning the patient's mental health. In addition, psychotherapy may be unproductive if environmental causes are at work. Labeling a patient as having a psychiatric illness may be pejorative from the perspective of an employer, co-workers, and family. That psychiatric records are kept separate from the medical records of patients is no accident. In the event that psychoactive drugs are used, unraveling an environmental cause or contribution to the patient's underlying condition may be greatly complicated." N. Ashford and C.S. Miller, *op. cit.,* p. 141.

46. C.S. Miller, "Chemical Sensitivity: symptom, syndrome or mechanism for disease?" p. 84.

47. J. Blondell and V.A. Dobozy, *Review of Chlorpyrifos Poisoning Data.* Environmental Protection Agency (January 14, 1997). As reported in C. Duehring, "EPA Dursban Review Finds MCS—Dow revises marketing," *Medical and Legal Briefs,* 2, #6 (May/June 1997) 10.

48. N. Ashford and B. Hinzow, *Chemical Sensitivity in Selected European Countries: An exploratory study,* Ergonomia, Ltd. (November 1995). As quoted in C. Duehring, "Overview of Biologic Research," *Medical and Legal Briefs,* 2, #6 (May/June 1997) 1–5. p. 1.

49. S. Sontag, *Illness as Metaphor* (New York: Doubleday, 1978) 83.

50. *Ibid.,* p. 54.

51. *Ibid.,* p. 55.

52. *Ibid.*

53. *Ibid.*

54. *Ibid.*, p. 57.

55. *Ibid.* See also the *Book of Job* in which Job's "friends" tell him that he deserves all the physical calamities that have befallen him.

56. "California Requires Warning Posted in Dental Offices," *News Bites* (January 1997).

57. *Ibid.*

58. *Nation's Health* (October 1997) 8.

59. *Ibid.*

60. Z. Bankowski, ed., *International Ethical Guidelines for Biomedical Research Involving Human Subjects* (Geneva, Switzerland: Council for International Organizations of Medical Sciences [CIOMS] 1993) 63. p. 10.

61. M. Lappé, *A Toxics Bill of Rights.* Center for Ethics and Toxics (1996). Article 2.8.

62. C. Van Strum, *A Bitter Fog: Herbicides and Human Rights* (San Francisco: Sierra Club Books, 1983) 288+x. p. 238–9.

63. Oregon HB 3281 was considered in early 1998.

64. C. Van Strum, *op. cit.*, p. 236.

65. *Ibid.*, p. 237.

66. *Ibid.*, p. 239–40.

67. Work by researchers at the University of Arizona found that "'significant numbers' of dangerous human disease organisms infect even treated sewage sludge." Quoted in J. Stauber and S. Rampton, *Toxic Sludge Is Good for You: Lies, Damn Lies, and the Public Relations Industry* (Monroe, ME: Common Courage Press, 1995) 236+iv. p. 119. See also T.M. Straub "Hazards from Pathogenic Microorganisms in Land-Disposed Sewage Sludge," *Reviews of Environmental Contamination and Toxicology*, 132 (1993) 55–91.

68. J. Stauber and S. Rampton, *ibid.*, p. 104.

69. *Ibid.*, p. 113.

70. Quoted *ibid.*, p. 107.

71. *Ibid.*

72. *Ibid.*, p. 108.

73. *Ibid.*

74. *Ibid.*, p. 120–21.

75. Quoted *ibid.*, p. 121.

76. *Ibid.*, Chapter 8.

77. *Ibid.*, p. 122.

78. *Ibid., passim.* See also D. Wilson, "Fear in the Fields," *Seattle Times* (July 4–5, 1997) A1ff. Mr Wilson won the prestigious Goldsmith Prize in Investigative Reporting for 1997 for his "Fear in the Fields" story revealing how industrial wastes were being recycled into fertilizers to be spread on crop fields, usually without the farmers' knowledge. The series explained that the practice was largely unregulated. "The Goldsmith Prize is awarded by Harvard University 'to the journalist whose investigative reporting in a story or series of related stories best promotes more effective and ethical conduct of government, the making of public policy, or the practice of politics.'" Staff, "Times reporter wins 2 national awards," *Seattle Times* (March 15, 1998). B1.

79. L. Gayle, *op. cit.,* p. 80–81.

80. Letter from Thomas Jefferson to William Charles Jarvis, September 28, 1820. Quoted in C. Van Strum, *op. cit.,* p. 241.

81. "Support for labels on gene-altered food," *Nature,* 385 (February 27, 1997) 762.

82. D.C. Vacco, *The Secret Hazards of Pesticides: Inert Ingredients.* New York State Department of Law, Environmental Protection Bureau (February 1991, 1996) p. 2.

83. *Ibid.,* p. 7–8.

84. *Ibid.*

85. *Ibid.,* p. 1.

86. *Ibid.,* p. 9–10.

87. *Ibid.*

88. C. Cox, "Dichlobenil," *Journal of Pesticide Reform,* 17, #1 (Spring 1997) 14–20.

89. D.C. Vacco, *op. cit.,* p. 5.

90. D. Fagin and M. Lavelle, *Toxic Deception: How the Chemical Industry Manipulates Science, Bends the Law, and Endangers Your Health* (Secaucus, NJ: Carol Publishing Group, 1997) 294+xxvi. p. 6.

91. R. Greene, "Inert pesticide ingredients lose EPA secrecy privilege," *Oregonian* (October 19, 1996).

92. See N. Ashford and C.S. Miller, *op. cit.,* p. 62.

93. "Plans for protecting food safety, regulating pesticides announced," *The Nation's Health,* 27, Number 4 (April 1997) 5.

94. *Ibid.*

95. *Ibid.*

96. *Ibid.*

97. A State Department notice—on behalf of the various U.S. agencies involved—which explains the effort to develop a consistent worldwide hazard communication system and requesting public comment was scheduled to appear in the April 3, 1997 Federal Register.

98. D. Kearns, *EPA's 1995 Toxics Release Data Includes First-Ever Reporting on 286 New Chemicals* EPA, May 20, 1997.

99. M. Lappé, *op. cit.* Article 2.7. This article should probably also include endocrinological effects among those to be thoroughly evaluated before a product is allowed to come to market.

100. APHA, "Policy statement 9606: The precautionary principle and chemical exposure standards for the work place," *American Journal of Public Health,* 87, Number 3 (March 1997) 500–501.

101. *Ibid.,* p. 501.

102. Again, new pesticides are the exception, though we may question how well they are tested for both immediate and long-term health effects.

103. In the case of pharmaceuticals and medical devices, developers must prove the product to be both safe and effective.

104. C. Duehring, "Plaintiff Awarded $4.2 Million Against DuPont in Toxic Carpet Suit," *Medical and Legal Briefs,* 2, No. 4 (January/February 1997) 1–4. p. 1.

105. See T. Svoboda, "Every Breath She Takes," *Utne Reader* (March-April 1987) 59–63.

106. C. Duehring, "Plaintiff Awarded $4.2 Million Against DuPont in Toxic Carpet Suit," p. 2.

107. *Ibid.*, p. 3.

108. *Ibid.*, p. 1.

109. C. Van Strum, *op. cit.*, p. 16–17.

110. C. Hignite and D.L. Azarnoff, "Drugs and drug metabolites as environmental contaminants: chlorophenoxyisobutyrate and salicylic acid in sewage water effluent," *Life Sciences*, 20, Number 12 (January 15, 1977) 337–41.

111. P. Montague, "Drugs in the Water," *Rachel's Environment and Health Weekly*, 614 (September 3, 1998).

112. *Ibid.*

113. *Ibid.*

114. Quoted in C. Van Strum, *op. cit.*, p. 231.

115. A.W. Nichols, "Amending the United States Constitution to Include Environmental Rights," *The Nation's Health* (September 1997) 18–19. p. 18.

116. *Ibid.*

117. *Ibid., passim.*

118. Failure-to-warn statutes should be enhanced and made applicable to manufacturers and distributors of products (and byproducts) containing potentially harmful toxicants. This means simply that anyone who is harmed by exposure to industrial byproducts or by exposure to toxicants in consumer products should be able to sue manufacturers, transporters, distributors, marketers and applicators for a failure to warn them of possible health effects associated with being exposed to their products or industrial byproducts.

119. This may even, in some cases, require developing separate standards for certain ethnic groups if those groups are shown to be more vulnerable to certain kinds of toxicants.

120. APHA, "Policy statement 9606: The precautionary principle and chemical exposure standards for the work place." *Passim.*

121. *Ibid.*

122. *Ibid.*, p. 501.

123. C. Duehring, "Overexposure from legal pesticiding: a generation at risk," *Medical and Legal Briefs*, 3, No. 6 (May/June 1998) 1–4. p. 1.

124. Quoted in S. Lewis, "Promoting Child Health and the Convention on the Rights of the Child," *Health and Human Rights*, 2, Number 3 (1997) 77–82. p. 78.

125. Quoted *ibid.*, p. 79. By the term "traditional practices," the drafters of this paragraph were probably referring to practices such as female genital mutilation (see *ibid.*, p. 79), and yet the document clearly refers to any traditional practices that put the health of children at risk. Some traditional practices in schools, such as the unannounced indoor spraying of pesticides, for example, while not as gory as female genital mutilation, do in fact put children at risk of adverse health effects, and should therefore be dealt with under this provision of the *Convention on the Rights of the Child*.

126. "Healthier schools focus of WHO report," *The Nation's Health* (February 1997) 24.

127. Reported *ibid.*

128. Quoted in D.J. Rapp, *Is This Your Child's World? How You Can Fix the Schools and Homes That Are Making Your Children Sick* (New York: Bantam, 1996) 635+xix. p. 196.

129. "[C]hildren can encounter pesticides in drinking water, the home, schools, day-care centers, lawns, gardens, playgrounds, ball fields, golf courses, swimming pools, in paints, and in treated lumber." P. Montague, "1997 Snapshots—Part 2," *Rachel's Environment and Health Weekly*, #579 (January 1, 1998).

130. For a summary of some sources of indoor pollutants in both schools and homes, see W.R. Ott and J.W. Roberts, "Everyday Exposure to Toxic Pollutants," *Scientific American* (February 1998).

131. See, for example, *ibid.*

132. D. Hallaby, "Australia's Chemical-Free School," *Our Toxic Times*, 8, No. 2 (February 1997) 6.

133. The University of Notre Dame, my own alma mater, is the example with which I am most familiar.

134. At a 1997 conference of college and university housing officers, one presentation discussed the necessity of providing chemically safe living environments for students as a way of minimizing students' toxic load, and maximizing their ability to learn and function well mentally.

135. N. Ashford and C.S. Miller, *op. cit.,* p. 165.

136. The TESC policy was implemented approximately one year before the NSCC policy.

137. For a discussion of exposure to toxicants in our indoor work spaces, see W.R. Ott and J.W. Roberts, *op. cit.*

138. APHA, "Policy statement 9606: The precautionary principle and chemical exposure standards for the work place," p. 500–01.

139. *Ibid.,* p. 501.

140. *Ibid.*

141. M. Wadman, "Study discloses financial interests behind papers," *Nature*, 385 (January 30, 1997) 376.

142. *Ibid.* According to Wadman, *JAMA* does require financial disclosures by its authors.

143. *Ibid.*

144. P. Montague, "Follow the money," *Rachel's Environment and Health Weekly*, #581 (January 15, 1998).

145. *Ibid.*

146. H.T. Stelfox, et al., "Conflict of Interest in the Debate over Calcium-Channel Antagonists," *New England Journal of Medicine*, 338, Number 2 (January 8, 1998).

147. *Ibid.*

148. *Ibid.*

149. K. Kerr, "Study: Doctors who backed heart drug had ties to makers," *Seattle Times* (January 4, 1998). A4.

150. Quoted in M. Wadman, *op. cit.*

151. H.T. Stelfox, et al., *op. cit.*, as quoted in P. Montague, "Follow the money."

152. M. Wadman, *op. cit.*

153. R. Marcus, "Judges take free trips in conflict of interest," *Seattle Times* (originally in the *Washington Post*), April 9, 1998, A3.

154. *Ibid.*

155. Several of these epidemiological studies have been summarized in N. Ashford and C.S. Miller, *op. cit.*, p. 232–34.

156. *Ibid.*, p. 233.

157. *Ibid.*, p. 232.

158. The NRC did not indicate in its report, however, what information this estimate was based on.

159. C. Duehring, "Manteca Hospital develops MCS accommodation policy," *Medical and Legal Briefs*, 4, Number 1 (July/August 1998) 9.

160. S. Steingraber, *Living Downstream: An Ecologist Looks at Cancer and the Environment* (Reading, MA: Addison-Wesley Publishing, 1997) 357+xvi. p. 115. In 1996 the APHA passed a resolution calling for health care facilities to phase out their use of polyvinyl chloride PVC plastics, and urging that these plastics be replaced with less toxic alternatives, especially considering that companies such as Nike, Volvo, Saab, Braun, Ikea and others are already taking steps to reduce their use of (and thus their customers' exposure to) PVC plastics. C. Cray and M. Harden, "PVC & Dioxin: Enough Is Enough," *Rachel's Environment and Health Weekly*, 616 (September 17, 1998). This resolution and others may be found on the web at: http://www.apha.org/science/policy.html. A list of potential alternatives to PVC plastics may be found at: www.greenpeaceusa.org/campaigns/toxics/pvc_dist.htm.

161. S. Steingraber, *ibid.*

162. C. Duehring, "Tort Claims Allowed for Workplace Fetal Injury," *Medical and Legal Briefs*, 2, No. 4 (January/February 1997) 10.

163. Snyder v. Michael's Stores, Inc., Calif Ct App, No. F024076, 9-23-96.

164. C. Duehring, "Tort Claims Allowed for Workplace Fetal Injury."

165. M. Lappé, *op. cit., passim.*

FOUR

———— Brick Walls ————

The image of a runaway train seems for some people to accurately represent the direction our planet is moving when it comes to the release of synthetic chemical compounds into the environment. The train, according to this image, is enormous, it weighs several thousand tons, and it has lost its brakes. It is careening faster and faster down a steep mountainside, completely out of control. At the bottom of the mountain is a village which will be almost completely obliterated when the train crashes into it at full speed.[1]

This image seems to be a common one in the minds of people who are acutely aware of environmental issues, including some of those issues we have been discussing in this book. Many of these environmental activists feel themselves to be in a position similar to that of the mythic Cassandra who had been cursed by the gods with the power to see into the future, but whose warnings were destined to not be believed. As one activist writes, "I firmly believe that we are on the brink of disaster, and that we must be very forceful if we are to stop the destruction before there is no 'us.' We have to ... start fighting as though our lives depended on it. Because they do."[2]

Most toxicant induced illnesses are, after all, anthropogenic and are therefore preventable. "If society caused it, society can prevent it."[3] And the measures for prevention would include the modest proposals outlined in Chapter Three.[4]

It will also be important to remember that when we are dealing with these toxicant induced illnesses, we are clearly dealing with human rights issues. As Sandra Steingraber, a professor and environmental activist, reminds us,

> cancer, as a preventable disease, is a human rights issue. Laws exist to prevent and punish other forms of criminal victimization; legislation that prevents and punishes victimization by environmental poisoning could dramatically reduce the incidence of cancer.[5]

And what holds true for cancer holds true for other toxicant induced illnesses.

In light of this, an awareness is growing of how important it is to do everything that can be done to prevent these toxicant induced illnesses. There is an emerging belief that the measures necessary for prevention will require societies and their governments to be willing to assess the *future* damage that toxicants are likely to cause, and then to take anticipatory measures to prevent those damages from occurring. After all, "the potential magnitude of damage to the environment that humans are now able to cause, and the speed with which such damage can occur, are such that it is now necessary for the impact to be assessed and action taken *before* the damage occurs rather than afterwards."[6]

And yet, unfortunately "[h]umans have rarely anticipated environmental pollution; action and pollution control have generally followed on from environmental disasters or unacceptable pollution damage."[7] If this reactive pattern continues in which societies and governments only *react* to environmental disasters which are already under way, then the runaway train will continue to loom as a very apt analogy.

I am not myself certain whether the sense of inevitability that is such a large part of this image is an accurate representation of the planet's future or not. John Cairns, a spokesperson on ecology for the National Institute of Environmental Health Sciences' *Environmental Health Perspectives*, is not certain either. He suggests that "unless we make fundamental changes in behavior and lifestyle, the possibility exists that we will be unable to reverse the trend of decline in environmental quality and life."[8]

Whether the decline is inevitable or not, I do know that the obstacles we will have to overcome in order to prove this image wrong are colossal and will sometimes seem insuperable. But I believe they *can* be overcome.

We turn our attention now to examining what some of these obstacles, these challenges, have been and will likely continue to be. We begin with the fact that the problem of toxics is not confined to any specific nation or region, but is in fact global.

1. Globality

Success in dealing adequately with toxics will require both a global perspective and global action.

As David Satcher, Director of the CDC, has written, "[P]ublic health in the 21st century must be global in its perspective and approach."

> As disease knows no borders [nor do toxics], the health of all human beings on the planet must be the concern of every person in public health. We are *already* a global village. We believe that, in the 21st century, to raise a child will take not only a village, but a *global* village.[9]

This means that, in our efforts to protect individuals and communities from the adverse health effects of ambient environmental toxicants, we must consider the issues involved from a global perspective, and we must recognize that ultimately the most beneficial actions will be those that will have a global impact.

The difficulty here, of course, is that regulatory laws and public policy are made within the boundaries of nation states, and therefore are implemented and have force only within those boundaries. Toxics, on the other hand, have no respect for artificial national boundaries. Pesticides can drift many hundreds and even thousands of miles, and are also carried via the food chain to locations many thousands of miles distant from the point of origin.[10] They can be transported on foodstuffs, on clothing and other textile products, and are frequently sprayed liberally on many materials being transported by truck, ship, and air. If the global human community is to be made safe from overuse of pesticides and other toxics, policymaking will clearly need to be transnational.

Fortunately, some steps in this direction have already been made. A piece in *Environmental Health Perspectives* highlights one.

> Thanks to a process initiated a few years ago by the United Nations, more than 100 countries, including the United States, are set to forge an international treaty that would ultimately prohibit use of some of

the world's most dangerous persistent organic pollutants (POPs). These chemicals ... can survive for decades and travel thousands of miles from their source—characteristics that enable them to contaminate the environment as well as accumulate in the fatty tissues of humans and animals.[11]

At a meeting in Nairobi, Kenya in January 1997, the United Nations Environment Program passed a resolution that called for international negotiations to begin early in 1998 "leading to a treaty banning or restricting the use of POPs [which is] to be in effect by the year 2000."[12]

The United Nations and the World Health Organization do have a history of helping in the formulation of international treaties and agreements concerning health policy. Halfdan Mahler, former Director-General of the World Health Organization, believes that "global health cooperation today is, in my opinion, in pretty bad condition." He does believe, however, that despite all its weaknesses, "WHO is the intergovernmental organization that truly must be the key player in improving global health collaboration."[13]

The challenges facing global health policy are enormous, but at least an awareness is growing that much more cooperation among nations will be necessary if the public health is to be well served.

2. Multinational Chemical Corporations

Corporations can and do sometimes effectively hinder or corrupt the making of sound environmental policy and law. We have watched the tobacco companies shape policy for decades, even despite a certain level of public disapproval of their conduct. The chemical manufacturers have been doing precisely the same thing for decades too, but there has been far less social awareness of their practices to date.

Dr. Thomas Stockman is the hero of Henrik Ibsen's classic drama, *An Enemy of the People*. The play is set in "a small Norwegian town." Dr. Stockman is the town's physician and sole scientist. The town's primary source of income is Kirsten Springs, a kind of health spa that people from all over Europe come to visit for its alleged health enhancing effects. The springs (before the action of the play begins) have recently been renovated and it is expected that there will be many visitors to them during the coming summer, providing the town with much needed income. Early in the play's action, however, Dr. Stockman discovers that tests he has independently conducted indicate that the water of the springs is dangerously polluted.

Officials in the town do not wish it to be known that the springs are polluted. If the pollution were to become common knowledge, the popularity of Kirsten Springs as a place to come for healing would diminish, and the town would suffer economically. The town officials thus need to discredit Dr. Stockman and his claim that the springs are polluted. Ibsen's play is the story of how Dr. Stockman and all his evidence are effectively contradicted and derailed by political influences, by the power of the press, and by the uninformed will of the great majority, "the people." (At one level, Ibsen's play is an illustration of Alexis de Tocqueville's concept of "the tyranny of the majority.") The drama very effectively portrays the power of the forces that oppose the doctor's revelation. Dr. Stockman, despite his ingenuous enthusiasm for discovering and publishing the truth about the adverse health effects of the Springs, is eventually successfully undermined by the opposing forces in the town and is formally declared to be an enemy of the people. The springs, therefore, despite being polluted, remain open.

This story takes place late in the 19th century, about the time the germ theory of disease has begun to be established and has become largely accepted by the medical community. The germ theory is nonetheless still somewhat new at that time and is not so completely accepted that it has the force of a foregone conclusion. The theory has not yet become part of popular culture.

At what stage of acceptance today is the theory that low doses of toxicants can be pathogenic? Probably not as far along in its acceptance as the germ theory was in Ibsen's drama. Therefore, those who today point out that toxicants in our air and water are making people sick, and who argue for protections against exposure to these toxicants, have a much more difficult time of it than did Ibsen's Dr. Stockman. They can expect the powers of the corporate world, the powers of the public relations industry, and perhaps even sometimes the powers of government regulatory agencies, to oppose them in their efforts to tell the community that "the springs are polluted." Many want to continue advertising and drawing people to the springs as paying customers. They want to continue to make money from the springs, even though they know it will make some people sick. As Dr. William Foege says of the corporate tobacco interests, "there are people [who] knowing that their decision to advertise and promote tobacco is going to kill people ... [are] still willing to do it."[14] This estimation may be true of some people in the chemical corporations as well.

A well-documented and clearly detailed account of how much effort chemical corporations are willing to expend to avoid taking responsibility for chemical contamination can be found in Jonathan Harr's highly readable 1995 bestseller, *A Civil Action*.[15] This book details the events and legal battles surrounding the discovery of a leukemia cluster among families who drank water from severely chemically contaminated wells in Woburn, Massachusetts. Those leukemia sufferers undertook a civil suit against the most obvious and probable polluters, W. R. Grace Co., and Beatrice Food Co. The trial spanned the second half of the 1980s and, despite the enormous amount of time, energy, and money that went into the efforts of the plaintiffs, the outcome clearly favored the corporations. Charles Nesson, one of the attorneys for the plaintiffs was (and still is) a professor at Harvard Law School. He has sometimes referred to the Woburn case in his law courses, saying

> I used to believe in the idea that justice would prevail if you worked hard enough at it.... I thought if judges saw cheating right in front of them, they'd do something about it. The Woburn case gave me a depressing dose of reality.[16]

His depressing dose of reality came in discovering that sometimes corporations, with their enormous financial resources, have enough power in these matters to avoid being held responsible by government agencies for what they have done. Two other researchers, Fagin and Lavelle, say it this way in their book, *Toxic Deception*:

> With millions—maybe even billions—of dollars to spend on lawyers, scientists, PR firms, campaign contributions, secrecy orders, and millions of pages and years of seemingly unlimited patience in litigation challenging the outmanned, underfunded government's every regulatory move, the chemical industry has managed to continue manufacturing what are generally considered to be harmful agents.[17]

Corporations, after all, despite their legal status as human persons, are neither biological entities nor spiritual and moral entities of the sort that have a conscience. They are only legal entities, and thus are obviously not capable of having any of the feelings characteristic of human beings, such as compassion, concern, or guilt.

They are much more like machines in that regard, churning along in their effort to produce profits. Unlike human persons, the modern corporation also has an essentially limitless lifetime, and thus has "the capacity to grow without limit."[18] Furthermore, as Peter Montague points out in a *Rachel's* article,

> After they grow large, corporations cannot feel pain. For example, the Exxon Corporation was fined $5 billion for the Exxon Valdez oil spill. On the day that enormous fine was announced, Exxon's stock price rose because investors realized that Exxon was invincible. No matter how odious its behavior, human institutions have no capacity to curb the excesses of a large transnational. Similarly, the day the government of India imposed an $800 million fine on Union Carbide for its role of negligence in the Bhopal disaster, Carbide's stock rose.[19]

This inability of corporations to feel any serious pain may have serious implications. Pain, after all, is a powerful teacher that clearly helps motivate human persons to modify their behavior. Montague continues:

> As infants, if we try to crawl through a solid door, we hit our forehead and are brought up short by painful reality. As toddlers, if we strike another person, we may be struck in return; thus we learn that violence is not necessarily the best policy. Eventually, external pain becomes internalized into a conscience and we become civilized adults. Under law, corporations are formally denied this civilizing impetus. As a result, corporations tend to behave like sociopaths.[20]

In these ways, while corporations have been granted many of the rights accorded to human persons, they do not have many of the constraints and controls—such as conscience, the ability to feel pain, having only a finite lifetime, and so on.

Corporations do, of course, have human beings employed in them and we might imagine that those human beings would sometimes be inclined to follow the dictates of their personal and social consciences. Unfortunately, however, the primary mandate of those human beings in their jobs as executives and employees is to serve the interests of the corporation. In fact, even socially conscious, environmentally aware, and ethically well-intentioned managers are legally very limited in what they would be entitled to do as employees. As Jerry Mander points out in his book, *In the Absence of the Sacred,*

No corporate manager could ever place community welfare above corporate interest.... U.S. corporate law holds that management of publicly held companies must act primarily in the economic interest of shareholders. If not, management can be sued by shareholders and firings would surely occur. So managers are legally obliged to ignore community welfare ... if those needs interfere with profitability.[21]

Thus, even though corporations do have human beings in their employ, many of whom would probably even be considered ethically good people, those human beings are nonetheless legally constrained in the kinds of choices and decisions they are allowed to make as corporate managers and executives. Their position and function as officers of the corporation is purely to serve the interests of the corporation's shareholders rather than the interests of their local (or global) communities, the interests of the public health, or even the dictates of their own consciences.

It is important to remember that just as the entire raison d'être of a lawnmower is to mow lawns, the entire raison d'être of a corporation is to return a profit to those who have invested money in it. A corporation, we can therefore conclude, although it is made up of human beings, is not itself a human being and is therefore entirely "incapable of feeling remorse for the irreversible damage it is doing to life on Earth."[22] As Peter Montague points out in another *Rachel's* article:

Corporations cannot voluntarily curb their misbehavior because they have only one duty: to return a profit to investors, no matter what the costs may be to others. So long as poisoning is legal, corporations will poison (and if poisoning is profitable, they will spend millions on election campaigns to make sure poisoning remains legal.)[23]

So, even though corporations may perhaps be managed by some good individuals, the corporations themselves have their own clear one-dimensional economic mandates. They have not been incorporated to serve the interests of communities, or to serve the public health, or for any other purpose than a single one: to earn profits and distribute them to their shareholders.

Of course, intending to make a profit is not in itself wrong at all. Machiavelli isn't the only one who would remind us that, "It is truly a natural and ordinary thing to desire gain."[24] Profit is laudable and is sought by many a good person. However, when a person's or corporation's *sole* intention is to make a profit and that goal is not complemented by the qualities of fairness, justice, concern for the well-being of others, social conscience and all the other moral and social values that hold societies and peoples together, that is when the profit motive is not laudable: that is when it becomes destructive.

Real living human persons generally have a multiplicity of purposes operating in their lives at any given moment. They are striving, for example, to be fair and just with their fellows, to be happy, to be approved of in their social groups, not to be punished or penalized for bad behavior, to love their friends and family, to earn a living, and so on. Corporations, on the other hand, have one purpose only, so their behaviors and actions are not modified by any other motives. When that is the case—when profit becomes the sole source of motivation—then the words of Sophocles are more likely to become true.

> Nothing is worse than money.
> Money lays waste to cities, banishes
> Men from their homes, indoctrinates the heart,
> Perverting honesty to works of shame,
> Showing men how to practice villainy.[25]

We will look at just one instance among the many which might have been chosen to show how a corporation's drive for profits can override the sense of responsibility to the larger community, to the public health, or to the right of individual citizens to know the nature of the products they purchase.

Since February of 1996, according to a third article by Montague in *Rachel's*,

> Monsanto has been marketing various genetically-engineered crops that are "Roundup-ready" in an effort to boost sales of Roundup, the herbicide responsible for a large proportion of Monsanto's annual profits. The idea is to douse Roundup-ready crops with Roundup to kill weeds, leaving the genetically-engineered crop intact.[26]

These genetically engineered crops will therefore allow a much heavier agricultural application of Roundup to the nation's (and world's) food crops, and this, of course, is expected to increase the sales of Roundup and therefore increase Monsanto's profits. Whether the increased production and use of Roundup, and the consequent increase in human exposure to this herbicide—via drift, runoff, and residues in food and water—will be detrimental to human, animal, or environmental health is of much less consequence to Monsanto than is the potential for increased profits in coming quarters. And, whether there may be potential for adverse human health effects from long-term exposure to genetically engineered food crops is also of less concern to them than the potential for increased profits.

Monsanto has also developed a genetically engineered potato, named the New Leaf Superior, which has been designed to express the same insecticidal protein that is expressed by Bt (*Bacillus thuriengensis*).[27] This protein is especially toxic to the Colorado potato beetle (as well as to some other insects), which is why Bt has often been used as an insecticide to deal with these insects. Because the New Leaf Superior secretes this toxin from all its cells, it has itself been classified as a pesticide. Although this genetically engineered vegetable has been in grocery stores in the U.S. since 1994, shoppers who buy it have not been informed that they are purchasing and eating potatoes that have been designated as a pesticide. The New Leaf Superior has not been regulated by the FDA because it *was* classified as a pesticide and the FDA does not have regulatory control over pesticides. Nor has the EPA required that the new potato be formally labeled so that consumers know what they are buying, because the potato is also a food, and food regulation is the charge of the FDA. One Monsanto official was asked (by the *New York Times* reporter who broke the story) whether he believed the potato to be safe for human consumption. "Monsanto should not have to vouchsafe [sic] the safety of biotech food," answered Phil Angell, Monsanto's director of corporate communications. "Our interest is in selling as much of it as possible. Assuring its safety is the FDA's job."[28]

Consequently, it will be in Monsanto's best interests not to have consumers becoming worried about the possible risks of purchasing genetically engineered foods to feed to their families. Monsanto, therefore, seems to feel that it is not appropriate to identify these genetically engineered foods with explicit labels which distinguish them from traditional or natural foods on the grocery shelves and in the produce bins. It has strenuously opposed all legislative efforts to require that such genetically engineered foods be clearly labeled so that consumers can make their own choices about whether to purchase them. Monsanto does not want people to have that freedom, even if they themselves want it. As a result, consumers do not have the ability to intelligently choose which foods to feed their families.

On the other hand, Monsanto is very clear when it comes to the

contract requirements that farmers must satisfy when they choose
to use Monsanto's genetically engineered, Roundup-ready crop seeds.
For example, according to a *New York Times* editorial, any farmer
who chooses to use Roundup-ready soybeans

> must pay an additional "technology fee" of $5 per 50-pound bag of
> seed. He must also sign a licensing agreement that requires him to let
> Monsanto agents inspect his fields, prohibits him from using any
> glyphosate herbicide but Roundup and prevents him from saving seed
> for future planting. He also consents, implicitly, to the further cen-
> tralization of agricultural control.[29]

Some analysts are concerned, as is the author of the *New York
Times* editorial quoted above, about the increasing power of corporations such as Monsanto to control matters related to production of food crops. Others are more concerned about the increasing
power of corporations to influence legislation.

The power that corporations exercise to influence legislation
and public policy has unfortunately been seriously underrated by
the public. Most of us have very little appreciation of the extent to
which corporations shape our lives. If more of us were aware of this,
we may feel some consternation that unelected powers like Monsanto, E. I. DuPont, and Dow Chemical are allowed to have such a
large influence over in lawmaking in a democratic government.

Halfdan Mahler, former director-general of the World Health
Organization based in Geneva, believes that there has been too little legislation and regulation supporting the health rights of human
beings around the world. "I see a frightening global laissez-faire
mentality in our increasingly amoral world, which is allowing global
casino economics to ride roughshod over political, civil, social, economic, and cultural rights."[30] The corporations simply have too
much power and influence over legislators and regulators.

More radical analysts believe that the fundamental problem lies
with the very nature of the corporation itself, and that none of the
problems associated with corporations (such as environmental pollution and neglect of the public health) will ever be significantly
improved until the form and structure of the corporation itself is
changed. After all, says one critic, Peter Montague,

> Corporations have limited capacity for self-restraint. They want it all
> and they want it now and they don't want anyone telling them what
> they can and cannot do. Until we recognize this—the nature of the

corporate form—as the key problem of our time, the environment and human health will continue to deteriorate.[31]

Because corporations are the nonmoral kinds of entities they are, it will be necessary for them to arrange matters so they can be perceived by the public as compassionate and humane. They want to be seen as institutions which care about the effects of their activities and products on health and the environment, and not as institutions which see predictable death and disability simply as necessary costs of doing business. Because of the inherent challenges in trying to create a favorable public image under such circumstances, most corporations spend heavily in enlisting the help of the equally powerful and influential public relations industry.

3. Public Relations

It is the greatest art of the devil to convince us he does not exist.
—Baudelaire

Public relations firms can sometimes exert powerful forces to dramatically influence public perceptions, policymaking, and even legislation. They see their main work to be the subtle, undetected, shaping of public opinion—the "manufacture of consent."

Dr. Stockman's discovery that Kirsten Springs was polluted constituted—at least in the eyes of the town officials who stood to profit from the springs—a serious public relations crisis. The contaminated wells in Woburn, Massachusetts, constituted a public relations crisis for W. R. Grace and Beatrice Foods. The spill of the Exxon Valdez in Prince William Sound was seen as a public relations crisis by the Exxon Corporation. The Surgeon General's declaration that smoking tobacco was dangerous to health was perceived as a public relations crisis by the tobacco industry.

It is worth noting that neither the Norwegian town fathers, nor W. R. Grace and Beatrice Foods, nor the Exxon Corporation, nor the tobacco companies, perceived their problem as a health crisis, a community crisis, an environmental crisis, or even as a personal crisis for the families involved. They saw all these events instead only as public relations crises for their municipal or corporate images.

Many public relations firms, fortunately at least for these corporations, offer a service to their clients that they term "crisis management."[32] This service is offered to help corporations manage the devastating impact on their corporate image and profits that can sometimes result from such public relations "crises." The tobacco industry, for example, with the growing public awareness that tobacco is responsible for so much cancer and cardiovascular disease, has faced an ongoing "public relations crisis" for the past several decades. In the face of it, the public relations firms that have been hired by the tobacco industry managed to wage "the longest-running misinformation campaign in U.S. business history," according to the *Wall Street Journal*.[33] Perhaps the tobacco industry's efforts should rather more accurately be characterized as only the longest running misinformation (or public relations) campaign *of which the public has so far been made aware*. Numerous other public relations campaigns have been just as effective as, perhaps more effective than, that of the tobacco industry partially *because* the public has not yet become fully aware of them. After all, "'The best PR is never noticed,' says the proud unwritten slogan of the trade."[34]

The public relations firms that have been hired by the chemical and pesticide manufacturing corporations, for instance, have waged long-running PR campaigns[35] that have arguably been even more effective than those of the tobacco industry. This would be evidenced by the fact that the public seems to still believe that most consumer toxicants and most pesticides are completely safe for general human use. This alone is powerful testimony to the efficacy of a well done PR effort.

PR firms also offer to their clients the service of managing crises of a more short-term nature. The crisis management plans they offer are believed to be most successful when they have been thought out and made ready ahead of time so that when an actual crisis develops, the plan can be deployed immediately.

To illustrate how such a crisis management plan would work, we might look at one that was actually developed for the Clorox Company by the Ketchum Public Relations firm in 1991. This plan was devised at a time when the activist organization Greenpeace was calling for a global phaseout of production of all chlorine products (a more radical version of the chlorine proposal I have recommended in Chapter Three). The Clorox Company was understandably concerned about what might happen to their image and profits if Greenpeace's recommendation caught on in the public mind, an eventuality which they would definitely consider a public relations crisis. So they hired Ketchum, one of the premier "greenwashing" PR firms, to help them manage the problem.[36]

In Ketchum's report to Clorox, they outlined some of the possible "worst case scenarios" that could develop, some of the key objectives that the Clorox Company would want to achieve in the face of these scenarios, and finally, some promising strategies for achieving those objectives.

In the words of the Ketchum report, one of the worst (for Clorox) case scenarios might look something like the following:

> The movement back to more "natural" household cleaning products is gaining momentum as consumers are eagerly looking for ways they can contribute to a cleaner planet.... A prominent newspaper columnist targets the environmental hazards of liquid chlorine bleach in an article, which is syndicated to newspapers across the country. The columnist calls for consumers to boycott Clorox products. Local chapters of Greenpeace take up the cause.... A dramatic drop in sales of Clorox products within several weeks.... Congress schedules hearings on the environmental safety of liquid chlorine bleach products....[37]

This series of events, though probably beneficial from the point of view of environmentalists and public health experts, would almost certainly be viewed as a public relations crisis by the Clorox Company. Some objectives that Clorox would probably want to achieve in the face of this crisis would be: (1) "Restore Clorox's reputation and that of the product as quickly as possible."[38] (2) "Prevent [the] issue from escalating and gaining credibility."[39] (3) "[F]orestall any legislative or regulatory action."[40] (4) "Maintain customer and consumer loyalty."[41]

Ketchum suggested several strategies that Clorox should use to achieve some of these objectives:

- An independent scientist is dispatched to meet with the columnist and discuss the issue.
- Teams of scientists, independent or from Clorox or both, are dispatched ... to conduct media tours.
- Arrange for sympathetic media, local, state and national governmental leaders, and consumer experts to make statements in defense of the product....
- Advertising in major markets, using Clorox employees and their families who will testify to their faith in the product....
- Advertising campaign: "Stop Environmental Terrorism," calling on Greenpeace and the columnist to be more responsible and less irrational.
- Video and audio news release to affected markets.

• Enlist the support of the union and the national union leadership, since jobs are at stake.
• Determine if and how a slander lawsuit against the columnist and/or Greenpeace could be effective.
• Mass mailings to consumers in affected cities.
• If the situation truly grows desperate, the team agrees to consider the possibility of pulling the product off the market, pending a special review, assuming the review can be done quickly.
• Survey research is conducted daily to measure public reaction, changing attitudes, perceptions, etc....
• Through the Chlorine Institute, third-party scientific experts are brought to Washington to testify....[42]

In addition: "Where possible, ignore Greenpeace and don't give it credence.... Help people understand that Greenpeace is not among the serious players in this issue...."[43]

Ketchum Public Relations is a firm which also offers "environmental public relations" services, i.e., services to help a client corporation give the public appearance of being environmentally responsible. The term "greenwashing" is sometimes used by critics to describe this service. The Clorox Company would clearly hope to benefit from Ketchum's greenwashing PR services.

Given what is known about the toxic effects of chlorine and chlorinated compounds, it is not impossible that such a "worst case scenario" could actually come to pass in the not too distant future. For public health and the environment, it might well be considered a beneficial development. Corporate interests, however, would fight it tooth and nail, with the aid of public relations firms like Ketchum. This would, of course, be entirely legal, even understandable. Most corporations, faced with such a situation, would "attempt to deflate the impact of anticipated public discourse about its products."[44] The problem is that the public health is involved, and thus so is the well-being of families and communities.

In reality, corporate interests are actually very well positioned to deal with such a threat to their image, should it occur. Stauber and Rampton quote Frank Mankiewicz, vice-chairman of Hill and Knowlton Public Relations, speaking at a gathering of PR executives:

The big corporations, our clients, are scared shitless of the environmental movement.... [However, I think t]he corporations are wrong about that. I think the companies will have to give in only at insignificant levels. Because the companies are too strong, they're the establishment. The environmentalists are going to have to be like the mob in the square in Rumania before they prevail.[45]

Unfortunately, Mankiewicz may well be correct about this. It might be that no environmental health reforms will actually take place without enormous efforts on the part of those working for the protection of the public health. Corporations, particularly when they use the powerful methodologies of the PR firms, have every intention of protecting their own (and their stockholders') economic interests, even at the potential expense, if necessary, of the environment and public health. As we have seen above, U.S. corporate law formally requires that officers of a corporation act solely in the economic interests of their shareholders, even if that means ignoring the interests of the environment and of public health.

Therefore, one of the biggest challenges facing those who are working to protect the health of the public from toxicant induced pathologies has been, and will continue to be, the economic power of the corporations, and the persuasive power of the PR firms that so successfully serve them.

As a final aside, it might perhaps be suggested that those on the public health side who are interested in forwarding the goals of environmental health should perhaps themselves consider hiring public relations firms to help them achieve their ends. Public health initiatives usually involve some attempt to modify certain public behaviors or attitudes and this is clearly an arena in which public relations firms are highly expert.

A recent article published in the *American Journal of Public Health* details some "advances" in public health communication,[46] but the article seems almost naive by comparison with the sophistication of public relations techniques. It suggests methods such as "social marketing" and "media advocacy" to help achieve public health goals, as if these methods might not normally be familiar to people in public health. These methods, and much more sophisticated ones, however, are the daily stock in trade of those working in public relations. So for this reason alone, some public health agendas *may* perhaps be well served by hiring them out to public relations firms.

In addition, something as simple as posting information on the Internet about industrial chemical releases, about the results from monitoring contaminants in air and water, about levels of toxics in various consumer products, and about local pesticide applications would at least increase the level of public awareness about exposures to toxics.[47] But of course, according a story in the *Wall Street Journal* in February 1998,

> A plan to post factory pollution risks on the Internet has drawn opposition from companies and state environmental officials. About 661 major industrial plants in the auto, paper, oil, steel and metals industries would be listed under the plan. The plan is known as the Sector Facility Indexing Project, or SFIP, and is part of an effort by Carol M. Browner to raise community support for the environment.... U.S. automakers have refused to cooperate with the plan.... Environmental groups, however, like the plan.[48]

A similar project, termed the "Chemical Scorecard" and undertaken by the Environmental Defense Fund, has been up and running on the worldwide web since early 1998.[49]

Probably, given the enormous power of corporations and their public relations firms, only the widest possible dissemination of toxics information to the public will offer any hope of effecting significant change in public policy regarding toxics.

4. Medical Paradigms

One of the key historical principles we have learned from Thomas Kuhn and his analysis of scientific revolutions,[50] is that scientific paradigms are amazingly persistent and conservative. Those who have been schooled in a given scientific or medical paradigm are often loath to modify it, and for this reason ways of thinking in medical practice, as in other fields, can sometimes be very slow to change.

In the present dominant medical paradigm, long-term exposure to low doses of ambient environmental toxicants, even of pesticides, is rarely suspected by clinicians of contributing in any significant degree to the variety of symptoms patients are suffering.

Part of the reason so few (and such inadequate) protective policies, laws, and regulations have been enacted, and part of the reason that there is such inadequate public disclosure of risks, is that many traditional medical practitioners have yet to fully recognize that low levels of toxicants could be responsible for any important adverse human health effects.[51] This is the case even though large numbers of people have developed serious disabling conditions which, according to their own experience and according to much clinical research, are clearly associated with exposures to ambient toxicants.

Because of clinicians' loyalty to the current governing medical paradigm and its view of toxics, many toxicant induced pathologies go unrecognized in physicians' offices.

Communities in general, and scientific and medical communities in particular, are extremely cohesive and tenacious when it comes to conserving their own current working paradigms. These paradigms have, after all, worked effectively in their past, and it would not be wise (they probably believe) to question and undermine something that has appeared so right and useful.

Fortunately, there are precedents in the history of medicine that can help us understand how this reluctance to accept new theories has operated as such a powerful force. The medical community's slow acceptance of the germ theory, for example, offers interesting parallels with the slow recognition of toxicant induced illnesses such as MCS. Many 19th century medical practitioners did, after all, find that it stretched the bounds of credulity to believe the claim that such tiny microbes could cause such big diseases. And besides that conceptual difficulty, medicine's skepticism was nourished and fostered by local business interests who strongly opposed belief in the germ theory for their own reasons.

Let us look briefly at what exactly the germ theory of disease claimed. The germ theory of disease causation, as it emerged in the latter half of the 19th century, held that certain kinds of tiny, almost undetectable, xenobiotic microorganisms could, by some process of infection, amplification, or perhaps even by some release of biological toxins, be the cause of certain diseases in human beings, even some fatal diseases.

Over 100 years before Edward Jenner's vaccination experiments for smallpox and 150 years before Louis Pasteur linked microbes to disease processes, the Dutchman, Antony van Leeuwenhoek (1632–1723), who had taught himself to grind lenses, assembled the world's first precision microscope. It was composed of only a single double-convex lens which magnified up to 270 times, and with it van Leeuwenhoek examined a wide variety of intriguing microworlds, including magnified rainwater, the tartar between his own teeth, human semen, and sometimes even his own feces (on occasions when he was "troubled with a looseness").[52] Under his microscope, van Leeuwenhoek discovered what he called "wee animalcules," microbes that were active, obviously alive, and extremely numerous.[53] His discoveries also included the existence of red blood cells, spermatozoa, and the striation of voluntary muscles, as well as bacteria, protozoa, and spirochetes.[54] Van Leeuwenhoek had no idea what role these "wee animalcules" played in human affairs, if any; in fact, he considered them probably to be intriguing novelties only.

It was not until Louis Pasteur, in the middle of the 19th century, that any connection was made between the existence of these microscopic life forms and the natural history of human disease.[55]

Prior to this time, of course, the medical community did have a fairly clear understanding of the symptomology and natural history of many contagious diseases, but had no understanding at all of their etiology (that is, no suspicion that such diseases were caused by bacteria, viruses and parasites), and no understanding at all of the mechanisms of pathogenesis. It would take a full development of the germ theory—which emerged slowly over decades—to make sense of the connections between these microbial life forms and certain human diseases.

The germ theory, once accepted, would turn out to have enormous implications for many areas of public health policy. The theory held, for instance, that it would probably be possible to control some epidemic diseases by somehow controlling the transmission or growth of these microorganisms. Isolation of infected persons away from the community of uninfected persons might be one such public health control measure. Quarantine of foreign vessels newly arrived in local harbors might prove to be another. In general, then, it was thought that initiating some controls over the free social intercourse between persons (and markets) would probably be one method public health officials might employ for controlling the spread of infectious diseases, especially if those diseases were caused by the transmission of microbes.

Commercial interests in general strenuously opposed acceptance of the germ theory of disease causation mostly because of its potentially dire consequences to free trade (at least in the short term). Public health officials, they worried, could perhaps be given too much authority to quarantine vessels, to regulate marketplaces, to enact ordinances governing the gatherings of peoples, and to institute various other measures which could have a dampening effect on free commercial trade. In effect, merchants were suspicious of any theory of disease causation that might have a negative impact on their ability to do business freely.

Some medical men opposed the germ theory primarily because it seemed, *a priori*, to be somewhat beyond credibility, but also because the theory was new and untried. It did claim, after all, that miniscule, invisible, and virtually undetectable microbes were the key causal agent in some very large-scale physical human events, a number of which were fatal, and some of which were fatal to whole communities. Furthermore, there were as yet only fragments of scientific evidence with which to support the theory, and that evidence was new, still uncorroborated by independent researchers, and open to doubt. More research, in their minds, was definitely needed. And finally, the competing and older miasma theory—that bad air accounted for the emergence and spread of many diseases—seemed to them to account for the appearances well enough in their minds.[56]

The low dose toxicity theories of disease causation, emerging now in the late 20th and early 21st centuries, bear some interesting similarities to the germ theory of disease. They too hold that very small, virtually undetectable xenobiotic agents can, over time, by some physiologic processes at the cellular level, or by some direct action on the central nervous system, or by some pathologic disturbance of the detoxification pathways, or perhaps by some other mechanism not yet understood, cause certain disease processes in human beings that have the potential to be severely disabling.

These low dose toxicity theories of disease causation[57] hold that it would be theoretically possible to prevent, and perhaps even to treat, certain toxicant induced illnesses by initiating some relatively strict controls over the kinds and amounts of synthetic chemicals to which people are regularly exposed, and by controlling the kinds and amounts of toxicants that are regularly released into the environment. Regulating industrial release of certain chemical byproducts may prove to be one effective method for minimizing the incidence of such illnesses. Regulating the marketing, use, and consumption of certain kinds of toxicants may be another useful mode of disease prevention. Widely disseminating complete information about the nature and health effects of the toxicants to which people are exposed in their daily lives may be another effective measure for improving the public health.

The chemical corporations have generally been highly suspicious of the claims of low dose toxicity theories largely because of their potentially dire economic consequences (at least in the short term) to their sector of the market. One simple way for these corporate commercial interests to protect themselves against possible government regulation of the production, marketing and use of synthetic chemicals would be to throw doubt on these theories, and to discourage clinicians and researchers from accepting them.

Some medical practitioners have also been suspicious of the theories of low dose toxicity perhaps because the concept has seemed somewhat implausible to them. These theories do claim, after all, that extremely miniscule and virtually undetectable doses of certain ambient toxicants and toxicant mixtures can cause quite dramatic symptoms, sometimes involving a multiplicity of body systems and organs. In addition, the theories are still relatively new and moving toward fuller scientific clarification and validation. Furthermore, there is not yet enough irrefutable scientific evidence to demand assent in the usually intellectually conservative medical community. Finally, there are almost enough accepted explanations—if one cobbles together fragments of orthodox medical doctrines—to account for some of the manifestations of toxicant induced illnesses.

Medical understanding, early in the 21st century, of how low doses of ambient toxicants can impact human physiological systems, is at roughly the same level as understanding of the germ theory in the 1860s and 1870s. The germ theory had not then fully emerged and belief in it was still considered controversial.

In the case of both theories too—the germ theory and the low dose toxicity theory—the stage had already been set and much of the preliminary work accomplished decades before acceptance. In the case of the latter, Dr. Theron Randolph[58] and others, in the early 1950s, had already recognized the toxic effects on some people of long-term exposure to low doses of ambient petroleum-based toxicants. In fact, Randolph himself sometimes referred to the clinical conditions he was seeing as "the petroleum problem." And in the case of the germ theory, Leeuwenhoek had, 150 years before Pasteur, accurately described a wide variety of parasites, bacteria and spirochetes that were only later recognized as playing a key role in disease causation.

And just as the germ theory of infectious diseases represented an entirely new concept of disease causation, so too today's low dose toxicity theories.[59] Moreover, just as not all illnesses caused by germs exhibit the same symptomology, so too not all conditions caused by toxicants.

In any case, whether the theories of low dose toxicant induced disease represent a new medical paradigm or a significant addition to the old one, there is little doubt—as Thomas Kuhn observes[60]—that they will be strenuously resisted.

Both in the case of the germ theory and of the low dose toxicity theories, we see that intellectual conservatives prefer not to take on an entirely new medical paradigm, especially if the old paradigm seems to have worked tolerably well for them.[61] This becomes particularly true when the act of accepting the new paradigm could perhaps have some serious implications for major changes in clinical practice and in public health policy. And if the theories of low dose toxicity do in fact turn out to be valid, and if we do come to realize that some levels of environmental toxicants (levels which today are considered acceptable) are indeed capable of causing real disease processes in a certain portion of the population, then some significant changes in public policy (such as those suggested in Chapter Three) would probably be called for.

One other characteristic of the current medical paradigm perhaps deserves mention in this context: the medical reductionism that seems to operate so strongly in it. Reductionism, at least in its medical form, is an expression of "the philosophic view that complex phenomena are ultimately derived from a single primary principle."[62] This form of reductionism may work relatively well in the understanding of certain infectious diseases (though perhaps not in complex diseases like HIV/AIDS), but it will not work nearly so well in the attempt to understand toxicant induced diseases.

In the case of at least some toxicant induced illnesses, a variety of toxicants from a variety of environmental media may be responsible for the development of similar disease processes. Sometimes toxicants combine with each other, either out in the environment or inside the individual's body, and then either the toxicants or the breakdown metabolites from them may cause disease. Individual toxicants or their mixtures or metabolites may first affect one primary body system (e.g., the immune system or the endocrine system), and the dysfunction of that system may secondarily impact other body systems, leading to an entirely new array of symptoms. This complex string of causes and effects may also be influenced by an individual's compromised ability to synthesize the enzymes necessary to break down and excrete certain chemicals. It may also be influenced by certain uniquely inherited physical characteristics, and perhaps even by exposures that may have occurred as many as three or four decades earlier. The presence of certain kinds of microbes may even turn out to play some role in the complex web of bodily events that result in toxicant induced illness. Certain kinds of physical or emotional stressors may play a part as well.

In other words, an illness that is the result of the interplay of a widely varied multiplicity of factors may not be amenable to adequate understanding within the confines of a medical paradigm that has become habituated to a reductionist view of causes and effects. The reductionist "one bug, one drug" theory—that is, the theory that wants to see one kind of microbe cause one kind of disease which can then be cured with one drug—will probably find it difficult to accept a theory of disease causality that is so multifactorial.

Therefore the current medical paradigm itself, or at least the reductionist character of its thinking, may need to be rethought.

And if Thomas Kuhn has taught us anything it is that in the history of human scientific thought, paradigms are essentially conservative and very slow to change. This may be especially true in the case of medical paradigms. Paradigms are likely to change only when people who have tenaciously held to the old paradigm eventually retire, and those who hold to the new one come into positions of influence. As Max Planck remarked toward the end of his distinguished career, "a new scientific truth does not triumph by convincing its opponents and making them see the light, but rather because its opponents eventually die, and a new generation grows up that is familiar with it."[63]

5. Others

Other obstacles to implementation of the proposals in Chapter Three would include the following.

DISABLED ACTIVISTS

Those who, because of their personal experience as sufferers of toxicant induced illnesses, would have become activists for changes in environmental health regulation, are often too disabled by their illnesses to stay in the fight.

(Perhaps the most useful comparison is with activism in causes related to HIV infection and AIDS, and the great accomplishments of some of those activists.)

PAUCITY OF RESEARCHERS

There is at present a severe paucity of environmental medicine practitioners and researchers.

Few medical schools in the U.S. offer specializations in occupational medicine, and I am not aware of any that have specializations in environmental medicine. Hence, not as much research is being done on issues related to the diagnosis and treatment of toxicant induced disorders as needs to be done. There is also, as a result, a severe shortage of physicians who have been properly trained to recognize, diagnose, and treat these disorders. Duke University's School of Medicine in North Carolina is one of the few schools offering a residency in occupational medicine. This lack of training in occupational or environmental medicine may partially account not only for the paucity of trained clinicians, but also, in a kind of vicious cycle, for the limited funding and opportunities for research on toxicant induced illnesses.

The American Academy of Environmental Medicine has only approximately 600 members in the U.S., a rather small membership compared to other American medical academies. One can only hope that these numbers will grow in coming decades.

These are some of the major challenges facing those who would like to see the implementation of the proposals outlined in Chapter Three. Until these obstacles are recognized and faced directly, it will be difficult to hope for an improvement in the environmental health of our communities.

Notes

1. Thanks to Mr. Keith McGuire of Merlin, Oregon, for articulating this image so clearly.

2. J. Winnow, "Lesbians Evolving Health Care: Cancer and AIDS," *One in Three: Women with Cancer Confront an Epidemic.* Ed. J. Brady (San Francisco and Pittsburgh: Cleis Press, 1991) 233–44. p. 244.

3. J. Brady, "The Goose and the Golden Egg," *One in Three: Women with Cancer Confront an Epidemic*, 13–35. p. 15.

4. "Any real 'fight against cancer' must take the form of prevention, becoming a fight against the industrial pollution of our world and the connivance of government with industry in the cover-up of that pollution." J. Brady, "The Goose and the Golden Egg." p. 30.

5. S. Steingraber, "We All Live Downwind," *One in Three: Women with Cancer Confront an Epidemic.* 36–48. p. 39.

6. J. Houghton, "Review of Stephen Schneider's *Laboratory Earth: The Planetary Gamble We Can't Afford to Lose*" (Basic Books, 1997, 174 p.) *Nature*, 386 (March 27, 1997) 345.

7. *Ibid.*

8. M. Dieter, "Sustainable Environment for all," *Environmental Health Perspectives*, 105, Number 11 (November 1997) 1162–3.

9. D. Satcher, "CDC's First 50 Years: Lessons Learned and Relearned," *American Journal of Public Health*, 86, #12 (December 1996) 1705–08. p. 1707.

10. T. Colburn, D. Dumanoski and J.P. Myers, *Our Stolen Future: Are We Threatening Our Fertility, Intelligence and Survival?—A Scientific Detective Story* (New York: Penguin Books USA, 1996) 306+xii. This work provides a convincing and detailed illustration of how a single PCB molecule travels through the environment and the food chain, from its place of origin in the Monsanto Chemical Works plant in Anniston, Alabama. Eventually, after a complex journey, it finds its way into the body fat of a female polar bear living on one of the Svalbard Islands off the coast of Norway, enters into her breast milk, and then is passed on to her newborn cub during nursing.

11. "Nations Move to Ban POPs," *Environmental Health Perspectives*, 105, Number 7 (July 1997) 693.

12. *Ibid.*

13. H. Mahler, "The Challenge of Global Health: How Can We Do Better?" *Health and Human Rights*, 2, Number 3 (1997) 71–75. p. 72–3.

14. Quoted in J. Galloway, "The health of nations," *Nature*, 385 (February 13, 1997) 594.

15. J. Harr, *A Civil Action* (New York: Random House, 1995) 500.

16. *Ibid.*, p. 493 of the Vintage paperback edition.

17. D. Fagin and M. Lavelle, *Toxic Deception: How the Chemical Industry Manipulates Science, Bends the Law, and Endangers Your Health* (Secaucus, NJ: Carol Publishing, 1997) 294+xxvi. p. xi.

18. P. Montague, "One Fundamental Problem," *Rachel's Environment and Health Weekly*, #582 (January 22, 1998).

19. *Ibid.*

20. *Ibid.*

21. Page 123, as quoted in J. Stauber and S. Rampton, *Toxic Sludge Is Good for You: Lies, Damn Lies, and the Public Relations Industry* (Monroe, ME: Common Courage, 1995) 236+iv. p. 203.

22. P. Montague, "Bad decisions again and again," *Rachel's Environment and Health Weekly*, #541 (April 10, 1997).

23. For intriguing details regarding how the gasoline and lead industries dispersed millions of tons of neurotoxic lead into the environment from 1925 until 1989, see P. Montague, "Bad decisions again and again." P. Montague, "History of precaution, Part 2," *Rachel's Environment and Health Weekly*, #540 (April 3, 1997).

24. N. Machiavelli, *The Prince*, trans. Donno, Daniel (New York: Bantam Books, 1513, 1981) 90. p. 20.

25. Sophocles, *Antigone (in Three Theban Plays)*, trans. Banks, Theodore Howard, (New York: Oxford University, 1956) 144, lines 273–77 in *Antigone*. We might also in this regard consider William James' insight that narrow and short-sighted goals have always been seen as an indication of low intelligence. "In all ages the man whose determinations are swayed by reference to the most distant ends has been held to possess the higher intelligence. The tramp who lives from hour to hour; the bohemian whose engagements are from day to day; the bachelor who builds but for a single life; the father who acts for another generation; the patriot who thinks of a whole community and many

generations; and finally, the philosopher and saint whose cares are for humanity and for eternity,—these range themselves in an unbroken hierarchy, wherein each successive grade results from an increased manifestation of the special form of action by which the cerebral centres are distinguished from all below them." G.W. Allen, *William James* (New York: Viking, 1967) 556+xx. p. 213. According to this ancient notion, corporations—whose goals are focused on earning the maximum profits in the immediately upcoming quarters—would rank in the lower strata of quasi-intelligent beings.

26. P. Montague, "Genetic engineering error," *Rachel's Environment and Health Weekly*, 549 (June 5, 1997).

27. M. Pollan, "Playing God in the Garden," *New York Times Magazine* (October 25, 1998) 44–51, 62–3, 82, 92–3.

28. P. Montague, "Seeds of Destruction," *Rachel's Environment and Health Weekly*, #622 (October 29, 1998).

29. V. Klinkenborg, "Editorial: Biotechnology and the future of agriculture," *New York Times* (December 8, 1997). A22.

30. H. Mahler, *op. cit.*, p. 71.

31. P. Montague, "Right to know nothing," *Rachel's Environment and Health Weekly*, 552 (June 26, 1997).

32. Mark Dowie, in his Introduction to J. Stauber and S. Rampton, *op. cit.*, p. 3.

33. A.M. Freeman and L.P. Cohen, "How cigarette makers keep health questions 'open' year after year," *Wall Street Journal* (February 11, 1993) A1. Also: "Fighting desperately for its economic life, the tobacco industry launched what must be considered the costliest, longest-running and most successful PR 'crisis management' campaign in history." J. Stauber and S. Rampton, *ibid.*, p. 27.

34. Mark Dowie, in his Introduction to J. Stauber and S. Rampton, *ibid.*, p. 2.

35. See J. Stauber and S. Rampton, *ibid., passim.*

36. This story is detailed in Appendix B, *ibid.*

37. Quoted *ibid.*, p. 210.

38. *Ibid.*, p. 211.

39. *Ibid.*

40. *Ibid.*, p. 212.

41. *Ibid.*

42. Quoted *ibid.*, p. 211–12.

43. *Ibid.*, p. 212. For another detailed example of how corporations and the public relations firms that serve them can effectively use subtle and covert methods to accomplish their ends, see the following article. "This paper describes the strategies used by Philip Morris and other tobacco companies to promote a California initiative (Proposition 188) preempting local control of tobacco and those used by public health groups to defeat the initiative." H. Macdonald, S. Aguinaga and S.A. Glantz, "The defeat of Philip Morris' 'California Uniform Tobacco Control Act,'" *American Journal of Public Health*, 87, Number 12 (December 1997) 1989–96.

44. D. Fagin and M. Lavelle, *op. cit.*, p ix.

45. J. Stauber and S. Rampton, *op. cit.*, p. 123.

46. E. Maibach and D.R. Holtgrave, "Advances in Public Health Communication," *Annual Review of Public Health*, 16 (1995) 219–38.

47. A major step in this direction has been taken by the Environmental Defense Fund's "chemical scorecard," a website that displays documented industrial releases of TRI toxicants. See http://www.scorecard.org.

48. "EPA-pollution grading plan provokes opposition of companies, state officials," *Wall Street Journal* (February 17, 1998). B8.

49. http://www.scorecard.org.

50. T.S. Kuhn, *The Structure of Scientific Revolution*, 2nd ed. (Chicago: University of Chicago, 1962, 1970) 210+xii.

51. A recent Harris poll found that 82 percent of Americans believe that "ensuring that people are not exposed to unsafe water, air pollution or toxic waste is 'very important.'" Reported in [1997 #94].

52. C-EA. Winslow, *The Conquest of Epidemic Disease* (Madison: University of Wisconsin, 1943, 1980) 411+viii. p. 156

53. P. Radetsky, *The Invisible Invaders: The Story of the Emerging Age of Viruses* (Boston: Little, Brown, 1991) 415+xvi. p. 41

54. C-EA. Winslow, *op. cit.*, p. 157–59.

55. P. Radetsky, *op. cit.*, *passim*.

56. Much of the story of the emerging Germ Theory is outlined in the following sources: Rosen, 1958, 1993 #2; C-EA. Winslow, *op. cit*; P. Radetsky, *ibid*. See also the Foreword to Defoe, #9.

57. See, for example, N. Ashford and C.S. Miller, *Chemical Exposures: Low Levels, High Stakes*, 2nd ed. (New York: Van Nostrand Reinhold / John Wiley & Sons, 1998) 440+xxiii. See also W. Rea, MD, *Chemical Sensitivity* 4 (Boca Raton, FL: Lewis Publishers, and CRC, 1992–97) 2924.

58. See, for example, T.G. Randolph and R.W. Moss, *An Alternative Approach to Allergies,* revised edition (New York: Harper and Row, 1980, 1989) 337+viii.

59. See, for example, N. Ashford and C.S. Miller, *op. cit.*

60. T.S. Kuhn, *op. cit.*

61. See, for example, *ibid.*

62. G. Engle, "The Need for a New Medical Model: A Challenge for Biomedicine," *Science*, 196 (1977) 4286, p. 130. As quoted in S. Kroll-Smith and H.H. Floyd, *Bodies in Protest: Environmental Illness and the Struggle Over Medical Knowledge* (New York: New York University, 1997) 223+xiv. p. 60.

63. Quoted in T.S. Kuhn, *op. cit.*, p. 151.

Conclusion

From the right to know and the duty to inquire flows the obligation to act.[1]

The challenges created by the emergence of toxicant induced illnesses are not simple, and whatever measures the world's nations eventually develop to meet will also not be easy. The methods of minimizing the prevalence of this class of illness, furthermore, will almost certainly not be exclusively medical, because the causes are not exclusively medical—they are social, economic, cultural and political as well.

Just as societies have developed a wide variety of public health measures to help control the spread of infectious diseases—closed sewers and septic systems, clean water and other sanitation measures, for example—so too will societies (including international organizations such as WHO) need to develop measures to help control the emergence and spread of these toxicant induced illnesses. Unfortunately, the measures necessary to deal with these newly emerging diseases may need to be even more comprehensive, and thus more challenging, than those devised to control infectious diseases.

Assume that most of what we learned in Chapter One of this book is true. That, effectively, is what Kroll-Smith and Floyd ask us to do in their book, *Bodies in Protest*:

Assume people really do become sick from exposure to a seemingly endless array of chemicals found in ordinary environments. Assume the chemicals that cause illness are [ubiquitously] present in the environment.... Moreover, assume that exposure to one chemical compound sensitizes the body to an array of unrelated chemical compounds. Finally, assume any body system is subject to the disease. If these assumptions are true, what is at stake is ... the vast process of chemical production, disability rights legislation, housing, commercial and public building construction codes, personal habits and codes of conduct, and local, state, and federal tolerance regulations, among other significant societal changes.[2]

The impact on the production, sale and use of chemicals and chemical-related products could therefore be dramatic. The Chemical Manufacturers Association has estimated that "approximately 80 percent of the commodities in this country are manufactured through some type of industrial chemical process."[3] Although this estimate is almost certainly overblown (considering its source), it is still clear that chemicals and chemical processes are a very large component of today's world economy.

Nonetheless, the economy is here to serve people; people are not here to serve the economy. The proposals outlined in Chapter Three of this book are intended to be modest, not radical. However, with an increase in public knowledge about contaminants in the consumer products we use, the air we breathe, the water we drink and the food we eat, we can expect that people will become more clear about what they want their economy to do for them and that may mean the emergence of proposals which are more radical and less modest. This may especially be the outcome with an increase in freely available public information about the health effects these toxicants often have on women, men, and children. We can certainly hope that with more and better information people will participate more knowledgeably in the public debates about chemicals and chemical exposures, and will be able to make wiser choices both in their purchasing and in their voting.

Nevertheless, we must not fail to keep in mind that the current assault on human and ecological health by the widespread manufacture and use of environmental toxicants is serious in the highest degree. It might even properly be termed an "eleventh plague," analogous in some ways to the plagues during the Hebrew captivity in Egypt.

The plagues in the Hebrew scriptures include the Nile turning to blood (so that the fish died and the water was undrinkable), hordes of flies, swarms of crop-destroying locusts, destructive hail and lightning, festering boils on humans and livestock, a fatal pestilence among all the animals, and the death of the firstborn in all families.[4] According to the tradition, these plagues were visited by God upon the Egyptians as a way of persuading the Pharaoh to free the Hebrews from their long slavery. The plagues eventually had their effect, and an exasperated Pharaoh finally allowed the Israelites to leave his land.

We might wonder how long today's eleventh plague must last and how severe it must become before the world's citizens will be moved to free themselves from the health endangering effects of their enslavement to toxicant production and usage. As Al Gore reminds us in his book *Earth in the Balance*, "The global environmental crisis is, as we say in Tennessee, real as rain, and I cannot stand the thought of leaving my children with a degraded earth and a diminished future."[5]

In all likelihood, this eleventh plague will continue to develop until the costs associated with ongoing adverse effects on human health and on the environment become fully evident and are recognized as intolerable. Part of the effort of good education is to help society become aware of these costs so that policymakers and legislators can muster the courage to begin changing course. After all, becoming aware of a problem, and learning about the present and future impact of that problem, is a large step toward a solution.

Niccolò Machiavelli, an author not often cited by ethicists (especially not favorably), recognized this principle long ago. In Chapter III of *The Prince*, he reminds political leaders that,

> By making provision in advance, princes may easily avoid such difficulties; but if they wait until they are near at hand, the medicine will not be in time, for by then the malady will have become incurable. In this matter the situation is the same as physicians report concerning hectic fever [tuberculosis]: in the beginning the disease is *easy to cure but hard to diagnose*; with the passage of time, having gone unrecognized and unmedicated, it becomes *easy to diagnose but hard to cure*. So it is with a state.[6]

So it is also with public health, and particularly with matters related to environmentally induced illnesses. When a physical or environmental condition is in its earliest stages it is more difficult to detect, so that only a few far-seeing visionaries may be able to discern what long-term effects are likely to emerge.[7] In these earlier stages, though the condition is more difficult to detect, it is also much easier to remedy. However, as the condition worsens and as its effects become much more evident to even the most short-sighted observers, it also becomes increasingly difficult to remedy.

With regard to the adverse human health effects of ambient environmental toxicants, the world is presently somewhere well along this spectrum of emergence, so that more and more observers are becoming increasingly aware of the risks to human health. Machiavelli, hard hearted pragmatist that he was, would probably urge our politicians to undertake all possible preventive measures early on, rather than wait till years or decades later when the developing problems may be almost insoluble. And if Martin Luther King is correct, there is indeed hope. "The arc of history is long, but it bends towards justice."[8] The question is only whether it will bend toward justice soon enough to prevent irreversible long-term damage to human health and the earth's ecosystem.

According to Dr. Paul Epstein, in a recent editorial in the journal *Health and Human Rights*, it is already becoming increasingly evident that "the costs of not changing course are beginning to rise."[9] Let us hope that this will also become increasingly evident to the world's peoples, to its governments' and even to the corporations which manufacture and use the toxicants that are at the root of the problem. Without this recognition, the earth and its citizens may be facing a developing catastrophe that could prove almost impossible to remedy.

Will we have the wisdom and the courage to make the kinds of choices that will benefit humanity in the long run, or will we continue to make the kinds of choices that satisfy only near-term needs? Again, the classical American philosopher William James states the principle involved most clearly:

> In all ages the man whose determinations are swayed by reference to the most distant ends has been held to possess the higher intelligence.[10]

James' point is simply that the wiser we are as decisionmakers, the more our thinking will be affected by reference to the largest and most all-encompassing ends. We will be less concerned with desires for immediate gain, comfort, or convenience, and more concerned with the whole scope of well-being for the community, the world, our whole generation, and generations to come.

As John F Kennedy stated so well in June of 1963: "In the final analysis, our most basic common link is that we all inhabit this small planet. We all breathe the same air. We all cherish our children's future. And we are all mortal."[11]

Notes

1. S. Steingraber, *Living Downstream: An Ecologist Looks at Cancer and the Environment* (Reading, MA: Addison-Wesley, 1997) 357+xvi. p. 117.

2. S. Kroll-Smith and H.H. Floyd, *Bodies in Protest: Environmental Illness and the Struggle Over Medical Knowledge* (New York: New York University, 1997) 223+xiv. p. 44–5.

3. *Ibid.,* p 44.

4. A recent UK television program suggested that these plagues may have had earthly as well as divine causes. It proposed the following sequence: "The trigger was a red algal bloom that killed much of the life in the Nile, especially the fish which normally kept the toad population under control. It was argued that this led, by plausible steps, to plagues of flies and midges and hence to animal and human plagues for which they were vectors. The final catastrophe arose from the storage of wet grain contaminated by locust droppings which led to the poisoning of human and animal food supplies with microtoxins." J. Lydon, "Was Moses the First Ecologist?" *Nature, 395* (September 24, 1998) 317.

5. A. Gore, *Earth in the Balance: Ecology and the Human Spirit* (New York: Houghton Mifflin Company, 1992) Quoted in J.B. Berkson, *A Canary's Tale: The Final Battle, Politics, Poisons, and Pollution vs. the Environment and the Public Health* (Hagerstown, MD: Self-published, 1996) 452+xviii. p. 156.

6. N. Machiavelli, *The Prince*, trans. Donno, Daniel (New York: Bantam Books, 1513, 1981) 90. p.18. My emphasis.

7. As Machiavelli says, "The man who does not recognize ills at their inception does not have true wisdom, and this is given to [only a] few." N. Machiavelli, *op. cit.,* p. 53.

8. Quoted in J. Mann, "Health and Human Rights: If Not Now, When?" *Health and Human Rights,* 2, Number 3 (1997) 113–20. p. 120.

9. P.R. Epstein, "Human Rights and Natural Laws," *Health and Human Rights,* 2, Number 2 (Spring 1997) 1–4.

10. This passage from James' classic, *Principles of Psychology*, is quoted in G.W. Allen, *William James* (New York: Viking Press, 1967) 556+xx. p. 213.

11. Quoted in J.B. Berkson, *op. cit.,* p. 98.

Appendix I

North Seattle Community College Indoor Air Quality (IAQ) Policy

(Very similar in structure and content to the IAQ policy of The Evergreen State College in Olympia, Washington, USA)

POLICY

In a spirit of cooperation and caring for our fellow campus community members, we present this policy as a starting point for addressing health and safety concerns related to air quality on the North Seattle Community College (NSCC) campus.

North Seattle Community College recognizes that the air is shared by all members of the college community and those who visit the campus; that suitable air quality is important in fostering a healthful and creative learning and working environment; and that maintaining suitable air quality requires continual attentiveness to mitigate or to eliminate unfavorable conditions.

This policy is undertaken in the context of NSCC's identity as a learning community, with a commitment to the ideals outlined in our Mission and Goals and Shared Vision statements. In the service of these ideals, and with a recognition that much remains to be learned about air quality issues, community members are expected to participate, with respect and civility, in informing, teaching, and learning from one another about matters related to this policy.

247

Selection of products for use on campus should be consistent with the goal of this policy, which is to reduce or limit exposure to airborne contaminants. Product selection should take into consideration factors such as effectiveness of alternatives, application process, location of use, extent of exposure, and cost.

NSCC supports the concept of a fragrance- and pollutant-free environment on its campus and in its programs. The college seeks to maintain the best possible air quality attainable within fiscal, legal, and regulatory constraints. In pursuit of that goal, the following procedures will be implemented.

PROCEDURES

1. Air Supply. NSCC community members are expected to exercise care when undertaking projects which may affect building air quality by mitigating or eliminating pollutants from, for example, idling vehicles, construction projects, sign-making, etc.

2. Approval/Adequate Notice. A product evaluation must take place whenever there is a potential for hazardous chemicals being present in any manner such that community members may be exposed to them. Plans for using potentially hazardous products or new applications of products which were previously approved must be submitted to the Health and Safety Committee for evaluation. Material safety data sheets (MSDS) must accompany the plans. (The Health and Safety committee, in the absence of adequate expertise on the committee, may need to seek outside assistance in the form of private consultants familiar with the issues of indoor air quality.)

Product evaluation will include any possible route of human and environmental exposure as well as physical hazards which could cause an accident or injury. Plans and MSDS must be submitted at least five working days in advance, with the understanding that approval may not be granted in that time period due to testing requirements, searches for alternative products, or a requirement that work be performed under special circumstances. When required, approval will be contingent upon the user notifying members of the NSCC campus community about the location of areas which may be affected.

3. Training and Educating. The Academic Vice President, in conjunction with Human Resources, will develop information and training for faculty, staff, students, and other members of the community who use college facilities. Subjects covered will include: the appropriate uses for and alternatives to chemicals; reduction of chemical exposure; multi-chemical sensitivity (MCS); and the effects of scented products, including personal care products, on sensitive individuals.

4. Information Posting. The Safety and Security Supervisor will post air quality guidelines on safety bulletin boards to be installed in each building.

5. Inspection and Updating. The Manager of Facilities Operations will ensure that air delivery systems are regularly maintained and inspected.

6. Use of Scented Products. NSCC community members are asked to refrain from using or wearing scented products while on campus. NSCC community members are asked to also respect the more strict requirement to not wear any scented products in classrooms which have been specially designated as scent-free.

7. Policy Dissemination. On a continuing basis, every office with purchasing authority will notify vendors and contractors about this policy. Quarterly the office of the Vice President for Student Programs will inform students, staff, and faculty about this policy, and will include this policy in the quarterly class schedule, as well as in the Student Handbook. Human Resource Services will provide all new employees with a copy of this policy.

8. Facilities' Use. Staff, faculty, and students who make arrangements for use of NSCC's facilities will provide non-college groups with written information about this policy. Groups using college facilities will be expected to observe this policy.

9. Monitoring. The Health and Safety Committee (or an IAQ subcommittee) will have the responsibility of monitoring campus procedures to ensure that provisions of this policy are adequately observed.

10. Complaint Process. A complaint process (below) is available for addressing air quality concerns.

Compliance Process

PURPOSE

The goals of these complaint guidelines are to improve communication and to effect fair, uniform, and timely resolution of air quality complaints and concerns.

Steps you may use are listed separately based on the source of the problem. Any of the persons receiving a complaint which requires other resources may call on other offices within the college.

ENVIRONMENTAL CAUSE AS SOURCE (CHEMICAL SPILL, ODORS)

In case of injury to a person, call 911 first (on campus phones, dial 9-911).

Call the Safety and Security Supervisor (xt xxxx) if a chemical spill occurs or if an odor is present which is causing health effects. The Safety and Security Supervisor will implement safety procedures, mitigate resulting harm from a spill or mishap, coordinate assistance of on-campus personnel, and notify appropriate authorities as is prudent and as required by law.

HEATING, VENTILATION, AND AIR CONDITIONING (HVAC) SYSTEM AS SOURCE

This refers to temperature and air draft problems, inadequate ventilation rates, and other problems that seem related to the air delivery and exhaust systems. Included are both minor problems that can be remedied easily, and more complex issues that may be difficult to define and resolve.

1. Report all HVAC problems to Facilities (xt xxxx). (This line is usually personally attended, but is sometimes used as a message line.)

2. When the problem is chronic, serious, or unusual, call the Facilities Manager (xt xxxx).

3. In case of emergency, call the Safety and Security Supervisor (xt xxxx), or call 911.

INDIVIDUAL AS SOURCE

This refers to a personal source, such as an individual who uses scented products that cause adverse health affects.

1. Approach the individual, explain the problem, and ask for consideration or changes in behavior that can improve the situation. (**This step is consistent with NSCC's Mission and Goals, and Shared Vision statements which affirm that NSCC will provide a safe and healthy working, teaching, and learning environment for its campus community.**) If no resolution results,

2. Request the assistance of your supervisor, faculty, or administrator. If no resolution is reached,

3. Report the problem to your Student Complaints Officer if you are a student, or to the Human Resources Representative if you are a staff member.

AFTER-HOURS EMERGENCY

Call Safety and Security (xt xxxx) or 911 for assistance.

• Other resources available are the Human Resources Representative, the Disability Services Office, The Students Complaints process, Union Shop Stewards, The Affirmative Action Officer, and the Health and Safety Committee.

• **Official forms for initiating the complaints process will be developed by the Health and Safety Committee (with expert consultation made available for their work). These forms will be distributed and made available in all campus Departments and Offices.**

• If the above process does not lead to a successful conclusion, contact the Human Resources Representative, who will establish a team to assist in finding a suitable resolution. The team will include the Human Resources Representative, the Manager of Facilities, the Student Complaints Officer, the Safety and Security Supervisor, and the affected person and his/her supervisor, faculty or administrator.

Appendix II

The Nuremberg Code (1947)

The great weight of the evidence before us is to the effect that certain types of medical experiments on human beings, when kept within reasonably well-defined bounds, conform to the ethics of the medical profession generally. The protagonists of the practice of human experimentation justify their views on the basis that such experiments yield results for the good of society that are unprocurable by other methods or means of study. All agree, however, that certain basic principles must be observed in order to satisfy moral, ethical and legal concepts:

1. The voluntary consent of the human subject is absolutely essential.

This means that the person involved should have legal capacity to give consent; should be so situated as to be able to exercise free power of choice, without the intervention of any element of force, fraud, deceit, duress, overreaching, or other ulterior form of constraint or coercion, and should have sufficient knowledge and comprehension of the elements of the subject matter involved as to enable him to make an understanding and enlightened decision. This latter element requires that before the acceptance of an affirmative decision by the experimental subject there should be made known to him the nature, duration, and purpose of the experiment; the method and means by which it is to be conducted; all inconveniences and hazards reasonably to be expected; and the effects upon his health or person which may possibly come from his participation in the experiment.

The duty and responsibility for ascertaining the quality of the consent rests upon each individual who initiates, directs or engages in the experiment. It is a personal duty and responsibility which may not be delegated to another with impunity.

2. The experiment should be such as to yield fruitful results for the good of society, unprocurable by other methods or means of study, and not random or unnecessary in nature.

3. The experiment should be so designed and based on the results of animal experimentation and a knowledge of the natural history of the disease or other problems under study that the anticipated results will justify the performance of the experiment.

4. The experiment should be so conducted as to avoid all unnecessary physical and mental suffering and injury.

5. No experiment should be conducted where there is an a priori reason to believe that death or disabling injury will occur, except, perhaps, in those experiments where the experimental physicians also serve as subjects.

6. The degree of risk to be taken should never exceed that determined by the humanitarian importance of the problem to be solved by the experiment.

7. Proper preparations should be made and adequate facilities provided to protect the experimental subject against even remote possibilities of injury, disability, or death.

8. The experiment should be conducted only by scientifically qualified persons. The highest degree of skill and care should be required through all stages of the experiment of those who conduct or engage in the experiment.

9. During the course of the experiment the human subject should be at liberty to bring the experiment to an end if he has reached the physical or mental state where continuation of the experiment seems to him to be impossible.

10. During the course of the experiment the scientist in charge must be prepared to terminate the experiment at any stage if he has probable cause to believe, in the exercise of the good faith, superior skill, and careful judgment required of him that a continuation of the experiment is likely to result in injury, disability, or death to the experimental subject.

from *Trials of War Criminals Before the Nuremberg Military Tribunals Under Control Council Law No. 10,* Vol. II. Nuremberg, Germany, October 1946–April 1949.

Appendix III

International Ethical Guidelines for Biomedical Research Involving Human Subjects

(CIOMS, WHO, Geneva, 1993)
(Basic guidelines only, without commentary.)

GUIDELINE 1: INDIVIDUAL INFORMED CONSENT

For all biomedical research involving human subjects, the investigator must obtain the informed consent of the prospective subject or, in the case of an individual who is not capable of giving informed consent, the proxy consent of a properly authorized representative.

GUIDELINE 2: ESSENTIAL INFORMATION FOR PROSPECTIVE RESEARCH SUBJECTS

Before requesting an individual's consent to participate in research, the investigator must provide the individual with the following information, in language that he or she is capable of understanding:
—that each individual is invited to participate as a subject in research, and the aims and methods of the research;
—the expected duration of the subject's participation;
—the benefits that might reasonably be expected to result to the subject or to others as an outcome of the research;

—any foreseeable risks or discomfort to the subject, associated with participation in the research;

—any alternative procedures or courses of treatment that might be as advantageous to the subject as the procedure or treatment being tested;

—the extent to which confidentiality of records in which the subject is identified will be maintained;

—the extent of the investigator's responsibility, if any, to provide medical services to the subject;

—that therapy will be provided free of charge for specified types of research-related injury;

—whether the subject or the subject's family or dependents will be compensated for disability or death resulting from such injury; and

—that the individual is free to refuse to participate and will be free to withdraw from the research at any time without penalty or loss of benefits to which he or she would otherwise be entitled.

GUIDELINE 3: OBLIGATIONS OF INVESTIGATORS REGARDING INFORMED CONSENT

The investigator has a duty to:

—communicate to the prospective subject all the information necessary for adequately informed consent;

—give the prospective subject full opportunity and encouragement to ask questions;

—exclude the possibility of unjustified deception, undue influence and intimidation;

—seek consent only after the prospective subject has adequate knowledge of the relevant facts and of the consequences of participation, and has had sufficient opportunity to consider whether to participate;

—as a general rule, obtain from each prospective subject a signed form as evidence of informed consent; and

—renew the informed consent of each subject if there are material changes in the conditions or procedures of the research.

GUIDELINE 4: INDUCEMENT TO PARTICIPATE

Subjects may be paid for inconvenience and time spent, and should be reimbursed for expenses incurred, in connection with their participation in research; they may also receive free medical services. However, the payments should not be so large or the medical services so extensive as to induce prospective subjects to consent to participate in the research against their better judgment ("undue inducement"). All payments, reimbursements and medical services to be provided to research subjects should be approved by an ethical review committee.

GUIDELINE 5: RESEARCH INVOLVING CHILDREN

Before undertaking research involving children, the investigator must ensure that:

—children will not be involved in research that might equally well be carried out with adults;
—the purpose of the research is to obtain knowledge relevant to the health needs of children;
—a parent or legal guardian of each child has given proxy consent;
—the consent of each child has been obtained to the extent of the child's capabilities;
—the child's refusal to participate in research must always be respected unless according to the research protocol the child would receive therapy for which there is no medically-acceptable alternative;
—the risk presented by interventions not intended to benefit the individual child-subject is low and commensurate with the importance of the knowledge to be gained; and
—interventions that are intended to provide therapeutic benefit are likely to be at least as advantageous to the individual child-subject as any available alternative.

GUIDELINE 6: RESEARCH INVOLVING PERSONS WITH MENTAL OR BEHAVIORAL DISORDERS

Before undertaking research involving individuals who by reason of mental or behavioral disorders are not capable of giving adequately informed consent, the investigator must ensure that:
—such persons will not be subjects of research that might equally well be carried out on persons in full possession of their mental faculties;
—the purpose of the research is to obtain knowledge relevant to the particular health needs of persons with mental or behavioral disorders;
—the consent of each subject has been obtained to the extent of that subject's capabilities, and a prospective subject's refusal to participate in non-clinical research is always respected;
—in the case of incompetent subjects, informed consent is obtained from the legal guardian or other duly authorized person;
—the degree of risk attached to interventions that are not intended to benefit the individual subject is low and commensurate with the importance of the knowledge to be gained; and
—interventions that are intended to provide therapeutic benefit are likely to be at least as advantageous to the individual subject as any alternative.

GUIDELINE 7: RESEARCH INVOLVING PRISONERS

Prisoners with serious illness or at risk of serious illness should not arbitrarily be denied access to investigational drugs, vaccines or other agents that show promise of therapeutic or preventive benefit.

GUIDELINE 8: RESEARCH INVOLVING SUBJECTS IN UNDERDEVELOPED COMMUNITIES

Before undertaking research involving subjects in underdeveloped communities, whether in developed or developing countries, the investigator must ensure that:

—persons in underdeveloped communities will not ordinarily be involved in research that could be carried out reasonably well in developed communities;

—the research is responsive to the health needs and the priorities of the community in which it is to be carried out:

—every effort will be made to secure the ethical imperative that the consent of individual subjects be informed; and

—the proposals for the research have been reviewed and approved by an ethical review committee that has among its members or consultants persons who are thoroughly familiar with the customs and traditions of the community.

GUIDELINE 9: INFORMED CONSENT IN EPIDEMIOLOGICAL STUDIES

For several types of epidemiological research individual informed consent is either impracticable or inadvisable. In such cases the ethical review committee should determine whether it is ethically acceptable to proceed without individual informed consent and whether the investigator's plans to protect the safety and respect the privacy of research subjects and to maintain the confidentiality of the data are adequate.

GUIDELINE 10: EQUITABLE DISTRIBUTION OF BURDENS AND BENEFITS

Individuals or communities to be invited to be subjects of research should be selected in such a way that the burdens and benefits of the research will be equitably distributed. Special justification is required for inviting vulnerable individuals and, if they are selected, the means of protecting their rights and welfare must be particularly strictly applied.

GUIDELINE 11: SELECTION OF PREGNANT OR NURSING (BREASTFEEDING) WOMEN AS RESEARCH SUBJECTS

Pregnant or nursing women should in no circumstances be the subjects of non-clinical research unless the research carries no more than minimal risk to the fetus or nursing infant and the object of the research is to obtain new knowledge about pregnancy or lactation. As a general rule, pregnant or nursing women should not be subjects of any clinical trials except such trials as are designed to protect or advance the health of pregnant or nursing women or fetuses or nursing infants, and for which women who are not pregnant or nursing would not be suitable subjects.

GUIDELINE 12: SAFEGUARDING CONFIDENTIALITY

The investigator must establish secure safeguards of the confidentiality of research data. Subjects should be told of the limits to the investigators' ability to safeguard confidentiality and of the anticipated consequences of breaches of confidentiality.

GUIDELINE 13: RIGHT OF SUBJECTS TO COMPENSATION

Research subjects who suffer physical injury as a result of their participation are entitled to such financial or other assistance as would compensate them equitably for any temporary or permanent impairment or disability. In the case of death, their dependents are entitled to material compensation. The right to compensation may not be waived.

GUIDELINE 14: CONSTITUTION AND RESPONSIBILITIES OF ETHICAL REVIEW COMMITTEES

All proposals to conduct research involving human subjects must be submitted for review and approval to one or more independent ethical and scientific review committees. The investigator must obtain such approval of the proposal to conduct research before the research is begun.

GUIDELINE 15: OBLIGATIONS OF SPONSORING AND HOST COUNTRIES

Externally sponsored research entails two ethical obligations:
— An external sponsoring agency should submit the research protocol to ethical and scientific review according to the standards of the country of the sponsoring agency, and the ethical standards applied should be no less exacting than they would be in the case of research carried out in that country.
— After scientific and ethical approval in the country of the sponsoring agency, the appropriate authorities of the host country, including a national or local ethical review committee or its equivalent, should satisfy themselves that the proposed research meets their own ethical requirements.

Appendix IV

Draft Declaration of Principles on Human Rights and the Environment (1994)

PREAMBLE

Guided by the United Nations Charter, the Universal Declaration of Human Rights, the International Covenant on Economic, Social and Cultural Rights, the International Covenant on Civil and Political Rights, the Vienna Declaration and Program of Action of the World Conference of Human Rights, and other relevant international human rights instruments,

Guided also by the Stockholm Declaration of the United Nations Conference on the Human Environment, the World Charter for Nature, the Rio Declaration on Environment and Development, Agenda 21: Programme of Action for Sustainable Development, and other relevant instruments of international environmental law,

Guided also by the Declaration on the Right to Development, which recognizes that the right to development is an essential human right and that the human person is the central subject of development,

Guided further by fundamental principles of international humanitarian law,

Reaffirming the universality, indivisibility and interdependence of all human rights,

Recognizing that sustainable development links the right to development and the right to a secure, healthy and ecologically sound environment,

Recalling the right of peoples to self-determination by virtue of which they have the right freely to determine their political status and to pursue their economic, social and cultural development,

Deeply concerned by the severe human rights consequences of environmental harm caused by poverty, structural adjustment and debt programmes and by international trade and intellectual property regimes,

Convinced that the potential irreversibility of environmental harm gives rise to special responsibility to prevent such harm,

Concerned that human rights violations lead to environmental degradation and that environmental degradation leads to human rights violations,

The Following Principles Are Declared:

PART I

1. Human rights, an ecologically sound environment, sustainable development and peace are interdependent and indivisible.

2. All persons have the right to a secure, healthy and ecologically sound environment. This right and other human rights, including civil, cultural, economic, political and social rights, are universal, interdependent and indivisible.

3. All persons shall be free from any form of discrimination in regard to actions and decisions that affect the environment.

4. All persons have the right to an environment adequate to meet equitably the needs of present generations and that does not impair the rights of future generations to meet equitably their needs.

PART II

5. All persons have the right to freedom from pollution, environmental degradation and activities that adversely affect the environment, threaten life, health, livelihood, well-being or sustainable development within, across or outside national boundaries.

6. All persons have the right to protection and preservation of the air, soil, water, sea-ice, flora and fauna, and the essential processes and areas necessary to maintain biological diversity and ecosystems.

7. All persons have the right to the highest attainable standard of health free from environmental harm

8. All persons have the right to safe and healthy food and water adequate to their well-being.

9. All persons have the right to a safe and healthy working environment.

10. All persons have the right to adequate housing, land tenure and living conditions in a secure, healthy and ecologically sound environment.

11. All persons have the right not to be evicted from their homes or land for the purpose of, or as a consequence of, decisions or actions affecting the environment, except in emergencies or due to a compelling purpose benefiting society as a whole and not attainable by other means. All persons

have the right to participate effectively in decisions and to negotiate concerning their eviction and the right, if evicted, to timely and adequate restitution, compensation and/or appropriate and sufficient accommodation or land.

12. All persons have the right to timely assistance in the event of natural or technological or other human-caused catastrophes.

13. Everyone has the right to benefit equitably from the conservation and sustainable use of nature and natural resources for cultural, ecological, educational, health, livelihood, recreational, spiritual or other purposes. This includes ecologically sound access to nature.

Everyone has the right to preservation of unique sites, consistent with the fundamental rights of persons or groups living in the area.

14. Indigenous peoples have the right to control their lands, territories and natural resources and to maintain their traditional way of life. This includes the right to security in the enjoyment of their means of subsistence.

Indigenous peoples have the right to protection against any action or course of conduct that may result in the destruction or degradation of their territories, including land, air, water, sea-ice, wildlife or other resources.

PART III

15. All persons have the right to information concerning the environment. This includes information, howsoever compiled, on actions and courses of conduct that may affect the environment and information necessary to enable effective public participation in environmental decision-making. The information shall be timely, clear, understandable and available without undue financial burden to the applicant.

16. All persons have the right to hold and express opinions and to disseminate ideas and information regarding the environment.

17. All persons have the right to environmental and human rights education.

18. All persons have the right to active, free, and meaningful participation in planning and decision-making activities and processes that may have an impact on the environment and development. This includes the right to a prior assessment of the environmental, developmental and human rights consequences of proposed actions.

19. All persons have the right to associate freely and peacefully with others for purposes of protecting the environment or the rights of persons affected by environmental harm.

20. All persons have the right to effective remedies and redress in administrative or judicial proceedings for environmental harm or the threat of such harm.

PART IV

21. All persons, individually and in association with others, have a duty to protect and preserve the environment.

22. All States shall respect and ensure the right to a secure, healthy and

ecologically sound environment. Accordingly, they shall adopt the administrative, legislative and other measures necessary to effectively implement the rights in this Declaration.

These measures shall aim at the prevention of environmental harm, at the provision of adequate remedies, and at the sustainable use of natural resources and shall include, inter alia,

* collection and dissemination of information concerning the environment
* prior assessment and control, licensing, regulation or prohibition of activities and substances potentially harmful to the environment;
* public participation in environmental decision-making;
* effective administrative and judicial remedies and redress for environmental harm and the threat of such harm;
* monitoring, management and equitable sharing of natural resources;
* measures to reduce wasteful processes of production and patterns of consumption;
* measures aimed at ensuring that transnational corporations, wherever they operate, carry out their duties of environmental protection, sustainable development and respect for human rights; and
* measures aimed at ensuring that the international organizations and agencies to which they belong observe the rights and duties in this Declaration.

23. States and all other parties shall avoid using the environment as a means of war or inflicting significant, long-term or widespread harm on the environment, and shall respect international law providing protection for the environment in times of armed conflict and cooperate in its further development.

24. All international organizations and agencies shall observe the rights and duties in this Declaration.

PART V

25. In implementing the rights and duties in this Declaration, special attention shall be given to vulnerable persons and groups.

26. The rights in this Declaration may be subject only to restrictions provided by law and which are necessary to protect public order, health and the fundamental rights and freedoms of others.

27. All persons are entitled to a social and international order in which the rights in this Declaration can be fully realized.

The Draft Declaration will evolve and the Sierra Club Legal Defense Fund therefore invites comments.

Please send comments to:

Appendix IV

INTERNATIONAL PROGRAM
SIERRA CLUB LEGAL DEFENSE FUND
180 Montgomery Street, 14th Floor
San Francisco, CA 94104-4230, USA
Telephone: (415) 627-6700
Facsimile: (415) 627-6740
email: scldfintl@igc.apc.org

Appendix V

Charter on Industrial Hazards and Human Rights (1996)

Permanent People's Tribunal (PPT), Via della Dogana Vecchia 5, 00186 Rome, Italy
Tel. + 396 654 1468 / Fax + 396 687 7774
PPT on Industrial Hazards and Human Rights, Hosted by The Pesticides Trust Eurolink Centre, 49 Effra Road, London SW2 1BZ
Tel. + 447 1274 8895 / Fax + 447 1274 9084.
Email: pesttrust@gn.apc.org

PREAMBLE

The Permanent People's Tribunal on Industrial Hazards and Human Rights,

Having convened four Sessions in New Haven, Bangkok, Bhopal and London since 1991 to receive testimony and deliberate on issues relating to the right to life, occupational health and safety, environment protection, risk management and damage reduction in the wider global context of hazardous production;

Having drafted over a period of four years a charter of rights designed to reflect the views and concerns of persons injured and distressed by industrial hazards, and having issued on the second day of December 1994 a Draft Charter for comment and discussion among individuals and non-governmental organizations, including trade unions;

263

Following the *Universal Declaration of the Rights of Peoples*, the *Universal Declaration of Human Rights*, the *International Covenant on Civil and Political Rights*, the *International Covenant on Economic, Social and Cultural Rights*, the *Convention on the Elimination of All Forms of Discrimination Against Women*, the *United Nations Convention on the Rights of the Child*, the *Vienna Declaration and Programme of Action of the World Conference of Human Rights* and other relevant international human rights instruments;

Guided by the Rio *Declaration on Environment and Development*, Agenda 21, the Draft *Declaration of Principles on Human Rights and the Environment*, the Draft *Declaration on the Rights of Indigenous Peoples* and other relevant instruments for prevention of industrial and environmental hazards;

Guided further by International Labour Organisation conventions and recommendations, including the Convention on Freedom of Association and Protection of the Right to Organise, the Convention on the Right to Organise and Collective Bargaining and the Convention Concerning the Prevention of Major Industrial Accidents;

Gravely concerned by the widespread diffusion of hazardous products and processes resulting in industrial practices which cause human, social and environmental destruction, threatening in particular the habitat, life, economy, society and culture of indigenous peoples;

Deeply concerned by the frequency of small-scale but harmful hazardous events, as well as the magnitude and nature of major industrial accidents, including the incidents in Seveso, Chernobyl, Bhopal, Basel and elsewhere;

Concerned by the ineffectual national and international system of hazard prevention, post-disaster relief, medical and legal assistance and legal accountability which in their current forms have failed both to adequately prevent occupational and environmental hazards and to bring to account those responsible for world-wide deaths and injuries;

Noting that urgent action is needed to prevent future degradation to human life, animal life and the environment and to adequately remedy the harms caused by industrial hazards;

Recognising that the personal experience and repeated demands of community members and workers affected by hazards provide the most sound basis for the enunciation of rights;

Cognizant of the inherent limitations of national and international law, as well as the vital role of community organisations and people's movements in preventing and ameliorating industrial hazards;

Convinced that new national and international systems of prevention, relief and legal accountability must be formulated and established;

DECLARES THE FOLLOWING:

Part I Rights of General Application

ARTICLE 1   NON-DISCRIMINATION

1. Everyone is entitled to all the rights and freedoms set forth in this Charter, without distinction of any kind, such as race, colour, sex, language, religion, nationality, political opinion or affiliation, ethnic or social origin, disability, age, property, sexual orientation, birth, income, caste or any other status.

2. On account of the particular discrimination faced by women, both as waged and unwaged workers, attention should be given to the specific application of the rights stated below where women may be affected.

3. On account of their vulnerability and exploitation in the labour market, special protection should be accorded to children exposed to industrial hazards.

4. On account of the connection between low wages and hazardous working environments and the disproportionate impact of industrial hazards on racial and ethnic minorities, special protection should be afforded low income groups and racial minorities.

ARTICLE 2   RELATION TO OTHER RIGHTS

The rights in this charter and other human rights, including civil, political, economic, social and cultural rights, are universal, interdependent and indivisible. In particular, freedom from hazards, including the right to refuse hazardous employment and the right to organise against hazards, depends upon the full implementation of social and economic rights, including the rights to education, health and an adequate standard of living.

ARTICLE 3   RIGHT TO ACCOUNTABILITY

All persons have the right to hold accountable any individual, company or government agency for actions resulting in industrial hazards. In particular, parent companies, including transnational corporations, shall be liable for the actions of their subsidiaries.

ARTICLE 4   RIGHT TO ORGANISE

1. All community members and workers have the right to organise with other local communities and workers for the purpose of seeking to ensure a working environment free from hazard.

2. In particular, the right to organise includes:

    (a) the freedoms of expression, association and peaceful assembly;
    (b) the right to form local, national and international organisations;
    (c) the rights to campaign, lobby, educate and exchange information;
    (d) the right to form trade unions;
    (e) the right to strike or take other forms of industrial action.

ARTICLE 5 RIGHT TO APPROPRIATE HEALTH CARE

1. All persons have the right to appropriate health care.
2. In particular, the right to appropriate health care includes:

(a) the right of individuals and groups to participate in the planning and implementation of health care;
(b) the right of equal access of individuals and families to health care the community can afford;
(c) the right to relevant health care services, including where appropriate access to hospitals, neighbourhood clinics, specialist clinics, as well as the services of general practitioners, other medical professionals and health care workers drawn from the affected community;
(d) the right to independent information on the relevance and reliability of health care services and treatments including allopathic, homeopathic, nutritional, physiotherapeutic, psychotherapeutic, indigenous and other approaches;
(e) the right to health care systems which recognise and take account of the different ways in which hazards affect women, men and children;
(f) the right to health education;
(g) the development of national, regional and international networks to facilitate sharing of information and experience.

ARTICLE 6 RIGHT OF REFUSAL

1. All communities have the right to refuse the introduction, expansion or continuation of hazardous activities in their living environment.
2. All workers have the right to refuse to work in a hazardous working environment without fear of retaliatory action by the employer.
3. The right to reject inappropriate legal, medical or scientific advice shall not be infringed.

ARTICLE 7 PERMANENT SOVEREIGNTY OVER LIVING ENVIRONMENTS

1. Each state retains the right of permanent sovereignty over the living environments within its national jurisdiction. No state shall exercise this right so as to injure the health or living environments of its people, nor to cause damage to the environment of other states or of areas beyond the limits of national jurisdiction.
2. Each state has the right and the obligation to regulate and exercise authority over hazardous and potentially hazardous enterprises in conformity with the interests and well-being of its people and their environment.
3. No state shall be:

(a) refused external finance or assistance on the grounds of its refusal to import or establish hazardous products or processes;

(b) Compelled to grant preferential treatment to foreign investment;
(c) Made subject to external threats or coercive measures, whether military, diplomatic, social or economic, intended to affect regulations or policies regarding hazardous production.

4. Transnational corporations and multinational enterprises shall not intervene in the internal affairs of a host state.

Part II Community Rights

ARTICLE 8 RIGHT TO LIVING ENVIRONMENT FREE FROM [INDUSTRIAL] HAZARDS

1. All persons have the right to a living environment free from [industrial] hazards. In particular, this right applies where hazards arise from:

(a) the manufacture, sale, transport, distribution, use and disposal of hazardous materials;
(b) any military or weapons application, regardless of national security.

2. Any person has the right to raise a bona fide complaint to the owner or occupier of an economic enterprise regarding activities of the enterprise which he or she believes are hazardous to the living environment.
3. Any person living in an environment from which it is impossible to eliminate a hazard shall have the right to protective safety systems necessary to eliminate any such hazard as far as possible. The owners or occupiers of the concerned hazardous enterprise may not refuse to provide the most effective systems available on the grounds of cost or inconvenience.

ARTICLE 9 RIGHT TO ENVIRONMENTAL INFORMATION

1. All persons have the right to be given reasonable notice of any proposal to establish, expand or modify a hazardous industry in such location or in such a manner as may put at risk public health or the living environment. To achieve the full realization of this right, the following steps shall be taken:

(a) All states shall ensure that communities, individuals and non-governmental organisations have the right of access to full information regarding the proposal. This right shall be effective well in advance of official authorization and shall not be abridged by claims of commercial secrecy.
(b) All states shall ensure that prior to official approval of any hazardous enterprise, independent and thorough assessments of the impact upon the environment and public health be conducted in consultation with the community. The methods and conclusions of such impact assessments shall be made available for public debate.

2. All persons have the right to be informed in their own language and in a manner which they are able to comprehend, of any possible hazards or risks associated with any product or process used by any enterprise with which they may come into contact.

3. All persons have the right to be informed of the safety record of any economic enterprises whose manufacturing or industrial processes could affect their living environment, including the number of accidents, the types of accidents that have occurred, the extent of injuries resulting from such accidents and any possible long-term adverse health effects.

4. All persons have the right to be informed of types and quantities of hazardous substances used and stored at the facility and emitted from the facility and contained in any final products. In particular, the right to information includes the right to regular toxic release inventories where appropriate. All persons living in the neighbourhood of hazardous facilities have the right to inspection of factory premises and to physical verification of hazardous substances and processes.

5. All persons who live in environments in which they may come into contact with materials or processes that are known to be seriously hazardous and which emanate from the activities of an economic enterprise, have the right to be examined regularly by an independent medical expert provided by the owner or occupier of the enterprise.

ARTICLE 10   RIGHT TO COMMUNITY PARTICIPATION

1. All persons have the right to participate in planning and decision-making processes affecting their living environment.

2. All persons have the right to planning and decision-making proceedings which are:

(a) public and open;
(b) accessible to all in timing and location;
(c) widely advertised in advance;
(d) not restricted by literacy, language or format of contributions.

3. All persons have the right to express their concerns and objections relating to hazards associated with establishing, modifying or expanding any economic enterprise.

4. All persons have the right to participate in the design and execution of on-going studies to determine the nature of any hazards to the living environment resulting from an economic enterprise.

ARTICLE 11   RIGHT TO ENVIRONMENTAL MONITORING

1. All persons have the right to regular and effective monitoring of their health and the living environment for possible immediate and long-term effects caused by hazardous or potentially hazardous economic enterprise.

2. All persons have the right to be consulted on the frequency, character and objectives of environmental monitoring. The right to organise non-professional monitoring strategies, such as lay epidemiology, shall

be protected. The rights of women, whose experience in providing health care may reveal otherwise unidentified consequences of hazards, are particularly affirmed.

3. Any person who bona fide believes that his or her community environment is endangered by the actions of any economic enterprise, has the right to an immediate and thorough investigation, to be carried out by an independent agency at no cost to the person acting bona fide.

ARTICLE 12   RIGHT TO COMMUNITY EDUCATION

1. All persons have the right to the effective dissemination of information regarding hazards in the community. This right extends to instruction based upon the best available information and standards, drawn from both national and international sources.

2. States shall take effective steps to provide for:

   (a) clear and systematic labeling of hazardous substances;
   (b) appropriate education of the community, including children, on hazardous products and processes;
   (c) training of police, medical professionals and other service providers on hazardous products and processes.

ARTICLE 13   RIGHT TO COMMUNITY EMERGENCY PREPAREDNESS PROCEDURE

1. All persons have the right to an appropriate emergency preparedness procedure. Such procedure shall include warning systems for impending dangers and systems for immediate relief efforts.

2. All states shall take steps to provide communities with adequate emergency services, including the provision of police, fire fighting, medical and paramedical facilities and disaster management services.

ARTICLE 14   RIGHT TO ENFORCEMENT OF ENVIRONMENTAL LAWS

1. All persons have the right to have their local environment adequately and frequently inspected by a trained environmental inspector who will rigorously enforce the law and take punitive legal action when serious breaches have taken place.

2. All persons have the right to environmental management legislation in compliance with the precautionary principle, so that where there are threats of serious or irreversible damage, lack of full scientific certainty shall not be used as a reason to postpone cost-effective measures to prevent hazards and environmental degradation.

ARTICLE 15 RIGHTS OF INDIGENOUS PEOPLES

1. Indigenous peoples have the right to protect their habitat, economy society and culture from industrial hazards and environmentally destructive practices by economic enterprises.

2. Indigenous peoples have the right to control over their land and resources management of their land which includes the right to assess potential environmental impacts and the right to refuse to allow environmentally destructive or hazardous industries to be set up on their land.

Part III Rights of Workers

ARTICLE 16   SPECIFIC RIGHTS OF WORKERS

In addition to their rights as members of the community, workers have specific rights applicable to their working environments.

ARTICLE 17   RIGHT TO WORKING ENVIRONMENT FREE FROM HAZARDS

1. All workers, both waged and unwaged, have the right to a working environment free from any existing or potential hazard arising directly or indirectly from the activities of any economic enterprise in particular from manufacturing or other industrial processes.

2. Any worker has the right to raise bona fide complaints to the employer or any outside parties regarding conditions or practices in the working environment that he or she believes are harmful or hazardous without fear of retaliatory action or other discriminatory action by the employer.

3. Any individual working in an environment from which it is impossible to eliminate any hazard, shall have the right to have provided, fitted free of charge and maintained in fully effective order, protective safety devices including personal protective equipment necessary to eliminate any such hazard as far as is possible. Employers may not refuse to provide the most effective equipment available on the grounds of cost or inconvenience.

4. All workers have the right to safe systems of work. All employers have the duty to devise, provide, maintain and regularly update safe systems of work based on the best available information at all times.

5. No worker shall be subjected to exposure to a chemical, product or process when a less hazardous one could be substituted.

6. Governments and employers are responsible for ensuring hazard-free working environments. The inaction by either employer or government shall not be an adequate excuse for a derogation of duty by the other.

ARTICLE 18   RIGHT TO HEALTH AND SAFETY INFORMATION

1. All workers have the right to be given reasonable notice of any proposed changes to their working environments which may pose a threat to worker health and safety.

2. All workers have the right to be informed in their own language and in a manner they are able to comprehend, of any known health hazard associated with any substance, material or process with which they come into contact during the course of their employment.

3. All workers have the right to be informed of the safety record of the work environment in which they are employed, including the number and type of accidents that have occurred, the extent of the injuries resulting therefrom and any known long-term adverse health risks that result from the substances, materials and processes used by the employer. Workers have the right to be regularly informed of the safety records of any economic enterprise affiliated by common ownership to the economic enterprise in which they work, and which uses any similar substance, material or process to that used in their work environment.

4. All workers employed in hazardous work environments have the right to be examined by an independent medical expert provided by the employer at the commencement of employment and thereafter at periodic intervals defined on the basis of the most conservative estimate of potential risks, but in any case not exceeding one year and to be furnished with the resulting medical information.

ARTICLE 19   RIGHT TO WORKER PARTICIPATION

1. All workers have the right to participate effectively in management decision-making affecting health and safety.

2. All workers have the right to elect safety representatives. Such representatives have the right to participate in joint committees, composed of worker and management representatives in equal number, which meet regularly to address health and safety matters.

3. All workers have the right to participate in the design and execution of ongoing health and safety studies in their working environments to determine the nature of any risks to health and safety.

4. All workers have the right to establish and associate with community hazards centres and information networks. Governments and employers have a responsibility to support such organisations and programmes.

ARTICLE 20   RIGHT TO HEALTH
AND SAFETY MONITORING

1. All workers have the right to a work environment that is regularly and effectively monitored for possible harmful effects to the health and safety of the workers employed therein.

2. Notwithstanding the duty of employers to monitor working environments, the right of workers to seek independent or worker-based monitoring shall not be infringed. This right includes the right to regular monitoring for possible adverse, long-term effects which may result from contact with the substances, materials or processes used in the working environment.

3. Any worker who bona fide believes that his or her health and safety is being or will be endangered by any substance, material or process used in the work environment has the right to an immediate and thorough investigation, to be carried out by the employer, an independent agency or by other means, at no cost to the worker.

ARTICLE 21　RIGHT TO
INSTRUCTION AND PRACTICAL TRAINING

1. All workers in contact with hazardous or potentially hazardous substances, materials or processes have the right to ongoing instruction and practical training regarding management of the hazard. The right to instruction and practical training based on the best available information, drawn from both national and international sources, is affirmed.

2. All workers and supervisors have the right to know and be fully instructed about the proper use and handling of any hazardous materials, the proper execution of any processes, the precautions necessary to protect health, safety and the living environment, and any procedures which should be followed in the event of an emergency.

ARTICLE 22　RIGHT TO WORKPLACE
EMERGENCY PREPAREDNESS PROCEDURE

1. All workers have the right to an emergency preparedness procedure appropriate for the conditions or practices in their work environment which shall include warning systems for impending dangers and systems for immediate relief efforts, with full scale emergency preparedness rehearsals and desk top exercises to be held frequently.

2. Emergency preparedness procedures shall take account of the particular needs of individual workers, including those with visual, hearing or mobility impairments.

3. All workers have the right to adequate emergency services, including police, fire fighting, medical and paramedical facilities and disaster management.

ARTICLE 23　RIGHT TO
ENFORCEMENT OF HEALTH AND SAFETY LAWS

1. All workers have the right to have their work environments adequately and frequently inspected by a trained health and safety inspector who will rigorously enforce the law and take punitive legal action when serious breaches have occurred.

2. All workers have the right to adequate planning control legislation in compliance with the precautionary principle, so that where there are threats of serious or irreversible damage, lack of full scientific certainty shall not be used as a reason to postpone cost-effective measures to prevent hazards and environmental degradation.

Part IV Common Rights to Relief

ARTICLE 24　RIGHT TO RELIEF AND COMPENSATION

1. All persons injured or otherwise detrimentally affected by any hazardous economic activity have the right to swift, comprehensive and effective

relief. This right applies to all persons affected by hazards or potential hazards, including persons not yet born at the time of injury or exposure, and those injured, bereaved or economically and socially disadvantaged, whether affected directly or indirectly.

2. This right includes the right to fair and adequate monetary compensation, paid to cover all costs associated with hazardous or potentially hazardous activities, including the costs of:

(a) drugs, tests, therapies, hospitalisation and other medical treatments;
(b) travel and other incidental costs;
(c) lost wages, bridging loans and other pecuniary loss;
(d) redundancy and unemployment in the case of plant shutdown;
(e) additional unwaged work, including health care, born by family and community;
(f) any purchase, measure or lost opportunity caused directly or indirectly by hazardous processes or products;
(g) environmental rehabilitation.

3. All persons affected by hazards have the right to effective and innovative policies to reduce, abate or compensate for hazardous activities. To achieve the realization of this right, the steps taken by states and businesses shall include:

(a) plant shutdown;
(b) pollution abatements or cessation;
(c) guarantee by liable defendants to keep assets unencumbered;
(d) forced liquidation of the assets of a corporation whose liability is equal to or greater than its measurable assets;
(e) placement of corporate assets in annuity funds controlled by the persons affected or their representatives for the interests of persons affected;
(f) fair and adequate compensation for the costs of the medical monitoring of symptoms;
(g) other remedies that may be deemed to be necessary for the benefits of persons affected.

4. Funds shall be established adequately to satisfy the claims for the persons affected and of those affected in future.

Article 25   Right to Immediate Interim Relief

1. All persons adversely affected by any hazardous economic activity have the right to immediate and adequate interim relief to alleviate their injuries and suffering during the time that liability and compensatory damages are being determined. States shall ensure that all hazardous or potentially hazardous enterprises provide financial resources, through insurance or other means, adequate to cover potential interim relief costs.

2. Where an economic enterprise fails to provide interim relief, it shall be the duty of the state to do so. Interim relief so provided will not be set-off against any final compensation allowed by the court.

ARTICLE 26   RIGHT TO MEDICAL INFORMATION

All persons immediately or subsequently affected by hazardous activities, including persons unborn at the time of the exposure to hazard, have the right to obtain relevant documents pertaining to injuries, including medical records, test results and other information. This right may be exercised at the earliest opportunity and may not be made subject to delay or non-compliance by either government or industry. Such disclosure shall not be made in a manner so as to prejudice the affected person's right of access to any service, insurance, employment or any social or welfare opportunities.

ARTICLE 27   RIGHT TO PROFESSIONAL SERVICES

1. All persons adversely affected by hazardous activity have the right of access to effective professional services, including the services of lawyers, journalists, scientific experts and medical professions.

2. Where questions of a scientific or medical nature are in dispute, all affected persons, or their representatives, have the right to genuinely independent advice, free from fear or favour. The right to seek independent or multiple advice is affirmed.

3. Professionals and experts shall refrain from:

(a) giving advice on the basis of inadequate information or expertise;
(b) obstructing the efforts of workers and communities to seek information, conduct research or gather data through lay epidemiology or other means;
(c) acting in concert against the interests of workers and communities.

4. All professionals having control of any information concerning the health of any injured or hazard-affected person shall have a primary duty of care towards the well being of that person. This duty shall at all times take precedence over any allegiance to any third party, including any government, professional organisation or commercial enterprise.

ARTICLE 28   RIGHT TO EFFECTIVE
LEGAL REPRESENTATION

1. All persons adversely affected by hazardous activities shall have the right to employ independent legal counsel.

2. All states shall provide free legal representation and legal assistance by an independent legal expert, in any case where the interests of justice so require.

3. In the determination of any suit, the persons affected shall be entitled to consolidate the claims under:

(a) the auspices of a workers' or community organisation; or
(b) class action laws in which the rights of any persons affected are determined in one action.

4. All persons bringing or attempting to bring legal action have the right to inspect any relevant legal files held by their legal representative.

ARTICLE 29   RIGHT TO CHOICE OF FORUM

1. All persons adversely affected by hazardous activities have the right to bring law suit in the forum of their choice against alleged wrongdoers, including individuals, governments, corporations or other organisations. No state shall discriminate against such persons on the basis of nationality or domicile.

2. All states shall ensure that in the specific case of any legal claims arising from the effects of hazardous activities, any legal rule otherwise impeding the pursuit of such claims, including legislative measures and judicial doctrines, shall not prevent affected persons from bringing suit for full and effective remedies. In particular, states shall review and remove where necessary, legal restrictions relating to inconvenient forum, statutory limitations, limited liability of parent corporations, enforcement of foreign money judgements and excessive fees for civil suits.

ARTICLE 30   RIGHT TO PRE-TRIAL DOCUMENTATION

All persons adversely affected by a hazardous activity and their representatives, have the right to seek and receive relevant documents, records or other information for submission in court or other independent tribunal or forum, for establishing individual, corporate, organisational or governmental liability during litigation.

ARTICLE 31   RIGHT TO FAIR PROCEDURE

All persons adversely affected by hazardous activities shall have the right to a fair and public hearing within a reasonable time by an independent and impartial tribunal established by law. Included in this right is the right to the due process of law, including:

(a) the right to opt out of class actions;
(b) the right to a reasonable notice and communication before an out-of-court settlement in a civil suit is reached;
(c) the right to bring lawsuit notwithstanding the period of limitation set by administrative, legislative or judicial or any other means.

ARTICLE 32   RIGHT TO FREEDOM
FROM FRAUD AND DELAY

All persons adversely by hazardous activities shall have the right to be protected against fraud by corporations, government or other organisations. Also prohibited is intentional delay or obstruction of the legal process, including:

(a) declaration of bankruptcy;
(b) abuse of the legal process to prolong adjudication;
(c) fabrication of evidence.

ARTICLE 33　RIGHT TO ENFORCEMENT OF JUDGEMENTS OR SETTLEMENTS

All persons adversely affected by hazardous activities and their representatives, shall have the right to enforce any judgement or settlement against the assets of the liable or settling party in any other countries and it shall be the duty of each state to provide under domestic law such comprehensive instruments as assist any of its citizens so affected.

ARTICLE 34　RIGHT TO SHIFT THE BURDEN OF PROOF

1. Where there is prima facie evidence that death or injury was caused by an industrial hazard, the hazardous economic enterprise has the burden of proving that it was not negligent.

2. No person adversely affected by hazardous activity shall be subjected to excessive documentation requirements or strict standards of proof in establishing that the hazardous activity caused their illness or symptoms. The link between hazards and illness shall be presumed if the affected persons establish:

(a) they suffer from symptoms commonly associated with any harmful substance, or any component thereof, which contaminated the environment; and
(b) either

(i) they were present within the geographical area of contamination during the period of contamination; or
(ii) they belong to a group of persons commonly identified as secondary victims, including the siblings, partners, children or close associates of the original victims of the hazard.

ARTICLE 35　RIGHT TO CORPORATE OR STATE CRIMINAL ACCOUNTABILITY

1. All persons who have suffered injury or death from industrial hazards, have the right to a full criminal investigation into the conduct of the economic enterprise, any concerned government officials and any other concerned individual or organisation. The investigation shall be both immediate and rigorous and shall include an assessment of whether potential criminal offences, including homicide or manslaughter, have been committed. Where sufficient evidence exists prosecution shall be pursued promptly and vigorously.

2. Where criminal liability of a company and or individual is proved, such fines and or prison sentencing are to be imposed as to have a punitive, exemplary and deterrent effect.

ARTICLE 36　RIGHT TO SECURE EXTRADITION

Where a person accused of a criminal offence in connection with hazardous activities resides or is located in a state other than that in which the trial is being or will be conducted, the right to demand and secure the extradition of the accused to the trial state is hereby affirmed.

Part V Implementation

ARTICLE 37   CORRESPONDING DUTIES

All persons, individually and in association with others, have a duty to protect the rights set out in this Charter. Employers and government officers are under a strict duty of care in vigilant application of the rights. Special responsibility for the realization of the provisions of this Charter lies with trade unions, community groups and non-governmental organisations.

ARTICLE 38   STATE RESPONSIBILITIES

All states shall respect and protect the rights of workers and communities to live free from industrial hazards. Accordingly, they shall adopt legislative, administrative and other measures necessary to implement the rights contained in this Charter.

ARTICLE 39   NON-STATE ACTION

The absence of state action to protect and enforce the rights set out in this Charter does not extinguish the duties of employers, trade unions, non-governmental organisations and individuals to protect and assert these rights.

This copy of the Permanent People's Tribunal Charter
was provided by the Australian Chemical Trauma Alliance.

Appendix VI

Twenty Most Common Chemicals Found in Thirty-One Fragrance Products

Study by U.S. Environmental Protection Agency (EPA), 1991
Reference: Lance Wallace, EPA; Phone 703.648.4287
Symptoms of exposure are taken from industry-generated
Material Safety Data Sheets (MSDS)
Compiled by Julia Kendall (1935–1997)
Distributed by Environmental Health Network

Principal chemicals found in scented products include

ACETONE (cologne, dishwashing liquid and detergent, nail enamel remover). On EPA, RCRA, CERCLA Hazardous Waste lists. "Inhalation can cause dryness of the mouth and throat; dizziness, nausea, incoordination, slurred speech, drowsiness, and, in severe exposures, coma." "Acts primarily as a central nervous system (CNS) depressant."

BENZALDEHYDE (perfume, cologne, hairspray, laundry bleach, deodorants, detergent, Vaseline lotion, shaving cream, shampoo, bar soap, dishwasher detergent). Narcotic. Sensitizer. "Local anesthetic, CNS depressant." "[I]rritation to the mouth, throat, eyes, skin, lungs, and GI tract causing nausea and abdominal pain." "May cause kidney damage." "Do not use with contact lenses."

BENZYL ACETATE (perfume, cologne, shampoo, fabric softener, stickup air freshener, dishwashing liquid and detergent, soap, hairspray, bleach, after shave, deodorants). Carcinogenic (linked to pancreatic cancer). "From vapors: irritating to eyes and respiratory passages, exciting cough." "In mice: hyperaemia of the lungs." "Can be absorbed through the skin causing systemic effects." "Do not flush to sewer."

BENZYL ALCOHOL   (perfume, cologne, soap, shampoo, nail enamel remover, air freshener, laundry bleach and detergent, Vaseline lotion, deodorants, fabric softener). "Irritating to the upper respiratory tract." "[H]eadache, nausea, vomiting, dizziness, drop in blood pressure, CNS depression, and death in severe cases due to respiratory failure."

CAMPHOR   (perfume, shaving cream, nail enamel, fabric softener, dishwasher detergent, nail color, stickup air freshener). "[L]ocal irritant and CNS stimulant." "[R]eadily absorbed through body tissues." "[I]rritation of eyes, nose and throat." "[D]izziness, confusion, nausea, twitching muscles and convulsions," "Avoid inhalation of vapors."

ETHANOL   (perfume, hairspray, shampoo, fabric softener, dishwashing liquid and detergent, laundry detergent, shaving cream, soap, Vaseline lotion, air fresheners, nail color and remover, paint and varnish remover). On EPA Hazardous Waste list; symptoms: "fatigue; irritating to eyes and upper respiratory tract even in low concentrations...." "Inhalation of ethanol vapors can have effects similar to those characteristic of ingestion. These include an initial stimulatory effect followed by drowsiness, impaired vision, ataxia, stupor...." Causes CNS disorder.

ETHYL ACETATE   (after shave, cologne, perfume, shampoo, nail color, nail enamel remover, fabric softener, dishwashing liquid). Narcotic. On EPA Hazardous Waste list. "[I]rritating to the eyes and respiratory tract." "May cause headache and narcosis (stupor)." "[D]efatting effect on skin and may cause drying and cracking." "[M]ay cause anemia with leukocytosis and damage to liver and kidneys." "Wash thoroughly after handling."

LIMONENE   (perfume, cologne, disinfectant spray, bar soap, shaving cream, deodorants, nail color and remover, fabric softener, dishwashing liquid, air fresheners, after shave, bleach, paint and varnish remover). Carcinogenic. "Prevent its contact with skin or eyes because it is an irritant and sensitizer." "Always wash thoroughly after using this material and before eating, drinking, ... applying cosmetics. Do not inhale limonene vapor."

LINALOOL   (perfume, cologne, bar soap, shampoo, hand lotion, nail enamel remover, hairspray, laundry detergent, dishwashing liquid, Vaseline lotion, air fresheners, bleach powder, fabric softener, shaving cream, after shave, solid deodorant). Narcotic. "[R]espiratory disturbances." "Attracts bees." "In animal tests: ataxic gait, reduced spontaneous motor activity and depression ... development of respiratory disturbances leading to death." "[D]epressed frog-heart activity." Causes CNS disorder.

METHYLENE CHLORIDE (shampoo, cologne, paint and varnish remover). Banned by the FDA in 1988! No enforcement possible due to trade secret laws protecting chemical fragrance industry. On EPA, RCRA, CERCLA Hazardous Waste lists. "Carcinogenic." "Absorbed, stored in body fat, it metabolizes to carbon monoxide, reducing oxygen-carrying capacity of the blood." "Headache, giddiness, stupor, irritability, fatigue, tingling in the limbs." Causes CNS disorder.

a–PINENE (bar and liquid soap, cologne, perfume, shaving cream, deodorants, dishwashing liquid, air freshener). Sensitizer (damaging to the immune system).

a–TERPINENE (cologne, perfume, soap, shaving cream, deodorant, air freshener). "Causes asthma and CNS disorders."

a–TERPINEOL (perfume, cologne, laundry detergent, bleach powder, laundry bleach, fabric softener, stickup air freshener, Vaseline lotion, cologne, soap, hairspray, after shave, roll-on deodorant). "[H]ighly irritating to mucous membranes." "Aspiration into the lungs can produce pneumonitis or even fatal edema." Can also cause "excitement, ataxia (loss of muscular coordination), hypothermia, CNS and respiratory depression, and headache." "Prevent repeated or prolonged skin contact."

Note: Julia Kendall had been unable to secure MSDS for the following chemicals: 1,8–CINEOLE; b–CITRONELLOL; b–MYRCENE; NEROL; OCIMENE; b–PHENETHYL ALCOHOL; a–TERPINOLENE

- Ninety-five percent of chemicals used in fragrances are synthetic compounds derived from petroleum. They include benzene derivatives, aldehydes and many other known toxics and sensitizers—capable of causing cancer, birth defects, central nervous system disorders and allergic reactions. "Neurotoxins: At Home and the Workplace," Report by the Committee on Science and Technology, U.S. House of Representatives, September 16, 1986. (Report 99-827).
- Chloroform was found in tests of fabric softeners: EPA's 1991 study.
- A room containing an air freshener had high levels of p-dichlorobenzene (a carcinogen) and ethanol: EPA's 1991 study.
- An FDA analysis (1968–1972) of 138 compounds used in cosmetics that most frequently involved adverse reactions, identified five chemicals (alphaterpineol, benzyl acetate, benzyl alcohol, limonene and linalool) that are among the 20 most commonly used in the 31 fragrance products tested by the EPA in 1991.
- Thirty-three million Americans suffer from sinusitis (inflammation or infection of sinus passages).
- Ten million Americans have asthma. Asthma and asthma deaths have increased over 30 percent in the past 10 years.
- Headaches cost $50 billion in lost productivity and medical expenses and 157 million lost work days in 1991. "Focus on Fragrance and Health," by Louise Kosta, The Human Ecologist, fall 1992.

A few related web sites:

<http://users.lanminds.com/~wilworks/ehnecohs.htm>Ecology House
Please respect the residents and their requests by following the instructions provided on our Ecology House page.

<http://users.lanminds.com/~wilworks/ehnindex.htm>EHN's home page

<http://users.lanminds.com/~wilworks/ehnfs.htm>Fabric Softeners
Health risks from dryer exhaust and treated fabrics

<http://users.lanminds.com/~wilworks/ehnlinx/index.htm
E-mail and WWW links

<http://users.lanminds.com/~wilworks/ehnglinx.htm
Government WWW links

<http://users.lanminds.com/~wilworks/ehnnr.html
The New Reactor

Bibliography

Allen, G.W. *William James*. New York: Viking Press, 1967. 556+xx.

Annas, G.J., and Grodin, M.A. "Medicine and Human Rights: Reflections on the Fiftieth Anniversary of the Doctors' Trial," *Health and Human Rights*, 2, No. 1 (1996) 7–21.

_____, and _____, eds. *The Nazi Doctors and the Nuremberg Code: Human Rights in Human Experimentation*. New York: Oxford University Press, 1992. 371+xxii.

APHA. "Policy statement 9606: The precautionary principle and chemical exposure standards for the work place," *American Journal of Public Health*, 87, Number 3 (March 1997) 500–501.

Arnold, S.F., et al. "Synergistic Activation of Estrogen Receptor with Combinations of Environmental Chemicals," *Science*, 272 (June 7, 1996) 1489–92.

Ashby, J., et al. "Synergy between synthetic oestrogens?" *Nature*, 385 (February 6, 1997) 494.

Ashford, N., and Hinzow, B. *Chemical Sensitivity in Selected European Countries: An exploratory study*. Ergonomia, Ltd., November 1995.

Ashford, N., and Miller, C. *Chemical Exposures: Low Levels, High Stakes*, 1st ed. New York: Van Nostrand Reinhold, 1991. 214.

_____, and _____. *Chemical Exposures: Low Levels, High Stakes*. Second ed. New York: Van Nostrand Reinhold / John Wiley & Sons, 1998. 440+xxiii.

Bankowski, Z., ed. *International Ethical Guidelines for Biomedical Research Involving Human Subjects*. Geneva, Switzerland: Council for International Organizations of Medical Sciences, 1993. 63.

Bell, I.R., Bootzin, R.R., et al. "A Polysomnographic Study of Sleep Disturbance in Community Elderly with Self-reported Environmental Chemical Odor Intolerance," *Biological Psychiatry* 40 (1996) 123–33.

Berkson, J.B. *A Canary's Tale: The Final Battle, Politics, Poisons, and Pollution vs. the Environment and the Public Health.* Hagerstown, MD: Self-published, 1996. 452+xviii.

Blank, D.M. "A Growing Sensitivity to What's in the Air," *New York Times,* February 22, 1998. BU 11.

Blondell, J., and Dobozy, V.A. *Review of Chlorpyrifos Poisoning Data.* Environmental Protection Agency. January 14, 1997.

"Book review of *HIV and the Blood Supply*," *American Journal of Public Health,* 87, Number 3 (March 1997) 474.

Brady, J. "The Goose and the Golden Egg," *One in Three: Women with Cancer Confront an Epidemic.* Ed. J. Brady. San Francisco and Pittsburgh: Cleis Press, 1991. 13–35.

Buchwald, D., and Garrity, D. "Comparison of Patients with Chronic Fatigue Syndrome, Fibromyalgia, and Multiple Chemical Sensitivities," *Archives of Internal Medicine,* 154 (September 26, 1994) 2049–53.

The Bulletin of the King County Medical Society, 73, #12 (December 1994) cover.

"California Requires Warning Posted in Dental Offices," *News Bites,* January 1997.

Carson, R. *Silent Spring.* Boston: Houghton Mifflin, 1962, 1994. 368+xxvi.

Charter on Industrial Hazards and Human Rights. Permanent People's Tribunal, 1996.

Colburn, T., Dumanoski, D., and Myers, J.P. *Our Stolen Future: Are We Threatening Our Fertility, Intelligence and Survival?—A Scientific Detective Story.* New York: Penguin Books USA, 1996. 306+xii.

Cox, C. "Dichlobenil," *Journal of Pesticide Reform,* 17, #1 (Spring 1997) 14-20.

Cray, C., and Harden, M. "PVC & Dioxin: Enough Is Enough," *Rachel's Environment and Health Weekly,* 616 (September 17, 1998).

Crisp, T.M., Clegg, E.D., and Cooper, R.L. *Special Report on Environmental Endocrine Disruption: An Effects Assessment and Analysis.* US Environmental Protection Agency. February 1997.

Cushman, J.H., Jr. "Group wants pesticide companies to end testing on humans," *New York Times,* July 28, 1998. A9.

_____. "U.S. Reshaping Cancer Strategy as Incidence in Children Rises," *New York Times,* September 29, 1997. A1 & A13.

Devlin, B., Daniels, M., and Raeder, K. "The Democracy of Genes," *Nature,* 388 (July 31, 1997) 468–74.

Dieter, M. "Sustainable Environment for All," *Environmental Health Perspectives,* 105, Number 11 (November 1997) 1162–3.

Draft Declaration on Human Rights and the Environment. United Nations, 1994.

Duehring, C. "EPA Dursban Review Finds MCS—Dow revises marketing," *Medical and Legal Briefs,* 2, No. 6 (May/June 1997) 10.

_____. "The global problem of MCS part one: overview of investigative reports' findings," *Medical and Legal Briefs*, 2, No. 5 (March/April 1997) 1–5.

_____. "'Golf ball liver' caused by herbicides," *Medical and Legal Briefs*, 4, No. 1 (July/August 1998) 6.

_____. "Gulf Vets' Injuries Echo MCS," *Medical and Legal Briefs*, 2, No. 6 (May/June 1997) 5–6.

_____. "Lupus Linked to Industrial Pollution," *Medical and Legal Briefs*, 3, No. 3 (November/December 1997) 5.

_____. "Manteca Hospital develops MCS accommodation policy," *Medical and Legal Briefs*, 4, No. 1 (July/August 1998) 9.

_____. "Nat'l Cancer Institute Statements Counteract Junk Science," *Medical & Legal Briefs*, 2, No. 4 (January/February 1997) 10.

_____. "Objective Sleep Abnormalities Found Even with Mild Chemical Sensitivities," *Medical & Legal Briefs*, 2, No. 4 (January/February 1997) 6–7.

_____. "Organochlorines linked with CFS and chemical sensitivities," *Medical and Legal Briefs*, 4, No. 1 (July/August 1998) 7.

_____. "Overexposure from legal pesticiding: a generation at risk," *Medical and Legal Briefs*, 3, No. 6 (May/June 1998) 1–4.

_____. "Overview of Biologic Research," *Medical and Legal Briefs*, 2, No. 6 (May/June 1997) 1–5.

_____. "Perfume Toxicity, Sensitivity, Accommodation and Disability—Part One: Evidence of Health Hazards," *Medical and Legal Briefs*, 4, No. 1 (July/August 1998) 1–6.

_____. "Plaintiff Awarded $4.2 Million Against DuPont in Toxic Carpet Suit," *Medical & Legal Briefs*, 2, No. 4 (January/February 1997) 1–4.

_____. "Plasticizers and Diesel Particulates Impair Sperm Motility," *Medical and Legal Briefs*, 3, No. 3 (November/December 1997) 6.

_____. "Sperm Density Decline Confirmed," *Medical and Legal Briefs*, 3, No. 6 (May/June 1998) 6.

_____. "Synergy Findings Withdrawn Re: Environmental Estrogens," *Medical and Legal Briefs*, 3, No. 2 (1997) 7.

_____. "Tort Claims Allowed for Workplace Fetal Injury," *Medical & Legal Briefs*, 2, No. 4 (January/February 1997) 10.

Ellington, C.P., et al. "Leading-edge vortices in insect flight," *Nature*, 384 (December 19/26, 1996) 626–30.

Engle, G. "The Need for a New Medical Model: A Challenge for Biomedicine," *Science*, 196 (1977) 4286.

"EPA—pollution grading plan provokes opposition of companies, state officials," *Wall Street Journal*, February 17, 1998. B8.

Epstein, P.R. "Human Rights and Natural Laws," *Health and Human Rights*, 2, Number 2 (Spring 1997) 1–4.

"Estrogens in the Environment," *Environmental Health Perspectives*, 105, Number 9 (September 1997) 910.

Fagin, D., and Lavelle, M. *Toxic Deception: How the Chemical Industry Manipulates Science, Bends the Law, and Endangers Your Health*. Secaucus, NJ: Carol Publishing, 1997. 294+xxvi.

Fielden, M.R., et al. "Examination of the Estrogenicity of 2,4,6,2',6'-Pentachlorobiphenyl (PCB 104), Its Hydroxylated Metabolite 2,4,6,2',6'-Pentachloro-4-Biphenylol (HO-PCB 104), and a Further Chlorinated Derivative, 2,4,6,2',4',6'-Hexachlorobiphenyl (PCB 155)," *Environmental Health Perspectives*, 105, Number 11 (November 1997) 1238–48.

Freeman, A.M., and Cohen, L.P. "How cigarette makers keep health questions 'open' year after year," *Wall Street Journal*, February 11, 1993. A1.

Fumento, M. "Allergic to Life," *Reason* (June 1996) 20–26.

Galloway, J. "The health of nations," *Nature*, 385 (13 Feb. 1997) 594.

Gayle, L. "Environmental Illness/Multiple Chemical Sensitivities: Invisible Disabilities," *Women and Therapy*, 14, Number 3/4 (1993) 171–85.

_____. "Mother's Milk—as Safe as Apple Pie?" *One in Three: Women with Cancer Confront an Epidemic*. Ed. J. Brady. San Francisco and Pittsburgh: Cleis Press, 1991. 79–87.

_____, Cheavens, J., and Warren, M.L. "Social Support in Persons with Self-Reported Sensitivity to Chemicals," *Research in Nursing and Health*, 21 (1998) 103–15.

Gore, A. *Earth in the Balance: Ecology and the Human Spirit*. New York: Houghton Mifflin, 1992.

Greene, R. "Inert pesticide ingredients lose EPA secrecy privilege," *Oregonian*, October 19, 1996.

Guralnik, J.M. and Leveille, S.G. "Comment: Environmental Racism and Public Health," *American Journal of Public Health*, 87, Number 5 (May 1997) 730–31.

Gurunathan, S., et al. "Accumulation of Chlorpyrifos on Residential Surfaces and Toys Accessible to Children," *Environmental Health Perspectives*, 106, Number 1 (January 1998) 9–16.

Hallaby, D. "Australia's Chemical-Free School," *Our Toxic Times*, 8, No. 2 (February 1997) 6.

Hanin, I. "GWS: Expanding knowledge on permeability of Blood-Brain Barrier," *Our Toxic Times*, 8, Number 4 (April 1997) 1–4.

Hardin, G. "Carrying Capacity as an Ethical Concept," *Lifeboat Ethics: The Moral Dilemmas of World Hunger*. Eds. G. R. Lucas Jr. and T. W. Ogletree. New York: Harper and Row, 1976. 120–31.

Harr, J. *A Civil Action*. New York: Random House, 1995. 500.

"Healthier schools focus of WHO report," *The Nation's Health* February 1997, 24.

Healthy People 2010. Office of Disease Prevention and Health Promotion, US Department of Health and Human Services, September 15, 1998.

Hertzman, C., et al. "Mortality and Cancer Incidence Among Sawmill Workers Exposed to Chlorophenate Wood Preservatives," *American Journal of Public Health*, 87, No. 1 (January 1997) 71–9.

Hignite, C., and Azarnoff, D.L. "Drugs and drug metabolites as environmental contaminants: chlorophenoxyisobutyrate and salicylic acid in sewage water effluent," *Life Sciences*, 20, Number 12 (January 15, 1977) 337–41.

Hill, A.B. "The Environment and Disease: Association or Causation?" *Proceedings of the Royal Society of Medicine*, 58 (1965) 295–300.

Ho, D.D., et al. "Rapid turnover of plasma virions and CD4 lymphocytes in HIV-1 infection," *Nature*, 373 (January 12, 1995) 123ff.

Hood, C., and JDK C, eds. *Accident and Design: Contemporary Debaters in Risk Management*. London: UCL Press Limited, 1996. 253+xiv.

Hooper, K., et al. "Analysis of Breast Milk to Assess Exposure to Chlorinated Contaminants in Kazakhstan: PCBs and Organochlorine Pesticides in Southern Kazakstan," *Environmental Health Perspectives*, 105, Number 11 (November 1997) 1250–54.

"Hormone disruptors require additional study, EPA says." *New York Times*, March 14, 1997. A26.

Houghton, J. "Review of Stephen Schneider's *Laboratory Earth: The Planetary Gamble We Can't Afford to Lose* (Basic Books, 1997, 174 pp)," *Nature*, 386 (March 27, 1997) 345.

Hume, D. *An Enquiry Concerning Human Understanding* (1748).

Jacobson, J.L. and Jacobson, S.W. "Intellectual Impairment in Children Exposed to Polychlorinated Biphenyls in Utero," *New England Journal of Medicine*, 335, No. 11 (September 12, 1996) 435–45.

Jerome, R., and Nelson, M. "Toxic Avenger." *People,* February 9, 1998, 113–15.

Kaiser, J. "New Yeast Study Finds Strength in Numbers," *Science*, 272 (June 7, 1996) 1418.

Kardestuncer, T., and Frumkin, H. "Systemic Lupus Erythematosus in Relation to Environmental Pollution: An Investigation in an African-American Community in North Georgia," *Archives of Environmental Health*, 52, Number 2 (March/April 1997) 85–90.

Kearns, D. *EPA's 1995 Toxics Release Data Include First-Ever Reporting on 286 New Chemicals*. EPA, May 20, 1997.

Kelly, E. "Fillet of methylmercury: Fish health warnings rise." *Seattle Times*, April 9, 1998. A8.

Kerns, T.A. *Ethical Issues in HIV Vaccine Trials*. New York: St. Martin's (Macmillan, Ltd., in the UK), 1997. 244 +xvi.

_____. *Jenner on Trial: An Ethical Examination of Vaccine Research in the Age of Smallpox and the Age of AIDS*. Lanham, MD: University Press of America, 1997. 104.

Kerr, K. "Study: Doctors who backed heart drug had ties to makers," *Seattle Times,* January 4, 1998. A4.

Kettles, M.A., et al. "Triazine Herbicide Exposure and Breast Cancer Incidence: An Ecologic Study of Kentucky Counties," *Environmental Health Perspectives*, 105, Number 11 (November 1997) 1222–27.

Klinkenborg, V. "Editorial: Biotechnology and the future of agriculture," *New York Times,* December 8, 1997. A22.

Kroll-Smith, S., and Floyd, H.H. *Bodies in Protest: Environmental Illness and the Struggle Over Medical Knowledge*. New York: New York University Press, 1997. 223+xiv.

Kuhn, T.S. *The Structure of Scientific Revolution*. 2nd ed. Chicago: University of Chicago Press, 1962, 1970. 210+xii.

Lappé, M. *Chemical Deception: The Toxic Threat to Health and the Environment*. San Francisco: Sierra Club Books, 1991. 360+xvi.

_____. *A Toxics Bill of Rights*. Center for Ethics and Toxics, 1996.

Lawson, L. *Staying Well in a Toxic World*. Chicago: Noble Press, 1993. 488.

Lerman, S., and Kipen, H. "Material Safety Data Sheets: Caveat Emptor," *Archives of Internal Medicine*, 150, #5 (May 1990) 981–4.

Lester, S., and Gibbs, L. *A Citizen's Guide to Risk Studies*. Citizens' Clearinghouse for Hazardous Waste, 1988.

Levy, B. "Conditions in which people can be healthy," *The Nation's Health*, 27, Number 4 (April 1997) 2.

Lewis, S. "Promoting Child Health and the Convention on the Rights of the Child," *Health and Human Rights*, 2, Number 3 (1997) 77–82.

Lorde, A. *The Cancer Journals*. San Francisco: Aunt Lute Books, 1980. 77.

Lydon, J. "Was Moses the first ecologist?" *Nature*, 395 (September 24, 1998) 317.

Macdonald, H., Aguinaga, S., and Glantz, S.A. "The defeat of Philip Morris' 'California Uniform Tobacco Control Act,'" *American Journal of Public Health*, 87, Number 12 (December 1997) 1989–96.

Mahler, H. "The Challenge of Global Health: How Can We Do Better?" *Health and Human Rights*, 2, Number 3 (1997) 71–75.

Maibach, E., and Holtgrave, D.R. "Advances in Public Health Communication," *Annual Review of Public Health*, 16 (1995) 219–38.

Mann, J. "Health and Human Rights: If Not Now, When?" *Health and Human Rights*, 2, Number 3 (1997) 113–20.

Marcus, R. "Judges take free trips in conflict of interest," *Seattle Times* (originally in the *Washington Post)* April 9, 1998. A3.

Masters, R.D., Hone, B., and Doshi, A. "Environmental Pollution, Neurotoxicity, and Criminal Violence," *Environmental Toxicology*. Ed. J. Rose. London and New York: Gordon and Breach, 1997.

McGue, M. "The democracy of genes," *Nature*, 388 (July 31, 1997) 417–18.

McKinney, J.D. "Interactive Hormonal Activity of Chemical Mixtures," *Environmental Health Perspectives*, 105, Number 9 (September 1997) 896.

Millar, H., and Millar, M. *The Toxic Labyrinth*. Vancouver, BC: NICO Professional Services, 1995. 301.

Miller, C.S. "Chemical Sensitivity: symptom, syndrome or mechanism for disease?" *Toxicology*, 111 (1996) 69–86.

_____. Personal communication. May 20, 1997.

_____. "Toxicant-induced Loss of Tolerance—An Emerging Theory of Disease?" *Environmental Health Perspectives*, 105, Supplement 2 (March 1997) 445–53.

_____. "White Paper: Chemical Sensitivity: History and Phenomenology," *Toxicology and Industrial Health*, 10, Number 4/5 (1994) 253-76.

_____, et al. "Empirical Approaches for the Investigation of Toxicant-induced Loss of Tolerance," *Environmental Health Perspectives*, 105, Supplement 2 (March 1997) 515–19.

Montague, P. "Bad decisions again and again," *Rachel's Environment and Health Weekly*, #541 (April 10, 1997).

_____. "Childhood Cancer and Pollution," *Rachel's Environment and Health Weekly*, #559 (August 14, 1997).

_____. "Drugs in the Water," *Rachel's Environment and Health Weekly*, #614 (September 3, 1998).

_____. "Fish Sex Hormones," *Rachel's Environment and Health Weekly*, #545 (May 8, 1997).

_____. "Follow the money," *Rachel's Environment and Health Weekly*, #581 (January 15, 1998).

_____. "Genetic engineering error," *Rachel's Environment and Health Weekly*, #549 (June 5, 1997).

_____. "History of precaution, Part 2," *Rachel's Environment and Health Weekly*, #540 (April 3, 1997).

_____. "Immune system toxins," *Rachel's Environment and Health Weekly*, #536 (March 6, 1997).

_____. "Infectious disease and pollution," *Rachel's Environment and Health Weekly*, #528 (January 9, 1997).

_____. "1997 Snapshots—Part 2," *Rachel's Environment and Health Weekly*, #579 (January 1, 1998).

_____. "One Fundamental Problem," *Rachel's Environment and Health Weekly*, #582 (January 22, 1998).

_____. "PCB exposure linked to low IQ," *Rachel's Environment and Health Weekly*, #512 (September 19, 1996).

_____. "Right to know nothing," *Rachel's Environment and Health Weekly*, #552 (June 26, 1997).

_____. "Seeds of Destruction," *Rachel's Environment and Health Weekly*, #622 (October 29, 1998).

_____. "Statement on immune toxins," *Rachel's Environment and Health Weekly*, #544 (May 1, 1997).

_____. "Toxics affect behavior," *Rachel's Environment and Health Weekly*, #529 (January 16, 1997).

_____. "Toxics and Violent Crime," *Rachel's Environment and Health Weekly*, #551 (June 19, 1997).

_____. "The Weybridge Report," *Rachel's Environment and Health Weekly*, #547 (May 22, 1997).

Moses, M. *Designer Poisons: How to Protect Your Health and Home from Toxic Pesticides*. San Francisco: Pesticide Education Center, 1995. 415.

The Nation's Health, October 1997. 8.

"Nations Move to Ban POPs," *Environmental Health Perspectives*, 105, Number 7 (July 1997) 693.

Nichols, A.W. "Amending the United States Constitution to Include Environmental Rights," *The Nation's Health*, September 1997. 18–19.

O'Brien, M.H. "The Need to Assess Alternatives to the Production and Release of Dioxin." A speech presented at the San Francisco Bay Regional Water Quality Control Board workshop, Oakland, CA. May 7, 1997.

Omenn, G.S. *Framework for Environmental Health Risk Management*. Presidential/Congressional Commission on Risk Assessment and Risk Management, January 1997.

Ott, W.R., and Roberts, J.W. "Everyday Exposure to Toxic Pollutants," *Scientific American*, February 1998.

"Panel urges medicine to stress prevention, public health," *The Nation's Health*, 27, No. 1 (January 1997) 3.

Pieper, J. *The Four Cardinal Virtues: Prudence, Justice, Fortitude, Temperance.* Notre Dame, IN: University of Notre Dame Press, 1966. 234+xiii.

Pimentel, D. "Ecology of Increasing Disease: Population Growth and Environmental Degradation," *Bioscience*, October 1998.

"Plans for protecting food safety, regulating pesticides announced," *The Nation's Health*, 27, Number 4 (April 1997) 5.

Pogoda, J.M., and Preston-Martin, S. "Household Pesticides and Risk of Pediatric Brain Tumors," *Environmental Health Perspectives*, 105, Number 11 (November 1997) 1214–20.

"Poll: Definition of public health unclear to most Americans," *The Nation's Health*, February 1997. 24.

Pollan, M. "Playing God in the Garden." *New York Times Magazine*, October 25, 1998. 44–51, 62–3, 82, 92–3.

Proctor, R.N. *Cancer Wars: How Politics Shapes What We Know and Don't Know about Cancer.* New York: Basic Books, 1995. 356+xii.

"Puberty Signs Evident in 7- and 8-Year-Old Girls." *USA Today*, April 8, 1997. 1A.

Radetsky, P. *The Invisible Invaders: The Story of the Emerging Age of Viruses.* Boston: Little, Brown, 1991. 415+xvi.

Randolph, T.G., and Moss, R.W. *An Alternative Approach to Allergies.* Rev. ed. New York: Harper and Row, 1980, 1989. 337+viii.

Rapp, D.J. *Is This Your Child? Discovering and Treating Unrecognized Allergies in Children and Adults.* New York: William Morrow, 1991. 626+.

_____. *Is This Your Child's World? How You Can Fix the Schools and Homes That Are Making Your Children Sick.* New York: Bantam, 1996. 635+xix.

Rastogi, S.C., Johansen, J.D., and Mennde, T. "Natural ingredients based cosmetics: content of selected fragrance sensitizers," *Contact Dermatitis*, 34, Number 6 (June 1996) 423–26.

Rea, W. *Chemical Sensitivity*, 4. Boca Raton, FL: Lewis Publishers, and CRC Press, 1992-97. 2924.

Repetto, R. and Baliga, S.S. *Pesticides and the Immune System.* Washington, DC: World Resources Institute, 1996. 100.

A Report on Multiple Chemical Sensitivity. Interagency Workgroup on Multiple Chemical Sensitivity. (Agencies represented on the workgroup included the Department of Defense, Department of Energy, Department of Health and Human Services, Department of Veterans Affairs, and the US Environmental Protection Agency.) August 24, 1998.

"Review of John Wargo, *Our Children's Toxic Legacy*," *American Journal of Public Health*, 87, Number 3 (March 1997) 473.

Richardson, K.A., et al. "Using electrical noise to enhance the ability of humans to detect subthreshold mechanical cutaneous stimuli," *Chaos*, 8, Number 3 (September 1998) 599–603.

Roe, D., et al. *Toxic Ignorance*. Environmental Defense Fund, 1997.

Rouché, B. *The Man Who Grew Two Breasts: And Other True Tales of Medical Detection*. New York: Truman Talley Books/Dutton, 1995. 197.

Rowat, S.C. "Integrated defense system overlaps as a disease model: with examples for Multiple Chemical Sensitivity," *Environmental Health Perspectives*, 106, Supplement I (February 1998) 85–106.

Satcher, D. "CDC's First 50 Years: Lessons Learned and Relearned," *American Journal of Public Health*, 86, #12 (December 1996) 1705–08.

Sellers, C. "Discovering Environmental Cancer: Wilhelm Hueper, Post-World War II Epidemiology, and the Vanishing Clinician's Eye," *American Journal of Public Health*, 87, #11 (November 1997) 1824–35.

Simeons, A.T.W. *Man's Presumptuous Brain: An Evolutionary Interpretation of Psychosomatic Disease*. New York: Dutton, 1960, 1961. 290.

Sontag, S. *Illness as Metaphor*. New York: Doubleday, 1978. 83.

"The state of the science on endocrine disruptors," *Environmental Health Perspectives*, 106, Number 7 (July 1998) A319–20.

"State seeking records for defunct smelter." *The Eugene Register-Guard*, March 26, 1997.

Stauber, J., and Rampton, S. *Toxic Sludge Is Good for You: Lies, Damn Lies, and the Public Relations Industry*. Monroe, ME: Common Courage Press, 1995. 236+iv.

Steingraber, S. *Living Downstream: An Ecologist Looks at Cancer and the Environment*. Reading, MA: Addison-Wesley, 1997. 357+xvi.

_____. "We All Live Downwind," *One in Three: Women with Cancer Confront an Epidemic*. Ed. J. Brady. Pittsburgh: Cleis Press 1991. 36–48.

Stelfox, H.T. et al. "Conflict of Interest in the Debate over Calcium-Channel Antagonists," *New England Journal of Medicine*, 338, Number 2 (January 8, 1998).

Stine, G. *Acquired Immune Deficiency Syndrome: Biological, Medical, Social and Legal Issues*. 1st ed. Englewood Cliffs, NJ: Prentice Hall, 1993. 462+xxxii.

Straub, T.M., et al. "Hazards from Pathogenic Microorganisms in Land-Disposed Sewage Sludge," *Reviews of Environmental Contamination and Toxicology*, 132 (1993) 55–91.

Stuller, J. "Golf gets back to nature, inviting everyone to play." *Smithsonian*, April 1997. 56–66.

"Support for labels on gene-altered food," *Nature*, 385 (February 27, 1997) 762.

Svoboda, T. "Every Breath She Takes," *Utne Reader*, March-April 1987. 59–63.

Swan, S.H., Elkin, E.P. and Fenster, L. "Have Sperm Densities Declined? A Reanalysis of Global Trend Data," *Environmental Health Perspectives*, 105, Number 11 (November 1997) 1228–32.

Swearingen, T. "Activist Mom Wins Goldman Prize," *Rachel's Environment and Health Weekly*, #542 (April 17, 1997).

"Times reporter wins 2 national awards." *Seattle Times*, March 15, 1998. B1.

Universal Declaration of Human Rights. United Nations, 1948. 6.

Vacco, D.C. *The Secret Hazards of Pesticides: Inert Ingredients.* New York State Department of Law, Environmental Protection Bureau, February 1991, 1996.

Van Strum, C. *A Bitter Fog: Herbicides and Human Rights.* San Francisco: Sierra Club Books, 1983. 288+x.

Varner, L.K. "Alarm over asthma," *Seattle Times,* February 22, 1998. E1,5.

Vergano, D. "Stress may weaken the blood-brain barrier," *Science News,* 150 (December 14, 1996) 375.

Vos, J.G., Younes, M., and Smith, E., eds. *Allergic Hypersensitivities Induced by Chemicals: Recommendations for Prevention.* London: CRC Press (on behalf of the World Health Organization Regional Office for Europe), 1996. 348.

Wadman, M. "Critics claim U.S. inquiry was 'irreparably flawed,'" *Nature,* 390, #6 (November 6, 1997) 4.

_____. "Study discloses financial interests behind papers," *Nature,* 385 (January 30, 1997) 376.

Wargo, J. *Our Children's Toxic Legacy: How Science and Law Fail to Protect Us from Pesticides.* New Haven, CT: Yale University Press, 1996. 380+xvi.

"WHO says chronic and infectious diseases are increasing worldwide," the *Nation's Health,* 27, Number 5 (May/June 1997) 11.

Wiesenfeld, K., and Jaramillo, F. "Minireview of stochastic resonance," *Chaos,* 8, Number 3 (September 1998) 539–48.

Williams, J.T. "The painless synergism of aspirin and opium," *Nature,* 390 (December 11, 1997) 557–58.

Wilson, D. "Fear in the Fields." *Seattle Times,* July 4–5, 1997. A1ff.

Winnow, J. "Lesbians Evolving Health Care: Cancer and AIDS," *One in Three: Women with Cancer Confront an Epidemic.* Ed. J. Brady. San Francisco and Pittsburgh: Cleis Press, 1991. 233–44.

Winslow, C-EA. *The Conquest of Epidemic Disease.* Madison: University of Wisconsin Press, 1943, 1980. 411+viii.

Winston, M.L. *Nature Wars: People vs. Pests.* Cambridge, MA: Harvard University Press, 1997. 210+x.

Index